Praise for
Primal Fat Burner

"Nora Gedgaudas was one of the early adopters of the low-carbohydrate, high-fat science and diet. She not only understands the science very well, she is able to simply and accurately explain it to the lay reader and health professional alike. From some fine science to its application, this book has much to offer for someone just starting out and wanting to dip their toes in the low-carb water or for those already better versed in the science. It is an entertaining and informative read, and I highly recommend it."

—Ron Rosedale, MD, founder of the Rosedale Center and the
Carolina Center of Metabolic Medicine and
author of *The Rosedale Diet*

"Gedgaudas deftly describes the link between what we eat and what we become. Millions of years of human evolution made us omnivores with well-muscled bodies and extraordinary minds that could not have developed without a diet rich in fat, including saturated fat! Read this book and you'll understand why much-maligned animal fat is so important to your health and why it is critical that it come from animals grazing on healthy land (and not confined to feedlots). I cannot recommend this book highly enough."

—Allan Savory, The Savory Institute

"*Primal Fat Burner* is always engaging and flawlessly referenced. For everyone who is interested in the science and practicality of prolonging the health span, this book is a must-read."

—Dan Murphy, DC, Professor, Life Chiropractic College West

"This unique book provides a much-needed big picture, addresses the state of humankind, the errant direction we have all taken, the dark influence of global corporations, and most important, how we can regain our power and embrace a truly healthy, sustainable future. Nora makes the case to focus on what we all share: a common biological design, and a need for a food economy that restores local, natural systems. In this way, we can take back what was once ours, and what is fundamentally our primal birthright."

—Helena Norberg-Hodge, author of *Ancient Futures*

"Gedgaudas's nutritional knowledge is about a decade ahead of 99 percent of US physicians, who are taught virtually zilch about healthful eating in medical school. Counterintuitive though it sounds, increasing your fat intake will promote weight loss. The real nutritional villain is sugar (a fact kept hidden from us by the sugar industry!). The low-carb, high-fat diet in *Primal Fat Burner* actually protects people from obesity and heart disease. When it comes to making the overweight and chronically ill American healthy again, *Primal Fat Burner* is destined to be a real game changer."

—David Edelberg, MD, author of *The Triple Whammy Cure*

"*Primal Fat Burner* has a wealth of new information and science showing the power of a ketogenic diet in addressing many health issues including obesity, diabetes, heart disease, neurological diseases, and cancer. Nora writes with passion, enthusiasm, and a warm sense of humor as she takes you on a life-changing, easy-to-implement journey to take control of your health by putting fat front and center! Should be read far and wide."

—Vicki Poulter, Director, Nourishing Australia and international advisory board of Price-Pottenger Nutrition Foundation

"If I could recommend only one book for the hungry, the lost, and the wounded, it would be *Primal Fat Burner*. A meticulous merging of science and storytelling, *Primal Fat Burner* is as satisfying as the food it champions. Gedgaudas makes the unassailable case for the centrality of animal fat in our history and our health. This is a book with a mission: to break the addictive, destructive spell of agricultural foods and restore us, body and mind, to ourselves."

Lierre Keith, bestselling author of *The Vegetarian Myth: Food, Justice, and Sustainability*

PRIMAL FAT
BURNER

Live Longer, Slow Aging, Super-Power Your Brain, and Save Your Life with a High-Fat, Low-Carb Paleo Diet

NORA GEDGAUDAS,
CNS, NTP, BCHN

Foreword by David Perlmutter, MD

ATRIA PAPERBACK

NEW YORK   LONDON   TORONTO   SYDNEY   NEW DELHI

ATRIA
PAPERBACK

An Imprint of Simon & Schuster, Inc.
1230 Avenue of the Americas
New York, NY 10020

Names and characteristics of some of the clients portrayed in this book have been changed.

First Atria trade paperback edition December 2017

ATRIA PAPERBACK and colophon are trademarks of Simon & Schuster, Inc.

For information about special discounts for bulk purchases, please contact Simon & Schuster Special Sales at 1-866-506-1949 or business@simonandschuster.com.

The Simon & Schuster Speakers Bureau can bring authors to your live event. For more information or to book an event, contact the Simon & Schuster Speakers Bureau at 1-866-248-3049 or visit our website at www.simonspeakers.com.

Interior design by Kyoko Watanabe

Manufactured in the United States of America

10 9 8 7 6 5 4 3 2 1

Library of Congress Cataloging-in-Publication Data
Names: Gedgaudas, Nora T., author.
Title: Primal fat burner : live longer, slow aging, super-power your brain, and save your life with a high-fat, low-carb paleo diet / Nora Gedgaudas, CNS, NTP, BCHN.
Description: New York : Atria Books, [2017]
Identifiers: LCCN 2016033323 (print) | LCCN 2016045502 (ebook)
Subjects: LCSH: Reducing diets. | Ketogenic diet. | Low-carbohydrate diet. | Prehistoric peoples—Nutrition. | BISAC: HEALTH & FITNESS / Nutrition. | HEALTH & FITNESS / Diets. | HEALTH & FITNESS / Healthy Living.
Classification: LCC RM222.2 .G43 2017 (print) | LCC RM222.2 (ebook) | DDC 613.2/833—dc23
LC record available at https://lccn.loc.gov/2016033323

ISBN 978-1-5011-1641-4
ISBN 978-1-5011-1642-1 (pbk)
ISBN 978-1-5011-1643-8 (ebook)

Dedicated to the pioneering work and memories of Mary Enig, PhD, George F. Cahill Jr., MD, and George V. Mann, MD, without whose courage, integrity, and important research we would all still be stumbling in the dark.

Also, for Lisa and for the wolves . . .

NOTE TO READERS

This publication contains the opinions and ideas of its author. It is intended to provide helpful and informative material on the subjects addressed in the publication. It is sold with the understanding that the author and publisher are not engaged in rendering medical, health, or any other kind of personal professional services in the book. The reader should consult his or her medical, health, or other competent professional before adopting any of the suggestions in this book or drawing inferences from it.

The author and publisher specifically disclaim all responsibility for any liability, loss, or risk, personal or otherwise, which is incurred as a consequence, directly or indirectly, of the use and application of any of the contents of this book.

Please note that while all readers should consult their doctor before implementing any of the suggestions in this book, the following is of particular importance for discussion with your doctor:

- If you are taking medication to control your blood sugar or blood pressure, your dosage requirements may change rapidly if you significantly restrict your carbohydrate intake.
- The diet outlined in *Primal Fat Burner* stresses the consumption of only moderate levels of protein and is not a high protein diet, for anyone who has serious kidney disease, any increase in dietary protein can potentially be a problem.

Note, however, that the dietary approach in this book also has the potential to benefit those with kidney-related issues.[1]

- If you have gallbladder attacks or gallstones, you should exercise extreme caution when increasing dietary fat.
- Anyone who has a serious illness such as unstable cardiovascular disease, cancer, or liver disease needs to exercise reasonable caution if making dietary changes.
- If you are pregnant or lactating, you should not overly restrict protein (or fat) intake. Babies, young children, and teens have much more demanding nutrient and caloric needs and should not have their protein or fat intake overly restricted. There is no established dietary requirement for carbohydrates (sugar or starch), but when pregnant you should use caution in changing your existing diet—other than eliminating junk foods.

CONTENTS

PART TWO

THE METABOLIC FUEL DUEL: SUGARS AND FATS DUKE IT OUT

Challenging Sugar's Top-Dog Status, and
Why Fat Doesn't Make You Fat

PART THREE

THE UNRIVALED POWER OF PRIMAL FAT BURNING

Optimizing Your Health, Preventing and Resolving
Disease, and Achieving Peak Performance

PART FOUR

THE PRIMAL FAT BURNER PLAN

FOREWORD

We all have a sweet tooth. It is as basic to our constitution as thirst. And for more than 99 percent of the time we have walked this bountiful planet, our sweet tooth has served us well and helped us to survive. The surge of insulin brought on by our deep desire for sugar flips biochemical switches that cause the human body to make and store body fat. And body fat, throughout the entire history of our species, has served as a supremely concentrated source of survival calories, allowing us to continue the tasks of hunting and gathering during times of food scarcity.

But times have changed. Coming upon a source of sugar, like a tree full of ripe fruit, is no longer a rare event that triggers life-sustaining fat deposition. For most people, sugar consumption, in all of its various forms, is a biochemical event culminating in the creation of fat tissue 365 days a year. A mechanism that graced us with survivability for millennia now threatens the functionality of every organ system in the body.

Dr. Robert Lustig, in his highly informative book *Fat Chance*, points out that "of the six hundred thousand food items for sale in the United States, 80 percent are laced with added sugar." Data suggests that close to *70 percent* of adult Americans are overweight or actually obese. And a powerful catchphrase that has supported the sales of these sugar-enriched products has often centered on their reduced levels of fat, as if that were somehow a health attribute.

In 2009, Nora Gedgaudas published her seminal book, *Primal Body, Primal Mind*, which confronted the well-accepted doctrine that so much of our ill health results from our consumption of dietary fat. Her detailed research revealed that while our Paleolithic ancestors did on occasion consume sugar and carbohydrates, the bulk of their calories, as much as ten times what we consume today, derived from fat.

Primal Body, Primal Mind eloquently presented the science supporting the role of healthful fats in keeping us healthy, especially when coupled with substantial reduction in sugar and carbohydrates. As a physician, I welcomed *Primal Body, Primal Mind* to my clinical practice, giving out hundreds of copies to fat-phobic patients whose health issues, including their obesity, clearly related to their consumption of sugar and carbohydrates coupled with a *lack* of adequate dietary fat.

In her new book, *Primal Fat Burner*, Gedgaudas writes from a position supported by a sea change in the scientific community. In these pages she underscores how, from an evolutionary standpoint, our body's relationship and response to specific foods have been finely honed over hundreds of thousands of years, how food actually informs our DNA about changes in our environment, and how current dietary choices threaten this intimate communication, paving the way for ill health.

The science presented in *Primal Fat Burner* is fascinating, as the narrative reveals how we have come full circle, back to a place of honoring the evolutionary gifts of our forebears. *Primal Fat Burner* leaves no doubt that much-maligned dietary fat is absolutely critical for health and longevity. But Gedgaudas carefully delineates the characteristics of healthful versus health-threatening fats. She shows how healthful fats serve to reduce inflammation, the cornerstone of all degenerative conditions, and how fat represents the most efficient fuel for each and every cell in the human body, creating energy while producing fewer damaging free radicals. She explores the important role of dietary fat in regulating hunger and explains how increasing dietary fat will actually open the door for weight loss.

But most important, the text is wonderfully actionable, compassionately taking the reader from "why" to "how." From vitamins to recipes, *Primal Fat Burner* leverages an incredibly robust body of science to create a life plan that will allow us to embrace our genetic legacy.

DAVID PERLMUTTER, MD, FACN
NAPLES, FLORIDA
JANUARY 2016

INTRODUCTION

In my first book, *Primal Body, Primal Mind*, I described how the primal lifestyle can lead to optimal health and longevity. In the seven years since its first publication, that book has reached more people than I could have ever imagined, many of whom have applied its principles and who have written me to say that their health and well-being improved significantly after changing what they eat. Many people asked that I put together a more structured eating plan along with additional information, recipes, and resources for primal eating. *Primal Fat Burner* does just that. But the book you are about to read isn't necessarily a weight loss book.

Fat—including saturated fat—is nowhere near the bad guy we used to think it was. Eating fat can make you thin. *Primal Fat Burner* helps you harness the best dietary practices of our ancestors with the most current scientific understanding of nutrition. With this knowledge you can use quality dietary fat and the rich abundance of critical nutrients contained within it to create total health and well-being.

I am not simply here to tell you that "fat isn't as bad as you might have heard," or "fats are okay, just as long as you keep them to a minimum," or "fats are okay just as long as you stick to strictly unsaturated fats." I am here to supply you with a mountain of compelling evidence that fats from animals that eat a natural diet not only are essential to your health but have served more than any other dietary adaptation to *literally make us human*.

In *Primal Fat Burner*, based on the latest science and research, I explain why eating foods rich in dietary fat (while avoiding the consumption of sugars and starch and moderating protein intake) is the best and most natural nutritional approach for your complete health and well-being. This book emphasizes (in part) a low-carbohydrate approach to eating. There is far more to the plan, but you will find that the fewer utilizable carbs you consume and the less insulin your body needs to produce, the better your long-term health will likely be.

Primal Fat Burner focuses on the single biggest factor in your health and longevity: the primal fat-burning diet, a modification of what is commonly known as a ketogenic diet. This approach to food is radically different from our current nutritional status quo—but in many ways it is the oldest form of nutrition in human history. A fat-based ketogenic diet has powered humans and our pre-human hominid ancestors through almost all of our three million years of evolution, and it is a critical tool that has the power to reduce weight, strengthen resilience, and reverse many of the chronic diseases of today.

As a clinical nutritionist and ancestral nutrition expert, I consult and lecture with health seekers around the globe. Countless times I've seen clients and audience members meet the word *ketogenic* with equal doses of fascination, trepidation, and misunderstanding: "Isn't that Atkins? Starvation? A medical treatment? For hard-core health nuts?" Having devoted my life to understanding the evolution of our metabolic functioning, I can assure you that a well-balanced ketogenic approach to eating is none of those things. Nor is it especially controversial. Surprise: the fat-burning ketogenic diet is actually our *norm*, and it is fundamental to our human design as breathing. It simply means using the energy from fats found in real foods, in the form nature intended them, as your primary source of fuel. When this is explained, what was once mysterious starts to become commonsense.

Over the fifteen or so years that I have followed a primal fat-burning protocol myself, I've worked with and counseled a remarkably diverse client population. At one end of the spectrum are those battling significant weight issues or serious ailments, from type 2 diabetes to early onset dementia. Often, the pain of the solutions they've been offered by medicine and mainstream nutrition exceeds the pain of the problem, so they come to primal fat burning in order to take things into their own hands. In the middle of the spectrum are women and men approaching middle age, or sometimes advanced age, who look healthy but who have discovered that they have underlying, unhealthy, and elevated blood sugar levels and other troubling blood test markers. They have been following seemingly balanced, carb-friendly ways of eating that have been invisibly ravaging their physiology—even though they still fit into their jeans.

At the far other end of the spectrum is a different crowd: people who are consciously eating what they consider to be a "paleo" diet (yes, I said "consider to be"—more on that later) but who have not gotten the results they are seeking; primal eaters who have drifted slowly from their low-carbohydrate goals and need help (or a swift kick in the pants) to reboot their program and to focus and dial in on their efforts; and elite or endurance athletes who are harnessing the energy from dietary fats to powerfully boost their performance.

If you've picked up this book piqued by the idea of becoming a primal fat burner, chances are you fall somewhere on this arc. You might have long struggled with diets that don't work, or despaired at ever achieving a lean physique. Like me, you might have a deeply personal experience with depression, anxiety, or low energy. Or maybe you are watching others in your family suffer from health issues you know to be genetic, and you want to do anything you can to avoid those diseases yourself. Women and men of all ages simply want to feel better, live longer, and look and feel younger, with a clearer mind and most certainly a leaner and more resilient body that they inhabit proudly. They want to enjoy every day of their lives—whether young, middle aged, or older—and they resist what is sold to us as the "inevitable" modern-day aging scenario of prescription drugs in their bathroom cabinet. They refuse to sign up for one of the so-called diseases of civilization—diabesity, depression, dementia and brain degeneration, heart disease, cancer. If this is "civilized," they are saying, they'd rather be primal!

For the Love of Fat

Fat has recently become the darling of the health world. In numerous peer-reviewed studies scientists are exonerating fat for health crimes it didn't commit. For fifty years, fat was vilified by an aggressive anti-fat campaign, which shunted it out of its rightful place on our plate to make way for excesses of carbohydrates.

While I am glad that fat has finally won some redemption, its acceptance has been a little begrudging and timid. Most experts are all open arms when it comes to fat-rich, plant-based foods. And they're pretty friendly with fish. They suggest modest little drizzles of this and splashes of this and that—and a quarter of an avocado, if you please.

As for me, please pass the lard. I wrote *Primal Fat Burner* to the beat of a much louder drum and with the intention of blazing a bolder path. This book is based on the fundamental scientific understanding that *all fats, especially fats from healthy animal sources and unrefined tropical oils, are paramount to the functioning of our physiology and to our robust health*. These formerly maligned fats must be wholeheartedly reclaimed as vital to our health. Animal-sourced fats provide sustaining energy and absolutely critical fat-soluble nutrients. Without them, we would not have become who we are as humans.

In *Primal Fat Burner* I will take you on a journey of discovery. I will show you how humans' ability to "run on fat" defined how our remarkable body and brain functioning evolved—and why the modern shift to "running on sugars" has been one of the most egregious missteps in human history. I will share why the natural fats found in wholesome real foods, in particular the fats from animals that eat a diet of grasses and other natural forage, are a match for your genetic makeup and help you achieve a stable weight and robust health—and how the lack of these things can dangerously erode your well-being. And I'll explain why naturally fat-rich foods, used correctly, are the foundation of an optimal way of eating that (with some minor tweaks in individual implementation) is relevant to everyone.

Then I take you further. I will give you tools that can help you become a lean and energized fat burner yourself.

In Parts One, Two, and Three, I share everything you need to know about how a fat-burning metabolic state functions and why it is your natural state. You'll discover that the cells of your body, in particular the cells of your heart and brain, thrive on fat. And you'll learn that not all calories are created equal. I explain how using *ketones*, the energy units of fat, instead of *glucose*, the energy from carbohydrates in the form of starches and sugars, gives you a life-changing (and potentially lifesaving) metabolic advantage. This advantage not only affects your entire quality of life but can be measured quantitatively on your blood work panels.

The real goal of *Primal Fat Burner* is to show you how to ignite your fat-burning metabolism—think of metabolism as the mechanism of converting food to fuel—by using a well-balanced and high-quality ketogenic diet. When you switch on your fat-burning metabolism and allow it to stay on continuously by maintaining this way of eating every day, the results can be tremendous. You create the conditions to achieve a healthy and stable weight, even if you are very overweight. That's because, once your body adapts to relying primarily on ketones and free fatty acids for energy, it starts using your fat reserves for fuel, instead of storing them on your belly, love handles, hips, and thighs. Your brain runs sharper and better, too—an effect

SWITCH ON A WELL-ADAPTED, FAT-BURNING STATE AND YOU LAY THE GROUNDWORK FOR:

- Easier weight loss, without excessive hunger or cravings, and long-lasting energy
- Reduced blood sugar issues, lower hemoglobin A1C and other metabolic markers associated with metabolic diseases such as obesity and diabetes
- An anti-inflammatory effect and a dampening of excess free radical activity (which causes harmful tissue damage and is a driver of disease and aging)
- Anti-aging effects, with improved cellular regeneration and repair mechanisms and healthier, younger-looking skin
- Improved sleep
- Improved immune function
- Reduced blood pressure
- Stabilized neurological functioning in the brain, which makes you less susceptible to migraines, panic attacks, mood swings, and seizures, and reduces your risk of neurodegenerative diseases . . . and more

that can stay with you for life. Imbalances in blood sugar and insulin as well as inflammation can be resolved, with the effect of stabilizing, reducing, or even eliminating chronic pain and disease.

And all these benefits come from making a basic but consistent modification to your diet, eating moderate protein from clean, sustainable, and nutrient-enhancing sources, ample fibrous vegetables and greens, and as much fat as you need to satiate your hunger. By the end of Part One, you'll come to an empowering understanding: you can decide whether to be a fat burner or sugar burner, simply by eating certain real, whole foods and avoiding others. This makes *you* the agent of your own well-being and longevity.

Then, in Part Four, I hand you the road map you need to make the metabolic switch yourself. To make it simple and achievable, I've outlined a 21-day plan that gives you step-by-step guidance. It includes sixty simple recipes for breakfast, lunch, dinner, and snacks; guidance on how to prepare, cook with, and store all kinds of healthy fats; and balanced weekly meal plans. It also lays out how to prepare yourself physically and how to avoid common pitfalls during the transition period.

Shifting to an effective and well-adapted fat-burning metabolism takes between three and six weeks for most people. Once initiated, this fat-burning metabolic state becomes a fairly effortless new norm. I'll also walk you through exactly what to do if fatigue or discomfort arises during this transition time.

When you are successfully using the energy of fat for fuel, you are in what I call a state of *effective ketogenic adaptation* (EKA). In this book, we'll be following a unique approach that combines a state of EKA with high-level nutrition derived from quality food sources and support against stress and toxicity. This is primal fat burning.

The effects of primal fat burning are:

Energizing. You benefit from enduring energy that takes
    you easily from one meal to the next without snacks or
    cravings.
Protective. Your mitochondria—the cellular powerhouses
    that supply energy and guard against aging, among other

important functions—are protected. The health of your
heart and brain is safeguarded, and those organs' efficiency
and function are greatly enhanced.[1]

Regulating. Your blood sugar and insulin levels are given the
conditions to normalize and function more efficiently, as
nature intended.[2] Excess weight that has been resistant to
diets can be regulated, as trapped fat stores get mobilized
for energy.[3]

Stabilizing. Brain function and moods normalize and stabilize
when the brain is fed with fat.[4] Emotional struggles around
food, such as cravings and even certain eating disorders,
can subside or be eliminated.

Anti-aging. Human longevity markers improve (including
thyroid efficiency), and overall disease risks related to
inflammatory markers, cholesterol (which tends to elevate
with inflammation), and more are naturally lowered.[5]

Completely safe. A fat-based ketogenic diet based on the
Primal Fat Burner Plan is safe for almost everyone—with
some possible exceptions, which I will explain in detail.
With guidance from a physician, it can also be modified
for specific needs, such as pregnancy or nursing, type 1
diabetics, the increased growth rates of children and teens,
and the demands of high-intensity athletics.

The Primal Fat Burner Plan has a varied and satisfying menu.
You'll eat grass-fed, fat-rich meat and wild-caught seafood; greens
and other fibrous vegetables and sprouts; nuts and a few seeds;
probiotic-rich, fermented foods; and homemade bone broth. You'll
find that the plan described in this book is also:

Achievable. It's refreshingly straightforward and simple to
execute.

Enjoyable and efficient. The tasty, satiating food is easy to
make for yourself and your family.

Familiar. It's a return to wholesome, traditional foods you may
already know and love.

Affordable. You'll consume fewer packaged, pre-made foods and snacks. You'll wisely use quality ingredients, including cheaper cuts of high-quality meat (and bones), and indulge in fewer pricey splurge foods and nutritionally empty treats.

Liberating. By shifting from primarily sugar as fuel (which is addicting and damaging) to mainly slow-burning fat, you are freed of urgent cravings and the sudden, intense need to eat (which come from a dependency on carbs). You'll discover a new relationship with farmers and other sources of health-giving food. Most important, your relationship to food and eating will become clearer, healthier, and more resilient. It is a far saner, happier way to be.

Some of the information that follows might seem radical at first. Stay with me: you will see that this approach to caring for your health is in fact quite rational. *Primal Fat Burner* is based on a deep understanding of our ancestral origins. It is a foundational way of eating with an unshakable basis in evolutionary science. Its primary principle is this: *If your body could choose its fuel, it would choose fat.*

Though we have been conditioned to believe that we are de-

Let's cut to the chase on one important subject: to maintain a fat-burning metabolism, you need to greatly minimize starches and sugars, every day. In our twenty-first-century society, with our obsession with instant gratification, this can sound shockingly rigorous. Yes, it requires a choice and a change. But that choice becomes self-reinforcing as you feel more energy, more clarity, and greater self-empowerment by the day as you throw off a dependency that was not doing you any favors. And when you choose to do this, your blood test results improve as well. If the thought of going low-carb strikes dread in your heart (and taste buds), know that anticipation is much worse than reality. You'll discover that the satiating qualities of good fats in each meal have an extraordinary power to quiet cravings for sugars.

signed to use glucose as our primary fuel, this is not exactly correct. The human glucose metabolism evolved to deliver short-term energy. Used in sustained or excessive ways, as occurs when you eat a carbohydrate-laden diet (and also one that contains too much protein), sugars damage cells. Over a lifetime, excessive glucose and other dietary sugars damage our health irreparably, causing obesity, neurodegeneration, and many chronic diseases. It also helps to create a cellular environment that's a little too friendly to cancer.

In fact, if you asked your body, it would tell you that it prefers ketones far more than glucose, because the fuel ketones deliver is steady and reliable—no spikes and crashes. Your body would tell you that it *needs* an abundance of quality fat to get critical micronutrients that its cells require for proper functioning. Oh, and it would tell you that eating fat does *not* make you fat—if done wisely, that is, with carbohydrates minimized. Two decades of clinical experience have shown me that a properly fed body can usually and almost effortlessly drop extra weight.

In the chapters to come, you'll find that there is a unique aspect to the primal fat-burning approach that makes it distinct from variations of paleo or primal nutritional advice you may already know. Eating the foods that our ancestors relied on as the most consistent available sources is just the starting point. The Primal Fat Burner Plan also assesses these original foods according to human longevity science to measure how optimally they fit our needs in the uniquely challenging world we live in today. For instance, we know that the high amounts of protein that our ancestors tolerated—perhaps thanks to their robust genome—are not suitable for us today. Despite what you may have read in some paleo guidebooks, there is no physiological justification for filling your supermarket cart with stacks of Styrofoam-encased, factory-farmed meat or piling your plate high with animal protein at every meal—an act that is both dubious healthwise and clearly unethical. You'll hear this a few times in this book: the Primal Fat Burner Plan is *not* a high-protein diet.

These days our bodies also need significantly more detoxification support to face the onslaught of pollution and stressors coming at us from every direction. That's why phytonutrient-rich, fibrous vegetables and greens are much more critical for us than they were for our predecessors. The toxic stressors we encounter every day are dangerous new selective pressures that compromise our human genome in ways our ancestors did not have to deal with. The alarming and unprecedented pollution pervasive in our air, water, soil, and food, and the constant presence of electromagnetic frequency pollution and radiation, motivate my quest to go beyond paleo. I will help you optimize your nutrition and keep your wits about you as you shop. The growing epidemic of autoimmune issues triggered by food sensitivities and environmental contaminants is something a foodie or cook might want to ignore but a true scientist cannot. Today we understand more than ever that the environment inside our cells, created by what we deliberately *and* unwittingly ingest and absorb, profoundly influences whether inherited tendencies toward illness are expressed or stay safely dormant. Bringing this consciousness to our plate is an important part of the Primal Fat Burner Plan; in fact, it may be as vital as the amount of fat and protein on your plate.

To protect and defend your health, the Primal Fat Burner Plan is built on a firm commitment to using only the most unprocessed, uncontaminated food sources. We need food that goes *beyond* being merely "natural" or coming from a health food store. We need food that actually comes from prime growing and raising conditions—the way nature intended food to be. That's why the plan is built on a foundation of humanely, healthfully, and sustainably pasture-raised animal products. It will help you find the best local produce you can. Only this way can you supply your body with the nutrients it needs to combat toxins and stress. The good news is that there *is* a way to do this affordably and wisely. Our great-grandparents did it, and so can we.

In the pages to come, these two aspects—ancestral roots and modern science—combine to create an optimized nutritional approach to your health and well-being that will give you back the power over your own health. Fair warning: this book *will* have you questioning authority and what you've come to know as "normal." It might have you questioning everyone who ever told you to finish your cereal, take two aspirin and call back in the morning, and avoid that evil, "artery-clogging" animal fat at all costs and replace it with margarine and canola oil instead. Let this be a motivating force: To help you switch on your fat-burning metabolism, free yourself from an unhealthful dependence on starches and sugars, and forge a more healthful alliance with nutritious, unadulterated fats. Serena Williams didn't get good at tennis by playing golf all day, any more than Tiger Woods mastered the game of golf by bowling. You cannot become good at burning fat by burning sugar all the time. To burn fat at a world-class level, you need to become a Primal Fat Burner and train your body to choose fat, not sugar, as your primary source of everyday fuel.

I've seen all kinds of people succeed in using the power of a fat-burning metabolism to transform their lifestyle and reclaim their good health, from the mother motivated to stay healthy for her children and dodge diseases that have taken her own parents to the septuagenarian who is able to put down his blood pressure and prostate medication and walk free of long-standing pain. The foundation to health that fat burning provides is universal. Of course, there may be some adjustments needed in order to target any uniquely personal vulnerabilities. But fat burning provides the firm ground on which to do that next level of work.

It really does all start with what you eat—and what you choose not to eat. When you restore your primal birthright of robust physical and mental health and a life unhindered by preventable pain and

WHAT DOES A PRIMAL FAT BURNER EAT?

In this way of eating, you will be enjoying roasted meats and poultry; creamy Thai coconut soup; colorful vegetables and greens that can be raw, steamed, sautéed, broiled, or cultured; seasoned ribs; pan-seared chicken livers with pastured bacon; ground beef salad; coconut-wrapped burritos; and succulent fish tacos; Thai salad with spicy dressing; lamb chops; steamed zucchini noodles with rich meat sauce; delicious and tangy cultured vegetables; burgers (with an extra-primal twist); coconut chicken salad; crispy pork belly; stuffed grape leaves; curries; and many other mouthwatering dishes.

disease, it is astounding how energized you feel to make and sustain change—and I mean that at every level. By the end of *Primal Fat Burner*, you will discover that it's really not as complicated as you might have thought.

Is Primal Fat Burning Right for You?

Given our common human design and our bodies' preference for running on fat, the short answer is universally yes! But use this quiz to check how it might specifically support you to feel your best and function at your peak.

Are you overweight? Do you experience:

Fatigue?
Mood swings?
Brain fog?
Chronic pain?
Food cravings or frequent hunger?
Memory issues or absentmindedness?
Problems focusing or thinking?
Morning stiffness?
Digestive problems?
Water retention or bloating?
Poor muscle tone?
Poor sleep?
Irritability or emotional reactivity?
Sleepiness after meals?
Feelings of helplessness and hopelessness about your health?
An awareness that things could and should be better?

If you answer yes to three or more of the questions, then you can be assured that *Primal Fat Burner* will offer you a powerful path forward to greater health and well-being. If you answered yes to fewer than three—or to none at all—read on anyway! The Primal Fat Burner Plan will increase your resistance to disease, improve

QUICK ASSESSMENT

If you have recent blood test results available, take a look at them now. If your results show any of the following, you are most definitely a prime candidate for the Primal Fat Burner Plan:

Fasting blood sugars above 90 mg/dL
Fasting triglycerides above 100 mg/dL
Hgb A1C above 5.5%
HDL below 55 mg/dL
CRP above 1.0 mg/L
Homocysteine above 6.0 μmol/L
Fibrinogen above 423 mg/dL

See Chapter 10 for more information on blood test markers.

your cognitive functioning, offer better physical performance, and more. You do not need to be sick or unhealthy to benefit from this approach, any more than you need to be out of shape in order to benefit from exercise!

PERSONAL PREFACE:
DISCOVERING A LONG-LOST KEY

"What are we meant to eat?" is a question that has inspired, provoked, challenged, and obsessed me for my entire life. For thirty-five years I've pondered it as a researcher, immersing myself in the study of anthropology and ancestral nutrition. And over my two-decade career practicing clinical nutrition and neurofeedback, I've pursued the subject in a hands-on way, seeking better results for my clients. But the roots of this inquiry go back further, to my own personal story of struggle.

The Canadian-born child of a prominent medical family, I grew up in the 1960s and 1970s in Minnesota. I followed the doctor-approved, heart-healthy diet of the time: low-fat food cooked in vegetable oils, potatoes topped with margarine, and low-sodium snacks from America's most trusted brands. My mother, a former ballet dancer, wanted to make sure we all stayed slim and healthy, and my father, a world-renowned radiologist with a specialty in cardiology, faithfully adhered to admonitions about avoiding evil fats and cholesterol and to recommendations about consuming superior grains and starches as reliable staple foods.

This way of eating, as it turned out, did not serve my beloved parents well. Their lives from late middle age onward were rife with medical interventions for everything from gallbladder disease, aneurysms, autoimmune disease, and cancer to, tragically, a fatal heart attack and Alzheimer's.

This diet also took its toll on me. As a child and young adult, I suffered from persistent depression. I struggled for years to understand why I felt this way, and I pursued every avenue of inquiry I could, encompassing mind, body, and soul. Slightly before I started study-ing premed at college, the emerging fields of nutritional research and supplementation captured my scientific mind. The cutting-edge work of longevity research scientists (such as life extension gurus Durk Pearson and Sandy Shaw) and amino acid researchers (such as Eric Braverman, author of *The Healing Nutrients Within*) hooked me with the promises that amino acid supplements and other natural substances could positively affect my brain chemistry. They did, to a point—sharpening my thoughts and lifting my dark moods. But these pricey supplements were more of a distraction than a cure, and in my excitement I didn't even realize I was missing out on a more fundamental piece of the puzzle: What *food* did my body and brain need to be well?

Being hip to the health trends of the eighties, I soon found my way to the "ultimate diet" according to the bestselling books of the time: vegetarianism. It lined up with what I'd heard all my life about the dangers of fat-rich, animal-source foods, so I faithfully followed the "healthful" path of whole grains, beans, and lentils—to my own detriment. Within a year I experienced deeper and longer depressive episodes, had pronounced anxiety and panic attacks, and developed an eating disorder. I began craving meat so much that, racked with guilt, I abandoned the vegetarian lifestyle before completing a second year. Fairly quickly my eating disorder evaporated and my depression and anxiety lessened. But rather than feeling proud that I had listened to my body, I struggled with feelings of shame and self-recrimination, thinking: *What is so wrong with me that I can't even succeed at being vegetarian?*

The answer, of course, was that there was nothing wrong with me; there was just something wrong with my diet. A life-changing invita-tion started to open my eyes. Famed wolf biologist Dr. L. David Mech offered me a coveted spot as his research assistant for a summer. Few people in my life at the time knew this but, along with bio-hacking and longevity research, I had an ardent passion for wolves. As a young child I'd read and reread Farley Mowat's classic book *Never Cry Wolf*, about his time observing the animals in the northern Canadian Arc-tic, and I had volunteered on wolf research projects in Minnesota in my twenties. So Dr. Mech's invitation was quite literally a childhood fantasy come true. We would live alone together on Ellesmere Island, less than five hundred miles from the North Pole, and closely observe a family of wild wolves. Days after my thirtieth birthday, and stocked with a summer's worth of personal provisions, I left civilization for the wilds of the Canadian High Arctic Archipelago.

The wolf pack that I would study lived 350 miles north of the closest village, the remote Inuit hamlet of Gris Fjord. These wild wolves were unique because they had never been hunted. As a result, they weren't afraid of humans, which allowed for unprecedented close-range observation of their otherwise elusive behavior. (They remain the subjects of ongoing research under the supervision of Dr. Mech, who returns each summer to observe this same pack.)

Known as Umingmak Nuna in the Inuktitut language, which means "land of musk ox," Ellesmere Island has a long history of native human habitation. According to archaeologists, the earliest Paleo-Eskimo inhabitants were made up of small bands of hunters drawn to the area for the abundant Peary caribou, musk ox, and a variety of marine mammals (including polar bears) starting about 2000 to 1000 BCE. The island holds remnants of the ancient Thule culture, ancestors of the Inuit. Strewn about ancient abandoned encampments were the bones and skulls of hunted animals. Stone hunting blinds topped hills from which ancient Thule hunters once ambushed musk ox. Stone circle outlines of what had been skin-covered summer shelters dotted the shoreline in clusters. A few artifacts were still lying out in the open as though their owners might be coming back for them. As I carefully stepped around the ancient animal skulls and bones, I made a startling observation: most of the skulls had been broken open for access to the nutrient-dense, fat-rich brains they had once housed, and numerous large femur bones from hunted land mammals had been cracked open for their precious marrow.

I had always felt an inexplicable connection to the peoples and the landscape of the High Arctic, and when I realized the cunning and ingenuity it had taken for the ancient Inuit to thrive in such a harsh climate, I was quite in awe.

Had any of them known about my dietary habits prior to arriving on Ellesmere Island, they would have thought them very odd indeed. My diet was primarily plant-based and dutifully low in fat, with some lean meat, seafood, and nonfat yogurt forming the occasional accents to my primary fare of salads and freshly made juices. (None of that felt incongruous with my fitness regimen of daily three-mile runs and some weight training—it was what "healthy" people did, after all.) Stepping off the Twin Otter cargo plane after arriving from Resolute Bay in my subzero boots, I was quite nervous about how I'd subsist up there, without any fresh fruits and vegetables or organic-food co-ops.

Ellesmere Island is a breathtakingly beautiful landscape that displays Mother Nature's grandeur in her barest, most raw, almost primordial countenance. Alive in its rich subtleties of colorful flora, it is a silent, dignified, and pristine land that time forgot. This land was not even glaciated during the previous Ice Age (the glacial movement that once covered most of North America had begun well south of this remote northerly place). The particular location on the island where Dave Mech and I spent the better part of our summer qualified as a "thermal oasis," with rich carpets of colorful greenery covering much of the hummocky landscape, rocky bluffs, and outcroppings, and small rivers and streams winding throughout the vast area. White glaciated mountains loomed in the distance, and the local fjord looked almost like a fairy tale of Arctic dreams, filled with ghostly, drifting icebergs, with the occasional thundering roar of calving glaciers some distance away. It is easily the most peaceful place on earth.

During my Arctic adventure, I spent long days sitting quietly upon the frozen tundra, closely observing a family of white Arctic wolves (*Canis lupus arctos*). Since the movement of humans can cause the wolves some distress, we respectfully maintained a quiet stillness. We did not interact with the wolves unless they initiated contact, but they treated our presence with a mix of curiosity and indifference, and frequently passed within inches of us. I once awoke from a nap to discover a huge paw print in the dust, one inch behind my head, where a wolf had sniffed my hair as I slept. The pups were always curious and frequently came close to us. Through this consistent, calm, and respectful behavior (and their long-term habituation to Dave during his many summers there), we earned their trust. We followed them on their hunts on ATV four-wheelers, to which they were accustomed.

While I occasionally took evening walks during the twenty-four-hour daylight, there were no real opportunities to go for a jog or lift weights. Nearly all my time was spent bundled up and just sitting on the frozen ground or on a four-wheeler on the tundra, observing the Arctic wolves. I was very well insulated and really never felt cold. My only other activity was eating. Constantly. And uncharacteristically for me, the one thing I craved above all else was *fat*. I ate copious amounts of nuts, cheese, and salami, plus some nut butter, but almost no fruits or vegetables (save some onions we had brought along to stir-fry in butter with the Arctic hare we were occasionally able to procure). It was the complete opposite of the diet I had been raised on.

In Farley Mowat's book *People of the Deer*, he documents his own life among the remote Ihalmiut people of northern Canada. In one section he recounts how he had become so mysteriously weak and ill that he couldn't even stand. His Ihalmiut companions rendered the fat of a caribou and forced him to drink the warm liquid tallow. He described his recovery as nearly miraculous and almost immediate. This particular account stayed with me, and during my silent research sessions, I wondered, *How could animal fat possibly heal like that?* I also recalled the writings of Vilhjálmur Stefánsson, an Arctic explorer who documented the Inuit way of life in the early 1900s. In his book *Arctic Manual* he attributed the Inuits' extraordinary physical prowess and mental constitution to their animal-source diet and documented the particular delicacies of the caribou—the marrow and in particular the fat behind the eyes, lower jaw, and kidneys. He also famously said that meat is a complete meal only when the animal you eat is fat. Nobody was offering *me* any caribou fat, but suddenly the logic of eating it started to make sense. I was certainly craving it!

Once a week Dave and I made a middle-of-the-night pilgrimage to a remote military weather station, which housed our extra supplies. With twenty-four-hour daylight in summertime, this isn't as strange as it sounds. Each of us would take a badly needed shower and make a fifteen-minute phone call to loved ones. The officer in charge would let us sneak into the mess hall, where food was set out for midnight snacks. The only thing I had eyes for was the enormous bowl of butter set out by the bread. I'd slather it onto a piece of toast— the mere vehicle for lashings of soft, creamy, salty-sweet fat—then repeat, indulging in as much of this heavenly ambrosia as I could.

You would think that someone doing nothing but sitting on her backside all day and eating such a diet would have gained a fair amount of weight over those couple of months. Yet when I arrived home at the end of that summer I had lost a good twenty-five pounds of body fat while developing an even leaner, more visibly muscular build. In fact, I looked so changed that my loved ones were concerned that I had been intentionally starving myself. Nothing could have been further from the truth! In fact, I felt transformed on multiple levels.

My body's changes that summer in the Arctic and my observations of the mostly subsistence-living Inuit peoples I had met in extreme northern Canada made me rethink everything I thought I knew about how to eat, and I started to seriously ponder what might actually constitute an optimal human diet. Some thermogenic effects may have helped my body burn more fat for warmth, at least in part, but I knew that there was more to the story than that. Why had I gotten healthier and leaner the more fat I consumed? And if eating fat doesn't make us fat, then what does?

A few years after returning from Ellesmere, as I continued to pursue a new passion for nutrition and refine my eating habits with good-quality, animal-sourced foods, I stumbled across the now-classic text *Nutrition and Physical Degeneration* by Weston A. Price. A dentist by trade and a pioneer in nutrition by passion, Price traveled the world in the 1920s and 1930s, covering more than a hundred thousand miles over ten years and chronicling the health and nutrition of numerous native and traditional peoples. His meticulous and exhaustive research ultimately concluded that, despite the varied nature of their diets, they all had two things in common. First, none of them ate strictly vegetarian or vegan diets; all of them consumed the many animal foods available to them. Second, in all of the cultures he studied, the most important and sacred foods were consistently those highest in fat and fat-soluble nutrients, regardless of whatever else they had available to eat. This was true whether these people lived on a remote tropical Pacific island, an African savanna, the hot, arid Australian outback, or the Arctic tundra. Dr. Price also observed that, when the first generation of these groups began eating processed and refined foods such as flour, sugar, and packaged foods, their health deteriorated. This was seen most visibly in their subsequent offspring's (and later descendants') cranial shape and dentition, and in emerging physical and mental problems. It was as if millennia of problem-free health were suddenly undermined—all by food.

Price's exciting findings about fat-rich ancestral diets offered tantalizing clues to a tightly woven relationship between human beings and fat that had been completely forgotten—or was it completely covered up?—in modern cultures. His research radically challenged the pervasive (some would say militant) anti-fat dietary dogma of the time and the paranoia about all things cholesterol-related. It hinted at serious problems with conventional paradigms and government-approved, starch-heavy food pyramids. But the many diets and foods of the global groups that Dr. Price surveyed didn't quite provide the fully foundational framework that I sought. I was searching for something that, most critically, would speak to our common physiological blueprint and provide a single way forward, relevant to us all.

To arrive at that answer, I engaged in a massive and complex investigation that took me thousands of generations further back in time than the relatively recent post-agrarian cultures in Dr. Price's studies. Combining my anthropological research with some of the most cutting-edge contemporary science and the stories from the clients I saw daily as a clinician, I would connect the dots to show that the missing key ingredient of our dietary health is fat.

It was the Inuit culture that inspired this radically different path for me—the group of people whose way of living seemed closest to the harsh conditions of our prehistoric Ice Age past, and whose fat-rich, nearly carbohydrate-free way of eating hinted at the longest-held patterns in human history. Unable to shake the stories of their robust constitution and the images of the shattered bones and skulls I'd seen, I peered back into the Ice Age and beyond, into our very origins and evolution as humans, seeking to uncover the roots of our basic physiological makeup and nutritional requirements toward a more universal and foundational approach to optimal health. I wondered, *Did the keys to our healthier future live in our primal past?*

PART ONE

Born to Run . . . on Fat

Why Our Ancestors' Persistent Search for Fat Is What Ultimately Made Us Who and What We Are (and Why Vegetarianism Is a Modern-Day Experiment)

L ook into the fossil record of our evolutionary antecedents, or explore the basic design of our human digestive system and physiological makeup, and you will find clues—distinct and clear clues—about how we evolved over roughly a hundred thousand generations to become fat burners. These principles formed the human blueprint and established the makeup of our very being, making us unique among all of the earth's life-forms. But we have more recently diverged from our ancestral norm in what is, evolutionarily speaking, the blink of an eye. What began as a backslide has become a dangerous, slippery slope. Today, humanity's very future lies in the balance . . . and clues to the ultimate solution may well lie in our evolutionary past.

CHAPTER 1

From Lucy to Tribal Hunter

HOW EATING MEAT—AND ESPECIALLY FAT—JUMP-STARTED OUR EVOLUTION FROM APELIKE TO HUMAN

The fresh kill left by the saber-toothed cats lay still in the dewy morning grass as the sun rose over the parched savanna. The heat was already beginning to rise as Lucy's eyes scanned the horizon for any sign of the predators that had brought down the giant, bloodied buck. The saber-toothed cats were busy chasing off hyenas, but they would soon return.

The smell of smoke from distant wildfires was a reminder that edible plant life in the area had been scarce since the long drought had set in. In the vast distance beyond the plain, a cloud of ash billowed high into the hazy sky from a looming volcano. Small particles of ash littered the landscape, smothering the few patches of green grass that were still growing. Only a few of the grazing animals that were still around were finding much to eat.

Lucy rose on her two legs to peer cautiously above the tall, dry grass for any sign of immediate danger and made her way a few feet to the kill. Her mate stood nearby, watching for the return of the cats.

The carcass was just too large and heavy to steal away, but Lucy had planned ahead. Her rough, leathery hand grasped a large, razor-sharp stone for carving flesh. With swift and powerful blows, she cut deeply into the partially eaten hindquarters and managed to disarticulate the large, meaty shank. She pulled and twisted it free from the rest of the carcass and quickly fled with her mate, scrambling for cover in the nearby brush. When they'd found a protected place, they ravenously feasted on that meat until all that was left was a femur and a smattering of smaller bones. Lucy raised her sharp stone tool and struck the bone repeatedly until it cracked open to yield the creamy contents within . . . rich, life-giving fat.

This scene, and others like it, took place about 3.39 million years ago. Not quite an ape and not quite human, Lucy has become something of a celebrity in paleoanthropology circles, the earliest hominin ever discovered. (She's a member of our hominid species group, but from a separate line called *Australopithecus afarensis.*) The unearthing of Lucy's partial skeleton in Ethiopia radically challenged the notion that our very earliest ancestors were herbivores. When it became clear that Lucy's kind used stone tools to cleave meat and marrow from animal prey, the practice of hominid meat eating became more deeply ingrained in history than previously thought—by a whopping eight hundred thousand years.[1]

When the global climate began to change and warm radically, less than a million years later, the earliest proto-members of our own human species finally emerged from the dwindling trees, forced by the change in climate to live out and exposed on the grass-filled savanna. The scarcity of edible plants pressured them to make meat and animal fat their primary food, with fruit and leaves becoming side dishes. This dependence on an extremely nutrient-dense food was a turbo-boost to this emerging brand of intelligent primate,[2] who learned to stand upright in order to better scan the horizon for predators, grasp and use spears (thanks to their opposable thumbs), and adapt to a hunting and scavenging way of life. Notably, they also learned how to scavenge brain tissue along with fatty bone marrow.

Before long, what anthropologists term "persistent carnivory"— the full-time dependence on meat eating—became our new consistent ancestral norm.[3,4] And it became the biological impetus for the development of a body that was very different from that of the apes that preceded us: our digestive tracts changed in order to process meat efficiently, and our stomachs developed the high acidity levels normally associated with scavengers in the wild.[5] Stomach acid is necessary to effectively digest animal protein, absorb minerals, and protect us from potentially harmful microbes. Our gallbladders evolved to handle significant amounts of fat and fat-soluble nutrients in the fatty animal foods we consumed. We also evolved the ability to absorb (and developed a distinct preference for) heme sources of iron, which come from blood and are found only in animal-source foods.[6] In addition, our heads and teeth evolved to meet our ever-greater carnivorous appetites, with skull, jaw, and teeth changes to accommodate the ripping and shearing of flesh.[7] Most dramatically, the hominin brain began to grow in size and sophistication at a rate that is unmatched in natural history. Our behaviors developed, our intelligence grew, and the first *Homo sapiens*—the humans we are today—began to emerge.

It's hard to overstate the significance of this dietary development. Though we often identify ourselves as "omnivores," able to consume a variety of food sources, the truth is that not all foods are created equal in the eyes of our physiological makeup. For most of our evolutionary history we have been mostly carnivores and scavengers—not only actively carnivorous, but actually even more so than the wolves, cats, foxes, and bears we lived among. We were cunning and sophisticated enough to procure *more* of our caloric intake from meat than they did, especially from the extra-large megafauna that were available to us until the end of the last glacial period. (This has been measured using high-tech devices called isotope ratio mass spectrometers, which can determine aspects of dietary composition from bone collagen samples of prehistoric humans and animals.)[8]

With apologies to vegetarians and those for whom *omnivorous* is shorthand for "just eat whatever you want," the fact is that it was a key dependency on meat and fat eating, and the development of increasingly sophisticated hunting practices, that allowed us to spread out of Africa and to adapt to new environments across the entire world.[9]

Selecting for Fat

To understand why we became fat burners, you need to factor in the environment we were living in for the majority of our evolution.

The past 2.58 million years are known as the Quaternary Ice Age (it hasn't ended yet, by the way), and for most of it, the global climate has been far less stable and friendly than it appears to us today. It has been marked by extreme bouts of climate change, including major periods of glacial advance alternating with (shorter) periods of glacial retreat. The key word here is *extremes*—extreme cold in some places and extreme heat in others, with drought, wildfires, and chaotic and quite frequent volcanic activity that destroyed plant-based foods in many regions, among other disruptive things. It was during one of the prolonged, colder, and more inhospitable periods roughly two hundred thousand years ago that our modern human physiology emerged more or less fully complete. We became humans by, quite literally, surviving catastrophes.

This means that the most powerful pressure we faced was the urgent need for nutrient-dense calories, enough to fuel our large, energy-hungry brain and to warm our fur-less bodies. (Though the majority of the world's humans were likely huddled closer to the equator, even those places experienced extreme, uncomfortable conditions—it can get perishingly cold even in a stormy jungle at night.)

Thus evolved what is perhaps the most critical but little-discussed aspect of our hunting and scavenging past: prehistoric humans didn't hunt and scavenge in the pursuit of meat per se but were driven by an urgent need for *fat,* the most calorically dense food. For several million years before the dawn of agriculture, our ancestors relied on abundant animal protein and fats of all kind—saturated fats and the delicate polyunsaturated fats known as omega-3s and arachidonic acid that exist alongside them in meat. We developed a dietary preference for large, fatty, and robust land animals and learned to use every part of them, nose to tail. This preference persisted even when, during the Mesolithic period—the transitional period of the Stone Age between the Paleolithic and the Neolithic periods from about twelve thousand years ago to roughly eight thousand years ago—humans began to eat more fish.[10]

In fact, this preference persisted even in post–Ice Age primitive, indigenous, and traditional societies wherever possible, even in the absence of the megaherbivores whose fat was far more plentiful.

When we scavenged carcasses, we created techniques to harvest the nutrient-dense parts that other predators could not—the juicy marrow inside the bones and the ultra-fat-rich brains. The saturated fats and key polyunsaturated fats we derived from them in turn fed *our* brains, which are fat-based and require animal-source fats as the critical building blocks. A positive feedback loop was created: the more animal fat we ate, the more our brains grew and intelligence developed, and the better we became at creating tools to procure even more meat and fat. When survival is at stake, you can't afford to get by on shreds of scavenged meat or wait for fruit trees to come into season. You want the most energy-dense food you can get. And the variety of fats from animal sources—immensely satisfying and nourishing in relatively small amounts—is exactly that.

It wasn't just any old animal sources of meat we sought. For prehistoric humans, the fatter and sassier the animal, the better the meal, and in Paleolithic terms, this meant *big*. Anthropologists call the extra-large land mammals of the time "megafauna"—these include woolly mammoths, mastodons, ground sloths, prehistoric bison (much different from today's hybridized buffalo), elephants, camels, Irish elk, and the giant auroch (the prehistoric ancestor of our cattle today). The larger the animals, the slower they moved, and the more body fat they accumulated. A woolly mammoth, for example, likely consisted of at least 50 percent fat (extrapolating somewhat from today's elephants), with stores of subcutaneous fat four inches thick—as well as a gigantic brain and megabones rich in marrow. It could weigh up to eleven tons, so taking it down required sophisticated technologies, bravery, and cunning—but the pursuit was worth it. Snag a full-size woolly mammoth, and you'd basically have a family barbecue—or maybe an all-you-can-eat buffet—that lasted for weeks. Early humans would have gorged on this fat-rich meat, seizing the opportunity to fill up their bellies when they got it. (This may also help explain the pronounced levels of hydrochloric acid in the human stomach, as compared with those of our other primate brethren: it takes a *lot* of hydrochloric acid to break down all that protein.)

Prehistoric people also hunted mountain sheep, beavers, bears, and wild pigs—all animals having high subcutaneous fat content.[11]

They weren't after the lean cuts of muscle meat; research has shown that both ancient and Neolithic hunters preferred tallow-rich fat in bison and camel humps and in nutrient-dense brains (which were 60 to 80 percent fat), tongues, kidney fat, and other organ meats.[12] Muscle meats—the cuts we tend to eat today—would have been dried and mixed with tallow to make energy-dense pemmican. At times the muscle meat got tossed down the food chain: according to stable isotopic analysis of Ice Age hunting tribes living in what is now the Czech Republic, humans ate the premium fatty mammoth meat, while the lean reindeer meat went to their dogs. Had Hanna-Barbera cartoonists understood all this, they would have depicted Fred Flintstone chowing on brain puree instead of Bronto Burgers at the Bedrock Stone Age drive-in.

Fueled by this food, our predecessors became master survivalists, able to persist despite the exceedingly challenging conditions throughout the Paleolithic era. In a feast-or-famine, climatically extreme world, fat came to mean survival—and *survival trumps everything else*. Our bodies, psychology, and biochemistry were forged around this basic principle, and we evolved inherent mechanisms for outlasting inevitable periodic famine, such as the fat-sensing hormone leptin (a subject covered at length in *Primal Body, Primal Mind*).

———

Today, we understand that fat was not only a preference but an absolute necessity.[13] We know that not only are animal-sourced fats the body's most efficient source of energy, but these fatty meats offer critical nutrients such as vitamin B_{12}, heme iron, zinc, and elongated omega-3 fatty acids that ensure the proper functioning of the brain and the entire nervous system, the health of our very cellular structure, and the strength of our immune system. Fats contain powerful anti-microbial properties to fight infection and fuel our most important system for homeostasis. They facilitate the absorption and utilization of protein, cushion our organs and keep us warm, and support the heart, bones, hormones, and lungs. And that's just the CliffsNotes version of everything fat does for us.

(An aside for foodies: Our ancestors developed a sophisticated sensory system designed to draw us irresistibly to fatty foods. Humans respond immediately to the smell, taste, and appearance of fat-rich foods because to survive, we had to be able to assess the energy content of foods with remarkable speed and accuracy. Next time someone laughs at your love of heirloom pork belly, tell them it's your evolutionary imperative at work.)

This veritable meat-fest was occurring during a relative dearth of usable plant foods. Not only would edible plants have been challenging to procure in this extreme climate, but gathering was time- and labor-intensive compared to hunting, with a low cost-to-benefit ratio in terms of calories acquired. It was also challenging due to the high level of toxicity in the very plants that could offer some protein or calories, such as wild legumes and wild potatoes. For survival, man needed nutrient density. The prehistoric mantra: meat, and especially fatty meat, is where it's at.[14]

Astonishing as it may sound to modern ears, eating all that fat did not make us fat. In fact, our ancestors were far leaner and more muscular than many professional athletes today. We ate lots of fat in the absence of carbohydrates, and this became the body's formula for optimal energy burning, sans the love handles, as you will discover. This is still the formula your body understands today.

Man, the Fat Hunter

About 12,800 years ago, things changed—suddenly, violently, and irrevocably.[15] A massive global cataclysm abruptly changed both the climate and growing conditions necessary for the survival of at least half the world's megafauna species, and these plus-sized creatures died out in the greatest mass extinction since the dinosaurs. Now living in a post-glacial recovery epoch—our world today, which anthropologists and geologists call the Holocene era—prehistoric humans were presented with a whole new challenge for procuring their primary food, fatty meat, in such volume. All of a sudden, hunting fare consisted mainly of smaller, leaner animals such as deer, elk, birds, and smaller game, which moved quickly and were harder to catch up to. This didn't change our preference for animal foods, however. To the contrary, it made hunting for fat an even more important focus, which forced us to further hone our hunting and observation skills.

Holocene humans became expert at selecting the fattest animals of the herd—bulls and females at the peak of maturity—through visual cues, such as the pronounced curves of the body and the sheen of the coat, and through seasonal selection, by tracking the animals' migration patterns.[16] To understand how remarkable this is and how different we are from other predators, consider that wild wolves always target the youngest or most infirm (often the leanest) animals in a pack. I have observed this firsthand many times: when wolves hunt, they aim for what is easiest for them to catch on foot. We, on the other hand, being the slowpoke predators we are, compensated for our physical limitations with lethally effective technology. Prehistoric humans also chose to do the opposite of what wolves and other predators do, risking their lives by targeting the healthiest, fattest, and sassiest animals in a herd. This demanded strategic thinking, communication, collaboration, and pushing ourselves to the limit—all things that unleashed our true, best, and unique human potential and rapidly grew our brains. And this was all made possible because our brains were supplied with the energy and the brain-essential nutrients found in animal fat.[17]

CHAPTER 2

Think Fat

If the notion that your very genome was built on delicacies such as mammoth meat and caribou tongue is a little hard to accept, don't blame me. Blame your brain. More than any other factor, its demands shaped the human affinity for fat in all its natural forms. The brain and fat go together like Fred and Ginger or Starsky and Hutch. They evolved to be in perpetual relationship. And not surprisingly, the health of our brains has suffered whenever we've deviated from satisfying that core need.

For an evolutionary scientist, the brain is the ultimate focus of study, because the speed of its evolution and growth in size, relative to that of any other species, is breathtaking. It is the organ that more than any other defines our humanness, with our extraordinary capacity for thought, feeling, language, philosophy, culture, and art. And it is the part of ourselves that we must protect, preserve, and optimize in order to build our resilience in the toxic modern landscape: smart choices, critical thinking, and empowered action have never been more crucial than they are today.

Unfortunately, today our brain is probably more under threat than any other part of us.

———

When I look at the brains of clients undergoing neurofeedback, via the squiggly lines of the EEG that depict the brain's electrical activity, I know that what underlies them are two mighty hemispheres made up of fat—up to 80 percent fat by dry weight, more or less. Of this, roughly half is protective saturated fat (seeing as our brain isn't refrigerated), containing fully 25 percent of your body's total amount of cholesterol. The brain has an extraordinary secret weapon of sorts, one that is unique in all of nature: the ability to rely on special units of energy from fat, called ketones, on an ongoing basis. Only human brains are capable of this.[1] And what does your brain do with all that fatty composition and unique fat-based energy? It can solve complex sophisticated problems at lightning speed, which no computer can match, and it can philosophically ponder the sophisticated origins of our vast universe and very existence.

What's extraordinary is that we acquired these incredible neurological machines because we put down the bamboo leaves and picked up the bones (and cracked them open). Without that fundamental shift, we might have just been another potbellied primate, foraging for fourteen hours a day along the forest floor and picking the tasty bugs off our neighbors' backs. Did our taste for meat and fat allow for that big, hungry brain? We don't know for sure (though it is likely), but we do know that humans allocate a *much* higher proportion of their energy expenditure to their brains than any other mammal or primate our size. And by developing (relatively) carnivorous digestive tracts and robust gallbladders, we were able to fulfill this energy need by digesting meat and animal fat instead of plant matter, thereby ensuring a calorically dense diet—something that hours of foraging leaves and plants could never provide.[2]

This theory is well established and accepted in paleoanthropology as the "expensive tissue hypothesis."[3] It posits that the increased energetic demands of a relatively large brain—the most "expensive" tissue in the body in terms of energy cost—are balanced by the reduced energy demands of a relatively small gastrointestinal tract that can efficiently process meat and fat. This digestive development, along with eating key long-chain polyunsaturated fatty acids (LC-PUFAs) that are critical to brain development, powered our cognitive quantum leap ahead of other primates. (Fatty acids are groups of fat molecules that can be absorbed into the bloodstream and used by the body.) To quote veteran ketogenic researchers George F. Cahill Jr., MD, and Richard Veech, MD, "Without this metabolic adaptation [to using fat as our primary source of fuel], *H. sapiens* could not have evolved such a large brain."[4]

A Tale of Two Brains

Rewind time to about two million years ago, and you would discover that our earliest ancestor of the genus *Homo* had a brain with a volume of about 900 cm³, two to three times the brain size of our closest primate cousin, the chimpanzee.[5] By the time that ancestor, *Homo erectus*, had become the anatomically modern *Homo sapiens*, his brain had increased 75 percent in size and was infinitely more sophisticated in functioning. This rapid encephalization—the technical term for brain growth—occurred over approximately 180,000 years, which is a relatively brief span of evolutionary time.[6] By contrast, the chimpanzee's much smaller brain hasn't changed at all in seven million years. This is largely due to our different diets, our different digestive systems, and the different way we obtain and synthesize fats.

I like to use the chimp-human comparison because there is a prevailing mythology that persists in some nutritional circles that we are all essentially primates—naked apes—and because primates eat primarily plants, so should we. Not so. Sure, we share most of our genes with our chimp cousins, and there are some notable similarities, but our differences are not as negligible as some think. On the similarity side, both human and chimp brains are constructed from fatty acids. But one brain is especially highly sophisticated, and the other is less so. Why? One major factor is the specific type of fat involved.

Picture the chimp's daily diet. It contains maybe an occasional bit of meat—mainly carrion, insects, and small animals—which donate some protein plus very little fat. The bulk of the diet, however, is plants, lots and lots of them. And what the chimp does with this vegetation is impressive: she processes it inside the incredible fermentation vats of her belly (which we lack), which accommodates about 60 percent more volume of large intestine than a human belly does. Microflora (gut bacteria) convert the plant material into short-chain saturated fatty acids. Through this fairly long and labor-intensive process (the labor being to eat, eat, eat and for her gut bacteria to ferment, ferment, ferment), she gets the calories she needs to supply up to 50 percent of her energy needs from saturated fat. Odd as it may seem, the carbohydrate in the sweet/starchy vegetation contributes just a small amount of energy.[7] The whole energy-making process is pretty inefficient, to say the least, but since the chimp's brain is fairly "cheap" (it only uses about 8 percent of her energy intake), this process suffices.

Human physiology evolved very differently. The large human brain is exceptionally hungry, or "expensive," requiring 20 to 30 percent of the body's available energy. These energy needs are even more pronounced in our early years. Babies' brains utilize up to 85 percent or more of the calories they consume, and in older children, the figure is 45 to 50 percent.[8] To meet this need, our digestive system got super-efficient in order to derive maximum energy directly from food, rather than by microbial fermentation. We evolved a hydrochloric acid–based digestive system, with a longer small intestine and shorter colon than other primates. This meant that we didn't need to—and actually couldn't—ferment vast amounts of plant matter to derive fatty acids and other nutrients; instead we have the ability to bypass the lengthy fermentation process and get our prefab fatty acids by eating animals that have already done the converting for us in the form of grass-fed, wild-ranged, healthy-as-it-comes meat—a process I describe below. And these fatty acids from animal meat included two complete game changers.

DHA: The Fatty Acids That Forged Our Intelligence

To build a brain takes more than mere calories; it takes building blocks of a variety of specific types of fatty acids, and a lot of cholesterol. Where chimps' brains use predominantly omega-6 essential fatty acids derived from plant foods as their building blocks, our human brains are structured using two critical long-chain fatty acids known as arachidonic acid (AA) and a key omega-3, docosahexaenoic acid (DHA), both of which are available only from (you guessed it) animal-source foods. This particular pair of pre-formed animal-source fatty acids accounts for many of the human brain's unique cognitive capacities.[9] They are the blocks that build our advanced brain structures with higher functions, such as our unique neocortex and prefrontal cortex. DHA in particular is the dominant storage form of omega-3s in the human brain; comprising fully one quarter of the brain, it is arguably the most critical fatty acid. We owe our human qualities in no small part to this wonder fat, which is found in meat that is 100% pastured and in wild-caught fish. (AA, by the way, is an elongated, animal-source omega-6 necessary for cognitive functioning, but it must be in just the right balance with sufficient omega-3s—which it is in wild and fully pastured animals.)

You might say, "But I get my omega-3s from flax oil" (or chia oil, or South American sacha inchi oil), "and the bottle says it is 'rich in omega-3'! What's not to love about that?" I hate to break it to you, but our brains actually don't have the capacity to make much use of the type of omega-3 derived from plant oils, called alpha-linolenic acid (ALA).[10] To become a building block for the brain, the ALA has to be elongated through a complicated biochemical process of enzymatic conversion (for the true geeks, the substances involved are called desaturase enzymes). Unlike chimpanzees and cows, humans have a very limited ability to do this. We have the capacity to convert *maybe* 6 percent of ALA into a substance called eicosapentaenoic acid (EPA), with a negligible amount converted into DHA. (Aside: Those of northern European, Celtic, and Native American heritage tend genetically to be unable to even achieve that much and simply cannot make these conversions at all, lacking the key first enzyme in the process, delta-6-desaturase.)[11]

Apart from being poorly converted (if at all) to the elongated omega-3s that your brain really needs, that pricey bottle of plant-based oil, whether flax, chia, sacha inchi, perilla, or walnut, has another downside: its contents will likely oxidize before you get halfway through it, as plant-based oils are very fragile and quickly go rancid when taken out of the seed or nut and exposed to air. Should you try to cook with them, you are almost guaranteed to render them oxidized and unusable—and even dangerous to your health. Consuming even high-quality plant sources of ALA in the amount you need to make better conversions (assuming no genetic or metabolic limitations) can easily flood you with tissue-damaging free radicals. Conversely, animal foods provide delicate omega-3s side by side with robust saturated fats that protect them from oxidizing and causing harm; the saturated fats actually help the omega-3s get safely to the areas where your body needs them, such as to combat inflammation or, of course, to build the brain. Nature designed them to occur together in a perfect nutritional package called 100% grass-fed, grass-finished meat.

The Food Chain Game

Cows, sheep, and goats are designed to graze. They are classified as ruminants, a name derived from the Latin word *ruminare*, meaning "to chew over again." Inside their bellies, large digestive systems comprising four stomach chambers allow them to swallow forage and then later regurgitate it, rechew it (called "chewing the cud") to break it down into smaller particles, and then swallow it again, where microorganisms ferment it, converting it into short-chained saturated fatty acids—mainly butyric acid, which they then use for up to 70 percent of their energy. (See, cows are fat burners too, though their brains can't typically run on ketones like ours.) Meanwhile, they also convert ALA from the chloroplasts of green plant cells into EPA and DHA and then store these in their tissues, something our position at the top of the food chain as hunters of grass-eating animals allowed us to exploit.

The takeaway: Consuming pre-formed, elongated omega-3s from animal-source foods—animals that ate fresh green grass/natural forage for their entire life cycle and were allowed to roam free, with plenty of sunshine—radically changed the way our brains operated and what we were capable of doing. And today our primal physiology hasn't changed, even while plant seed/nut oils galore are available on the shelves of health food stores. Fat-rich, raised-on-grass animal foods, rich in DHA, EPA, and sufficient AA (along with a plethora of other unique and critical nutrients), are nonnegotiable for your neurological system—grain-fed animals have a different fat profile, as we will discover—and the dearth of fully pastured fats in most people's diets is a little-discussed crisis.

CHOLESTEROL: YOUR BRAIN'S BEST FRIEND

The love story between brain and fat goes further. We need a huge variety of fat-based nutrients to function, and one of the most crucial is cholesterol. If you are protesting, "Surely not," please know that dietary cholesterol has been unjustly demonized; it was vital to the evolution of our sophisticated brain structure. Without enough cholesterol (or if you take statin drugs, which lower cholesterol), you risk memory problems, dementia, and worse. Without any cholesterol at all, your brain cannot function.

Fully 25 percent of all the cholesterol in the human body is concentrated in your brain, where it is needed to maintain healthy cognitive function and play myriad other important roles. It is required *everywhere* in the brain and delivered there by the unjustly dreaded LDLs (low-density lipoproteins, molecules that are carriers of cholesterol and other important fat-soluble nutrients). Cholesterol acts as an antioxidant,[12,13] it helps to insulate the neuronal membranes so that the neurotransmitters' activity is efficient, and it keeps the synapses between neurons structurally sound and functioning. In other words, cholesterol helps lay the very foundation of your neurological functioning. And what are the best sources of this necessary neural nutrient? Animal-source foods such as meats, organ meats, and eggs.

If you remember only one thing about this subject, remember this: if DHA is not in your diet, it's not in your brain.

Fat-Head vs. Potato-Head: Who Wins?

While the "expensive tissue" hypothesis is well validated, there still remains a school of thought that says we owe our big brains to starchy foods (in other words, preagricultural, wild-growing tubers and roots—the prehistoric versions of yams and carrots).[14] This "potato" hypothesis is predicated on a mistaken idea—one that this book refutes—that glucose, the energy from carbohydrate, is the human brain's primary and preferred source of fuel. As I will show you in the pages to come, this is true only if you have conditioned yourself for it to be true by training the brain to use glucose through a diet unnaturally high in sugar and starch. What the brain works best on, and what it needs not just to evolve in size but to function at its best every single day, is the energy and nutrients from animal-sourced fat. A quick look at the flawed "potato" hypothesis helps to illuminate a fundamental and very critical idea: humans could *not* have evolved by using plant food as a primary source of calories, even if other primates have happily subsisted on them, because there are simply not enough calories or brain-building fats and other brain-critical nutrients in starchy foods to supply our demanding brain.

You Say Potato, I Say Bacon

Vegans may not love me when I say this, but a solely plant-based diet simply goes against our evolutionary design. Any wild, fibrous, uncultivated plant tubers that our early ancestors came across would have been entirely indigestible, because when raw, their starches cannot be broken down or its nutrients absorbed by the small intestine. Starches in roots and tubers become digestible only after they have been cooked through prolonged exposure to high heat. Deriving energy from starchy roots and tubers during our early evolution would have required extensive cooking. The most current data suggest that our human ability to produce fire at will occurred only well after we had evolved into modern humans,[15] little more than 75,000 to perhaps 100,000 years ago.[16] By this time our uniquely dramatic brain expansion had already long since occurred. Interestingly, research shows that even habitual use of fire, including in more temperate regions where plant life was likely flourishing,[17] did not translate to a high consumption of plant-source foods.

Perhaps more critically, this would have required ample amylase, the enzyme that helps us to digest starch. Our species actually *lacked* the necessary genes to create much amylase until about two hundred thousand years ago, which was after we had already developed our big brains.[18] The adaption to significant starch consumption is not even a done deal today: modern people have highly variable capacities to digest fully cooked starches. This is because modern humans differ widely in the amount of amylase genes we carry, and may have anywhere from two to sixteen copies. (And there is no correlation with larger brain size in those with more copies.)

Roots and tubers—cooked or not—do not supply the critical nutrients that nourish the human brain. Even if our ancestors had been able to make use of starch calories in any significant way, they would have been getting substantially fewer calories and nutrients than they got in the dietary fat from the animals they hunted.

While we're at it, let's address the misconception that early humans roamed the earth munching on fruit, honey, and nuts galore. These edibles would have been merely a seasonal treat, and only in temperate regions. They would have certainly helped to fatten us up for the winter or in the possible event of food scarcity, helping us to develop an adaptive mechanism called mild insulin resistance, which actually supported us to store sugar as fat for the winter to come. But these plant foods would have been scarce, an occasional side dish at best, and not plentiful enough or fully nutritious enough to rely on to survive Paleolithic extremes. For vulnerable Ice Age beings, no matter what kind of ecosystem they lived in, dietary fat was the key to survival.

It boils down to this. Cooking didn't expand our brain. Eating potatoes or other carbohydrates didn't grow our brain. Eating dietary animal fat—and lots of it—is truly what provided the substrate for the highly sophisticated structure of our brain and ultimately made us human.[19]

Ketones: Your Natural IQ Fuel

The research of human metabolic expert George F. Cahill Jr., MD, presents an exciting confirmation of this theory: it turns out that humans are the *only* animal that can run virtually entirely on ketones, the energy units that come from fat. This unique, evolutionary adaptation was driven primarily by our brain! The cost of running our most expensive organ, the brain, is so high that we needed the most abundant, stable, reliable fuel source possible—fat. As you'll see in Chapter 4, the brain can use both glucose and ketones for energy—it's flexible—but it definitely prefers and performs better on the latter. In fact, fat is *so* preferable that, once your fat-burning state is fully switched on (i.e., when a healthy state of effective ketogenic adaptation is achieved), the ketones you produce stimulate the pathways that enhance the growth of new neural networks and protect neurons against multiple types of neuronal injury.[20] This is just one reason why the fat-burning or ketogenic approach to eating is used as a therapy for all kinds of neurological imbalances and diseases—often with rapid and remarkable results.

Here's a second fascinating insight: we are natural-born fat burners. Our earliest neurological functioning and development are powered by ketones. When an infant is nursing on mother's milk, it's the energy from the fat in the milk (in the form of ketones) that is *the* major fuel for brain development.[21] According to Dr. Cahill, "The larger the brain/body ratio, the more rapidly the ketosis develops, as in the newborn."[22] He went on in the same paper to say that "We are the only primate born fat, probably to furnish the caloric bank for our big brains." The sugars in the breast milk are important, too; they feed the lactobacillus bacteria in the baby's gut and are rapidly converted to subcutaneous fat, to give the baby a good insulating layer—in Ice Age terms, the chubbier the baby, the higher the odds of survival.[23]

The ketones derived from this stored fat and the DHA that comes with it, from mother's milk, are pivotal to feeding a rapidly developing human brain. The infant makes barely any starch-digesting amylase until at least five months of age. Nature very clearly intended for fat to be the fuel for the extraordinary development and functioning of our brains from the very start of life. Once we start feeding children sweet and starchy foods, we start to shortchange this critical development process . . . and they start craving sweets.

These scientific insights add more confirmation to the fat-burning hypothesis. To our primal physiology, ketones are the ultimate brain fuel. In terms of conferring brain benefits as we live and age, they leave the starch-based diet trailing in the dust.

The Incredible Shrinking Brain

Paleoanthropologists and other folks who like to investigate our ancestors have bad news for us: our brains are shrinking. They peaked in size about twenty thousand to thirty thousand years ago, as demonstrated by studies of Cro-Magnon remains—Cro-Magnons were the robust and powerful humans who were the first to live in cold, Ice Age conditions in what is now Europe—and our brains have been getting smaller ever since. The most rapidly evident shrinkage has taken place within the last ten thousand years—the era of agriculture, starch-based diets, and cultivated grains. If the "potato" hypothesizers were right, you would expect our health and brain function (and brain size and sophistication) to have improved significantly since agriculture helped us to adopt a starch-based diet. But the reverse is true.[24] As starch became our default food and nutrient-rich foods from wild animals were replaced, our brains started to shrink. Coincidence? I wonder.

How is it possible that we lost just over 10 percent of our brain volume in a mere ten thousand years? Did the abundance of grains and starches help us develop "improved brain efficiency," allowing us to do more from less (as potato-hypothesis proponents might argue)? In light of our evolutionary past, this seems more of a rationalization than a viable hypothesis.

The more compelling answer is that we shifted from a diet that contained close to 90 percent brain-building animal-source foods, rich in brain-building fats, to a diet that has as little as 10 percent of such foods today. As we did so, the brain lost its source of critical building blocks, such as DHA, as well as the fat-soluble nutrients that make it work optimally. Nature's design for our brain—to be built from fat, to function on fat, and to thrive on fat—got subverted. This has dramatic implications across the board, including, not surprisingly, how we age. As you'll see in Chapter 8, our post-agricultural diet is intricately connected to the modern crisis of neurodegenerative compromise, degeneration, and disease.

Rethinking Vegetarianism

Vegetable lovers can rejoice: the Primal Fat Burner Plan puts a strong emphasis on filling your plate with fibrous vegetables and greens (the non-starchy kind—think chard, asparagus, cauliflower, and cucumbers, not potatoes, rice, beans, peas, and corn) to get a steady supply of phytonutrients that our modern lifestyle and environment requires. But vegetarians, take heed: animal-sourced foods take their (moderate) share of the plate as well.

Having worked intimately with the human brain for twenty years as a neurofeedback practitioner, I've come to an undeniable—if somewhat politically incorrect—conclusion: by far the most damaged and intractable brains and nervous systems I encounter are those of strict vegetarians, and specifically vegans, who have spent years eating a low-fat, higher-carbohydrate diet. Whether they eat lots of whole foods or processed ones, the nutritional deficiencies from the lack of animal-source foods plus overreliance on antigenic and inflammatory grains and legumes can be very similar: the lack of fat-soluble vitamins, complete protein, essential fatty acids (EPA and DHA), and cholesterol compromises brain function and over time results in considerable mood lability and instability, from foggy thinking, irritability, agitation, insomnia, anxiety, and attention disorders to autoimmune issues and pronounced neurodegenerative symptoms.

On top of that, the damaging waves of glucose and insulin that result from their sugary, grain- and starch-filled diet unnaturally age the body and brain. By the time I see these clients, they often feel as if their health and mental clarity are eroding. They feel something is fundamentally wrong. From an ancestral health point of view, this is completely unsurprising. Nothing is more stabilizing to the brain than quality dietary fat, and nothing is more destabilizing than sugar and starch. From a modern statistical standpoint, the numbers are shocking: fully 75 percent of vegetarians and vegans abandon this way of life within ten years—and most do so typically because of health-related issues.[25]

Though you might not think it from reading this far, I actually feel a deep allegiance to these clients. They care deeply about planetary health, animal suffering, and restoring a healthy ecosystem, as I do. The world needs more people like this. But by cutting out all animal-source foods, they are sacrificing themselves to an ideal that has never existed in nature. On the occasions when I can influence a shift to a fat-burning way of eating with some quality animal-source foods, we often see significant improvements in stability, clarity, and total functioning—just as I personally experienced after my time in the Arctic—although the recovery is contingent, I'm sorry to say, on the length of time these compromises have existed.

I usually invite my vegetarian clients to ponder the greater philosophical question: when carbohydrate-based eating is your norm, and you invariably get mood and energy instabilities, cravings, and blood sugar spikes and crashes throughout the day, are you truly free to live your life as you like, or are you enslaved to being a grazer, constantly eating to fill a hunger that never quite dies? And in this era of Big Food, Big Agriculture, and Big Ag's best friend, Big Oil, who do you suppose benefits the most from us being in this (I have to say it: sheep-like) state?

A NOTE TO CURIOUS VEGETARIANS

The Primal Fat Burner Plan features a strong emphasis on sourcing foods that profoundly support ecosystem health, such as exclusively pastured meats raised in a truly sustainable manner—for more on this, see the Afterword—as well as ample health-promoting, organically grown plant-based foods. For those who have been following vegetarian and vegan diets and are ready to try transitioning to this way of eating, this book offers a moderate way to ease in, using easily digested and delicious bone broths for the first phase. Even as a full-blown fat burner you will never need to eat more than a small to moderate amount of actual meat, further helping ease any burden of potentially compromised digestion.

When we return to eating the way our primal bodies and brains are wired to eat, we reclaim not just better physical health but a healthy dose of independence and autonomy, too—we begin to know what our own body needs, and to take charge of the best way to fulfill that.

We haven't even gotten into the mechanics of fat burning, but I hope you can see how following a high-carb, low-fat, low-cholesterol diet—the exact prescription given out by decades of USDA food pyramids and erroneous factoids on the back of cereal boxes—is not only a scientifically unfounded proposition but the absolute opposite of what three million years of evolution intended for us.

CHAPTER 3

A Is for Agriculture and
Adapting to Glucose

By the time the Paleolithic era ended and the Neolithic era began some 11,500 years ago, humans had been evolving as nearly pure meat and fat eaters for more than a hundred thousand generations. The cataclysmic event that plunged the megafauna into extinction also melted the massive ice sheets of North and South America, wiped out coastal civilizations, and made procuring food substantially more challenging. Suddenly we were faced with a critical survival emergency and needed to adapt to changed circumstances.

Very rapidly (in evolutionary terms, at least), the majority of humans on planet Earth shifted from pure hunter-gatherers to semi-nomadic herders, and then to early farmers. By ten thousand years ago in what is now the Middle East, an entirely new, unprecedented form of food production got under way, the practice of agriculture. We hybridized and harnessed wild species of plants in a way that allowed for a constant, abundant, and stationary (albeit considerably inferior) food supply. Then once we figured out we could ferment and make beer from cultivated grains, there was no going back.

This period in human history is often called the dawn of higher civilization. But did we actually get elevated—or did we get crushed? Make no mistake: adopting an agricultural way of life changed everything for us, all right, but not all for the better. It opened the door to unprecedented, explosive population growth, although it allowed us to live in better-protected, safer, controlled environments. It also caused disastrous changes in human health and longevity and led to something else entirely new: ruling-class hierarchies, nation-states, and empires, in addition to full-scale war. And that may be understating it. In a groundbreaking and oft-quoted article published thirty years ago in the magazine *Discover*, Jared Diamond called agriculture "a catastrophe from which we have never recovered."[1] (As for the claim that agriculture marked "the dawn of civilization," it's worth pointing out that the oldest known structure ever discovered built by hunter-gatherers to date is Gobekli Tepe in what is now Turkey. This unique site was built in 9000 BCE, predating even ancient Sumeria, and its people lived a 100 percent hunter-gatherer lifestyle.)

The primary causes of death in Stone Age hunter-gatherers were accidents and infections. Their supposedly shorter life span was a statistical average attributable to circumstances relating to their comparatively hostile natural environment (and to estimated infant mortality, which significantly lowered the average). As long as we survived all that, odds were pretty good that we would make it to a healthy (if not *far* healthier than today) ripe old age.

But once the hunter-gatherer lifestyle began shifting toward growing and cultivating, human health and life span began to take quite a hit. There were much higher rates of infection from communicable diseases as humans lived in concentrated, stationary populations, and our reliance on plant foods increased our vulnerability to famine. A grain-heavy diet low in animal-source foods compromised our nutrition. In these early agriculturalists, cereal-based diets commonly led to numerous diseases associated with vitamin and mineral deficiencies, such as rickets, osteoporosis, and other bone disorders. Pellagra, scurvy, and beriberi, as well as deficiencies in vitamin A, iron, and zinc, were also rampant. Birth defects and degenerative diseases became more commonplace. And people became significantly shorter, too—implying some manner of nutrient insufficiency or adaptive conservation. (If you'd like to read more about the compromised health of early agriculturalists, I invite you to search my website for my article about a Neolithic-era man named Otzi—who provides us with remarkable insights into the results of switching from a strict hunter-gatherer diet to an agricultural one.)[2]

What we know today but didn't know then was that the minerals contained in grains are poorly available to us, if at all, due to the presence of a substance known as phytic acid—a fact that makes the oft-touted, government-sanctioned phrase "healthy whole grains" not only a misnomer but, from a human biochemical point of view, an outright fallacy. In fact, the protein in grains, known as gluten, *is not even digestible by any human*. The surprising truth is that human life expectancy actually declined by half—relative to our supposedly short-lived Paleolithic forebears—early on into the agricultural revolution. Stature (together with bone density) *and* life expectancy got shorter, while our brains got smaller—a bit of a bum deal, if you ask me.[3]

For anthropologists, one of the most telling signs of this nutritional compromise is the complex series of changes to the jaw that can be observed in the remains of grain-eating humans. Everything the hunter-gatherer ate, whether meat or the occasional side dishes of wild, uncooked vegetables, required vigorous chewing. Investigations of prehistoric skulls typically reveal a well formed cranium with a capacious jaw easily accommodating thirty-two teeth. By contrast, the sedentary farmer ate soft, cooked foods such as cereals and legumes, which required less chewing. Over some generations, in conjunction with depletion of nutrients that determine skeletal integrity, this led to a reduction in the size of the jaws without a corresponding reduction in the dimensions of the teeth. The increasingly cramped space for teeth led to high levels of malocclusion (misalignment of upper and lower teeth) and dental crowding—an abnormality seen even in remains of the world's earliest farmers some twelve thousand years ago in Southwest Asia,[4] and persisting since then. As Weston Price discovered, dental abnormality and jaw malformation are associated with seriously compromised physical *and* mental well-being—so much so that they are key indicators of nutrition and health, often used by paleoanthropologists to determine if a set of remains is from before or after the development of agriculture. Today, around one in five people in modern-world populations has these problems, which have been called a "malady of civilization."[5]

The Grain Drain

I could write an entire book about the unfortunate consequences we suffered by adopting a grain-heavy diet. But for the purposes of this chapter, let's just keep it simple. Grains provided a source of foods that our ancestors' stomachs couldn't digest and their immune systems didn't recognize. By relying on a year-round, largely starch-based diet for the first time in human history (along with gluten—a completely foreign protein in grains that our bodies couldn't really use and which automatically compromised our health), we began developing diseases that were ostensibly new to our species. The advent of grain consumption has been linked with allergies, food sensitivities, autoimmune disorders such as type 1 diabetes, Hashimoto's disease, asthma, psoriasis, and multiple sclerosis. It has been linked to essentially all autoimmune conditions, in fact, which so far number in excess of one hundred, with an additional forty diseases thought to have an autoimmune component. Other problems that began appearing after we shifted to agriculture include numerous cancers, pancreatic disorders, mineral deficiencies, arthritis, cardiovascular disease, celiac disease, epilepsy, cerebellar ataxias, dementia, degenerative diseases of the brain and central nervous system, peripheral neuropathies of axonal or demyelinating types, as well as autism and schizophrenia.[6] The name now commonly given to these unfortunate conditions, "diseases of modern civilization," almost makes them sound beneficially civilized (as is often the case with the word *modern*). This couldn't be further from the truth; they constitute a tragedy of epic proportions. And virtually *all* of these conditions have been linked in some way with the consumption of grains, and particularly gluten.

Further, with this shift to carbohydrate intake, blood sugar rose from the conversion of starches, and humans developed the internal need to lower blood sugar through the release of waves of insulin 24/7. Each rise in blood sugar is basically an internal emergency that the body has to deal with. So the body has to be on constant alert. This change, more than any other, has fueled our modern-day obesity epidemic.

To understand the magnitude of this shift, let's run a few numbers. Paleolithic hunters and gatherers derived around 90 percent of their caloric intake from the meat and fat of about one hundred to two hundred different species of wild animals. Small amounts of fibrous vegetables, greens, nuts, and fruits in season made up the rest. That is the natural diet of our species, and it was under these conditions that more than 99.99 percent of the human genome was forged.

Since the advent of agriculture, we have spent five hundred generations—*less than 0.4 percent of our evolutionary history*—eating a diet that is increasingly unnatural to our species. Things really started to get freaky about two hundred years ago, during the Industrial Revolution, in an acceleration that has now culminated in a monocultural agricultural diet of largely refined foods. Today, 90 percent of the world's food supply comes from seventeen species of plants (the ten most common are wheat, corn, rice, barley, soybeans, cane sugar, sorghum, potatoes, oats, and cassava), most of which were *not* present in the human diet during the majority of the time human evolution was occurring. Then factor in the rampant industrialization of post–World War II food production and the fact that most of these new staple food crops are grown with toxic chemicals, then processed and refined into products and by-products completely foreign to our physiology. They are packaged with preservatives for long shelf life (which increases commercial profit), further reducing any nutritional value. Today 90 cents of every food dollar spent in the industrialized world go for these nutrient-devoid, chemically laden Frankenfoods. The natural order of hunting and gathering could not be more subverted.

Our Paleolithic ancestors would have been baffled to see generations of modern humans diligently following a "food pyramid" built on a foundation of grains and legumes. Just as with grains, legumes are problematic, largely because of the nutrient-blocking phytic acid they contain compromising lectins, various thyroid-impairing and gut-irritating properties, and a high starch content (up to 60 percent). This follows an officially sanctioned directive that everyone should eat six to eleven servings of carbohydrates (grains) a day—for the first time in human history—in order to be healthy and slim. Paleolithic humans would have been equally baffled by the zealous mandates to avoid fat and cholesterol, especially saturated animal fat.

Our ancestors surely would have been astonished at our transformation from carnivores who hunt to live—lean, muscular, attuned to nature, cunning, and adaptable, with high endurance—into "carbovores" who acquire our nourishment from inferior foods produced by multinational corporations, constantly fight our weight, and are besieged with chronic health issues. We are a mere shadow of the robust, wild humans we once were.

Since the agricultural food system and industrialized way of life became our default, we have not been faring well. With each subsequent generation exposed to a deteriorating environment and food supply, the human genome gets compromised and harmed. Humans today are diagnosed with disease 33 percent (fifteen years) earlier than our grandparents were.[7] We are a far more fragile species today and more susceptible to compromise than our great-grandparents, our grandparents, and even our parents. Worse, it's now said that

THE HIGH COSTS OF CIVILIZATION

The number one cause of bankruptcy in the United States today is illness. The number of people who suffer from inflammation, debilitating chronic pain, mental health issues, cognitive problems, and metabolic disease is increasing. Obesity and its commonly associated/related metabolic disorders, including heart disease, diabetes, polycystic ovarian syndrome (PCOS), and stroke, are rampant today and growing in frequency. Conditions such as Alzheimer's, often referred to as "type 3 diabetes," and cancer are also growing. Major depression, the most common form of mental illness, which affects women more than men, is expected to be the second leading cause of disability worldwide by 2020— second only to ischemic heart disease, according to the Centers for Disease Control.[8] Today, researchers are redefining serious depression not as a disease of neurotransmitter deficiency per se but as a disease of inflammation.[9] Gluten immune reactivity and sugar addiction are certainly two viable culprits.[10,11]

today's children are the first generation who are not expected to live as long as their parents. Age thirty has become the new forty-five when it comes to the onset of chronic disease. This is one of the most telling signs of our departure from our primal birthright, and one that any clinician will likely acknowledge, regardless of the type of medicine or healing work practiced. This is all new, it is not normal, and it is intimately tied to our nutritional changes, our toxic environment, and our collective amnesia about the importance of naturally occurring fat as humans' original fuel and source of nourishment.

Losing Our Primal Potential: How We Diverged from Our Evolutionary Design (and How We Can Restore Order Again)

When it comes to defining the optimal human diet, there are a lot of different voices at the table, even—or is it especially?—within the niche of paleo and ancestral eating. Trying to achieve consensus in the paleosphere is like herding cats; everyone's priorities are different. These days, it seems that almost anything gets a free pass—"paleo" blueberry cheesecake, hand-pressed tortillas, even entirely non-paleo foods such as white potatoes and rice—as long as it fits under the very accommodating banner of "real food."

As you may have guessed, I don't subscribe to that approach— which doesn't always make me Ms. Popular in the paleosphere! Whether you enjoy the online debates, skirmishes, political posturing, and occasional head butting or not, it makes things extremely challenging for the average person to simply know what to do to stay or become healthy.

My intention in writing *Primal Fat Burner* is to provide you with a big-picture view of our genetic heritage as well as the specific challenges facing us today. I have distilled my research into a number of concise and relatively easy-to-grasp categories in order to cut through the confusion and mark a clear path forward that anyone can understand and follow.

From my point of view, there are five key ideas you must know about the ways we have diverged from our primal design and our original environment. These are the areas of compromise that we must address in order to restore balance and reclaim our primal birthright, because in nature, any time you go against your blueprint, some manner of disturbance and eventually chaos are sure to follow. If this sounds a little intimidating, please take heart: the Primal Fat Burner Plan will help you correct these five areas by making shifts in what is on your plate. These changes may be challenging, certainly, but you can do it. And you will derive transforming and empowering benefits as you reclaim your primal birthright of a healthy body, sound mind, and vital quality of life.

Restoring Your Primary, Originally Intended Metabolic Energy Pathway

One of the most devastating—and little-discussed—drivers behind our post-agricultural decline is the shift in our primary metabolic pathways. That might sound fairly innocuous, like changing your cell phone service provider. Far from it. The transition from burning mainly fats for energy to burning mainly sugars is a root cause of many of our ills. Prehistoric humans' meat-and-fat-rich, carbohydrate-minimal diet would have automatically given them a primary metabolic reliance upon fat; in other words, they would have largely been running on ketone bodies, the energy units from fat, along with free fatty acids. This metabolic function lets the body take advantage of fat's tremendous energy productivity—fat supplies roughly twice the caloric energy per gram that carbohydrates do (but many times more than that in the energy units known as ATP, or adenosine triphosphate). Fat burning allows us to store great quantities of fat on our bodies, even when we are thin. The capacity to burn stored fat is an evolutionary adaptation that allowed our ancestors to survive the lean periods in between successful hunts, as well as innumerable other challenges.

As a nutritionist and avid paleo diet researcher, I had always hypothesized that early humans must have been able to consistently burn fat for fuel. After all, if Paleo Woman had to stop to refuel every two hours, as is often the case on carb-dominated diets, how would she have survived at all? About fifteen years ago, one of the most hallowed pioneers in the field of ketogenic research, Dr. Richard Veech, added more scientific credence to this hunch. He declared in a groundbreaking article in the *New York Times Magazine* that fat burning is, physiologically speaking, "the normal state of man."[12] Veech called our ability to use ketones energy "magic." In a sense it is, creating steady and slow-burning energy even when there are gaps between meals, conferring protective benefits to the body, and enhancing the efficiency of the heart and brain by (according to Veech) a whopping 28 percent,[13] all while avoiding the damaging tidal waves of sugar and related hormones that lead to weight problems and disease.

Yes, humans can adapt to different conditions and find some way to compensate (for better or worse). When you restrict or eliminate dietary fat intake, for instance, your body will respond by becoming more efficient at manufacturing and storing fats from other things in the diet—mostly carbohydrate. As carbohydrate replaced fat in our diet, our bodies came to expect sugar as fuel and our fat-burning metabolism began to fall idle. Fat burning is your primary metabolism only if your diet is very low in sugars and starches.

Over the centuries, and of course particularly in the last half century as carbohydrates have become increasingly refined and stronger in their sugary impact, we have come to adapt ourselves metabolically to an unnatural dependence on glucose as our primary source of fuel. The results have been disastrous for us (though quite profitable for Nabisco, Kraft Foods, General Mills, Kellogg's, and other multinational Frankenfood cartels). Persistent weight gain is one of the more obvious and highly visible consequences of running on sugars, but metabolic disorders, tumor growth, autoimmune conditions, and neurological diseases are even more insidious, because they are less obvious, but just as debilitating or deadly, effects of these poor dietary choices.

The plan described in *Primal Fat Burner* retrains your body to do what it already knows how to do: flip on the fat-burning switch through a simple diet low in carbohydrates and high in healthy, natural fats, thereby restoring the metabolic advantage that we once enjoyed but have missed for far too long.

Making Peace with Fat

As we systematized our food sourcing, the newcomers to our diet (grains and starches) increasingly pushed the wise elders (healthful fats in their naturally occurring, intact state) off the table. But when combined with the new and unnatural carbohydrate overload, eating any fat was suddenly like throwing a match onto a keg of dynamite— it produced very harmful effects on almost every area of health, most notoriously cardiovascular health. First came the reduction of the variety of fats and fat-soluble nutrients we consumed as animal-sourced foods declined (it is critical for the body to get a wide variety of different fats and fat-soluble nutrients that serve and support different functions in the body). Then the rampant industrialization of food brought the twisted advent of refined and highly processed vegetable oils (which exploded our intake of omega-6s, rancid fats, and trans fats, while depriving us of needed omega-3s), leading to rampant inflammation, cardiovascular disease, even more cancer, and various forms of chronic pain.

In just the last fifty or sixty years, the wholesale demonization of naturally occurring fats, especially saturated fats, compounded these effects and created a collective fat-phobia from which we are only beginning to emerge. As it turns out, the idea that naturally occurring dietary fats cause cholesterol problems (as if naturally occurring cholesterol were a problem) and related disease processes is a colossal myth—and we're not talking the sweet Cinderella kind of fairy tale, but instead the dark and twisted Brothers Grimm kind.

I'll share more about the grievous errors of the heart-fat hypothesis in Chapter 8. Here's a preview: The experts and policy makers got it categorically wrong. *Fat is not, and never was, the bad guy.* Fat in its naturally occurring form, and eaten without carbs, does miraculous things for our bodies and brains. But man-made fats, including refined, hydrogenated, and interesterified vegetable and seed oils, plus the carbohydrates we now consume in vast and unnatural excess with dietary fats, are a different story. They are the villains that cause life-threatening diseases and illnesses.

The Primal Fat Burner Plan will guide you to eat more of the macronutrient that ultimately did the most to help our species survive and evolve: quality, natural, unadulterated fats from quality, unadulterated animals and a few certain plant foods (tropical oils, some nuts, avocados, and olives). And it will help you eat much less of the macronutrient that has caused so much unnecessary and unnatural suffering: carbohydrates from sugars and starches.

Resisting the Invisible Aggravators: Antigenic Foods

Our radical new reliance on foods we did not evolve to eat is taking a massive toll on our health. Grains and legumes, as well as commercial dairy (and for many people raw dairy, too) have "antigenic" (i.e., anti-genome, or anti-body) properties that can cause the body to fight them as if they are unwanted invaders, creating rampant inflammation. Every single time we hybridize grain, we create an average of 5 percent new proteins that our genome has never seen before and doesn't know how to recognize. Collectively, our inflammatory response to many post-agricultural foods—and this includes, but is certainly not limited to, gluten-containing grains—is a growing reality. In addition, we are dealing with genetically modified (GMO) foods that irritate and inflame the body in ways that we don't yet even fully understand.

The inflammatory influence of antigenic foods is associated with an epidemic of autoimmune disease,[14] including Hashimoto's disease, rheumatoid arthritis, autism, and multiple sclerosis (among so many others), as well as psychiatric disorders such as depression, anxiety, attentional disorders, bipolar disorder, and even Alzheimer's disease.[15] They are also linked to obesity and weight gain and to an unprecedented occurrence of chronic pain in young children and adolescents.[16] These foods can even damage or impair the gut's ability to absorb nutrients from food, so that we get even fewer nutrients from already compromised food sources.

In the Primal Fat Burner Plan, you will remove the most common antigenic and irritating foods and focus on eating foods *to which we are genetically better adapted*. This single step alone carries massive potential for reversing suffering. (You can read more about autoimmune conditions in Chapter 8.) Don't worry about being hungry: you will be eating plenty of nutrient-dense foods to provide for all your needs. Cravings will become mostly a thing of the past.

Compensating for Nutrient Depletion

The catastrophe that agriculture unleashed affected not just human bodies but also the environment. Count among the harsh costs of agriculture the following: the decimation of soils and ecosystem diversity, erosion that depleted soil further and altered landscapes, and the loss of innumerable healthy watersheds, leading to widespread desertification across close to two-thirds of our planet's landmass today. Factor in soil-depleting pesticides and chemicals, the development of mass feedlot operations that raise animals in unnatural, unhealthy, and inhumane ways, the widespread use of genetically modified cattle feed and human foods, and the fact that rapacious corporate interests have simply hijacked vast amounts of human food production (and laws governing it), and you end up with the troubling reality that much of the food people eat today is quite different, nutritionally speaking (if it is even definable as food any longer), from the real food of yesteryear.

The unprecedented deterioration of the quality of our soil, air, water, and food supply has led to a startling reduction of available micronutrient density.[17] It is an unfortunate paradox: with such an abundance of food available, we are increasingly less well nourished. This is not merely an inconvenience, as it has very serious consequences for our day-to-day vitality, to our resistance to disease, and ultimately, to the robustness of our genome.

As far back as 1936, the United States Senate stated, "The alarming fact is that foods . . . now being raised on millions of acres of land . . . no longer contain enough of certain vitamins and minerals. We cannot get all our daily essential nutrients from the food we grow and eat."[18] That was just a teaser: fast-forward to the start of the twenty-first century, and research showed you would need to eat ten servings of spinach today to get the same level of minerals you would have gotten from just a single serving about fifty years ago.[19] (Spinach is an extreme example, but not completely an outlier.) The National Academy of Sciences issued an alert in 2001 stating that it now takes twice as many vegetables to get the daily requirement of many nutrients than previously thought.[20]

Our modern practice of constant and intensive farming, combined with widespread use of pesticides and herbicides, has left our precious topsoil greatly weakened; it simply cannot feed the same level of nutrients to the plants, and therefore to us. Hybridization of plants has caused declines in nutritional value and increases in antigenicity. Food is picked days or weeks before it is fully ripe or ready, so that it can be shipped to consumers. Sometimes it is sprayed with preservatives and still called "organic." Even organic produce is not always significantly better if grown by massive industrial farming operations in depleted soils before traveling long distances to consumers.

And that's just talking about the plant foods. The fat and nutritional profile of animal-source foods has changed so much that I recommend that you eat meat from free roaming game and livestock that exclusively eat fresh grass outside in the fresh air and sun (what I call *exclusively pasture-raised*, or *grass-fed AND grass-finished* as the phrase "grass-fed" is now usually a catchall for "grass-fed and then grain-finished"). This meat is radically different from that of feedlot or factory-farmed animals that are contained and given agricultural feed for part or all of their lives. Fully pasture-raised animals are also the most unlikely kind to harbor pathogens, such as dangerous and sometimes deadly acid-resistant *E. coli*.[21] But only about 3 percent of beef sold in the United States is 100% grass-fed *and* grass-finished. That means the majority of meat eaten today is essentially degraded in nutrition and higher in risk-increasing anti-nutrients. Please avoid buying or consuming grain-fed or feedlot meat wherever possible.

Through the unnatural ways we grow and raise our food today, we have created a perfect storm of malnourishment. According to the World Health Organization, at least 30 percent of the world's population is suffering from iron deficiency anemia, and at least half of us are deficient in vitamin D, a critical fat-soluble nutrient. In fact, malnutrition has become the "new normal" and now affects a third of humanity, according to a study that warns of the devastating human and economic toll of undernutrition and obesity. The newly released 2016 Global Nutrition Report states unambiguously that "every country is facing a serious public health challenge from malnutrition."[22]

It's extremely common for people following all kinds of diets (including very-well-intentioned, plant-filled diets) to be deficient in most of the fat-soluble nutrients as well as minerals such as magnesium, iodine, and important B vitamins such as choline and B_{12}, which are essential for health, brain function and development, and overall wellness—not to mention deficiencies in the omega-3 fats EPA and DHA. We don't even fully know the extent of the decreases in other vitally important natural compounds such as natural folic acid, flavonoids, and other phytonutrients, because they were not measured in the past.

One effect of this nutritional starvation is obesity, paradoxical though it may seem. If the body is short on key nutrients that it needs in order to function, you may be compelled to keep eating, unconsciously seeking what is nutritionally missing. Your constant appetite frequently drives you toward "empty calories"—high-calorie foods with very little nutritional value. The result is a double negative; you come to weigh more and more over time, *and* your body is starved of nutrients that could help your metabolism work at its best and keep your immune system resilient.

In Part Four I will show you affordable ways to find meat that is raised in such a way that it has its intended nutritional profile and how to obtain fully organic vegetables from better soils. You will also learn to make cultured vegetables to provide key nutrients that other foods cannot offer.

Staying Strong in a Toxic World

We need abundant fat-soluble nutrients from quality animal-sourced foods, along with plentiful antioxidants and phytonutrients from healthfully raised plants, more than ever today in order to resist toxic stressors and detoxify from them. Virtually everything we consume or put on our bodies every single day contains compromising chemicals. That's an unprecedented burden for our primal bodies to bear. We need large servings of leafy greens and other non-starchy vegetables, as well as cultured vegetables, to fortify ourselves against environmental toxicity, radioactive fallout contaminants, pollution from electrical and magnetic fields (EMFs), and antibiotic-resistant superbugs. We need unadulterated foods from the purest sources possible. This means avoiding irradiated, chemically treated, and genetically modified foods as much as we can, supporting our local farmers and those raising animal foods ethically and sustainably.

If you've been reading closely, you may be wondering why I have not mentioned seafood more often as a source of key nutrients. As of this writing, I am far too concerned about contamination levels from methylmercury, PCBs, disastrous oil spills such as that in the Gulf of

---

**AT A GLANCE: THE FIVE PRINCIPLES
OF PRIMAL FAT BURNING**

1. Value the fats your ancestors ate and include in your diet a variety of quality, natural, unadulterated fats from both animals and certain plants like coconuts, olives, macadamia nuts, and avocados.

2. Eliminate the damaging effects of sugars by cutting out processed foods, sodas, fruit juices, grains, and starches, along with artificially sweetened foods, and replacing them with fibrous vegetables, greens, and a few whole fruits (mainly berries) and nuts.

3. Shift the ratios of dietary macronutrients so that you get the majority of your calories from fats, a modest amount from protein, and a *very* small amount of sugars and starches from large amounts of fibrous vegetables and greens, including cultured varieties.

4. Choose foods to which humans are the most genetically well adapted, and obtain them from the most naturally produced, highest-quality sources.

5. Enhance your detoxification capacity by eating an abundance of phytonutrient-rich vegetables, drinking purified water, and, when needed, using quality supplements.

Mexico (and the chemicals used in their cleanup), and innumerable other toxins, along with the current serious and growing threat of ocean radiation (from the still active Fukushima nuclear disaster), to condone significant seafood consumption. After painstaking research, I have arrived at the disturbing conclusion that seafood caught in the Northern Hemisphere may in fact no longer be safe. I am aware this commentary is something of an outlier and an unpopular one in the nutritional world today. It is a subject blatantly ignored by the corporate media. But from a purely rational, scientific perspective, fish eating currently has a big question mark over its head. But if you truly love seafood, seek out products from comparatively clean and safe sources (see "Nourishing Resources" on page 285).

In Part Four, you will find a balanced approach to animal-sourced foods based on moderate portions of meat, some eggs, and small and occasional (and optional) portions of quality fish. You will also enjoy plenty of foods that support your detoxification system, including lots of vegetables (cultured and otherwise), such as cruciferous ones loaded with anti-cancer indoles and glucosinolates, as well as certain kinds of sprouts, for their fresh, delicious taste and cleansing effects.

Eating for Joy, Eating for Stress

The way we relate to food psychologically and emotionally is another change from our evolutionary history. With day-to-day survival no longer at stake for the majority of us, and abundant food supplies fairly cheap, food has morphed away from its original purpose—sheer sustenance and quality nourishment—and has instead become a mere source of entertainment and comfort, and a way of filling our personal voids. The entire meaning of food has expanded, and as a result many gaps (or would that be booby traps?) have appeared, all too easy to fall into. Never before in our evolutionary history have we expected meals to be novel, convenient, and titillating. None of these things is entirely negative, but these expectations very often get in the way of making good choices. How often has someone subverted your nutritional goals by admonishing you to "live a little" and indulge in whatever dessert they like best? Emotion and rationalization can make all kinds of trigger foods or sabotaging foods momentarily acceptable!

As a clinical nutritionist, I advise clients to hold on to a bigger-picture perspective: is living about a getting a brief high from a fleeting indulgence, or is it about enjoying ongoing energy, clarity, and real symptom-free health because you made consistent, quality choices that actually support the health of your body and brain? And when it comes to the catchphrase "everything in moderation," by what (or whose) standard might the term *moderation* be defined . . . or rationalized? Who today can afford (much less enjoy) "moderate" inflammation, endocrine disruption, health, immune dysfunction, or health compromise?

Using food emotionally becomes even more dangerous in conjunction with stress—especially the chronic stress that is a norm for virtually everyone today, and which in and of itself leads to its own state of dysregulation. Blood sugar spikes from sugary or starchy meals, the resultant floods of insulin, and the constant high levels of cortisol from an overactivated fight-or-flight mechanism generate frequent, rapid surges and crashes that are inflammatory and anxiety-producing—causing more stress! All of this helps our sugar-burning metabolism to become *even more* firmly established, and makes our cravings for sugar (to deal with stress) even stronger.

Shifting to a principled primal fat-burning diet is supportive in multiple ways. You feel more satiated and more clear-thinking as you eat, able to automatically make better food choices along the way because your eating is no longer propelled by an uncontrollable appetite or cravings. An effective state of ketosis also stabilizes your nervous system and clears your emotional lens, allowing you to handle stress better, free of the constant overarousal of the nervous system. When irritating and antigenic foods are removed as well, this stable state typically gets even better.

And by the way, good, nourishing food full of healthy natural fat *is* titillating and extremely enjoyable to eat—try drizzling duck fat on your veggies or sinking a spoon into a rich coconut curry and tell me that it isn't! *Primal Fat Burner* helps you to make more consistently conscious, wise choices about the food you put inside your living matrix. It can help shift even a hardened carb- and junk-eating habit.

Pushing Back: Reclaiming Our Primal Birthright

Today's challenges to health and longevity can seem complex and overwhelming. The health of Americans is among the most compromised of any industrialized nation. Just a few short years ago the United States ranked twenty-sixth for life expectancy among industrialized nations, right behind Slovenia.[23] Now the United States spends much more on health care per capita than any other nation in the world, and yet today we rank an even more abysmal thirty-fourth in longevity! Yep—now we're tied with Costa Rica, which spends one-tenth of what we spend on health care per capita. Why are costs so much lower there? Maybe it's because the health care (read: disease management) industry in the United States prioritizes profits over health. The estimated annual economic cost to the US health care system of dealing with obesity and its related metabolic conditions alone has ranged from $215 billion to $300 billion in 2011[24,25]—and the cost is expected to double by the year 2030.[26]

And all of this is occurring despite the fact that enlightening new science is emerging every single day about the negative impacts of a carbohydrate-laden diet and the health-promoting potential of fats, along with many other areas of cutting-edge research into nutrition, disease, and longevity. Why hasn't this new information prompted a revolution and caused the masses to take back their health? How could something so simple as changing the food on our plates, a real choice that can save lives and prevent so much suffering and heartache, not have taken deeper root? Have our brains really shrunk so far or been so compromised by poor nutrition that the truth and reason cannot sink in, or are we too depressed (or addicted to nutrient-devoid sources of culinary entertainment) to act? Maybe so. But I'm here to tell you there is hope! Optimizing your nutrition still has the potential to ignite better thinking and decisive action.

Old mythologies die hard—especially when entrenched professional egos and corporate-influenced health authorities become invested in certain views in support of their own ends, and especially when their approaches have been wildly profitable for various multinational industries. When the profit-driven powers that be not only produce the food (or food-like substances) but make the messages that sell the food, influence the advisors and curricula who teach our nutrition, and make the medicine that cures the ills that came from all the bad advice, there is a lot of money to be made. The public is told to keep eating the very foods they are unhealthfully addicted to in the first place!

As I noted earlier, the number one cause of bankruptcy in the United States is a serious medical diagnosis such as cancer, diabetes, chronic illness, or other potentially life-threatening conditions.[27] It doesn't matter whether you have money or not, whether you are a Fortune 500 executive or flipping burgers at McDonald's, or whether you have great insurance or no insurance. The cost of being diagnosed with a serious illness—both the cost to your savings *and* the cost to your quality of life—is something that you cannot afford.

It's time to go against the grain (pun intended) of what our well-meaning but otherwise misguided neighbors, coworkers, family, and friends are eating and set a different example. Wouldn't it be better to see and treat food as the source of our fuller potential and fight consciously for our health by forging our own self-determined and enlightened path forward through today's unforgiving health landscape? (That's what Primal Man and Primal Woman would do, after all!)

The famous physicist Max Planck once said, "A new scientific truth does not triumph by convincing its opponents and making them see the light, but rather because its opponents eventually die, and a new generation grows up that is familiar with it." To paraphrase this, he is basically saying that science typically advances one funeral at a time.

We must be the new generation and awaken to new science. We must be willing to construct a new paradigm of health that makes sound scientific and evolutionary sense. It is not nearly as difficult as it sounds if we take control of what we can. We do this by ensuring that our bodies receive everything they need in order to be maximally resilient, and by avoiding unnecessary compromise wherever possible. The human body is miraculously capable of generating its own health and well-being, as well as (at times) even compensating for setbacks. When we maximize quality nutrients in alignment with our genetic compatibilities, we improve our odds of optimizing our health. So dig into that wilder, more primal urge within you to do things differently and challenge the norm—to evolve and discover a new, better way of being. Getting a little primal will pay off in more ways than you might imagine.

PART TWO

The Metabolic Fuel Duel: Sugars and Fats Duke It Out

Challenging Sugar's Top-Dog Status, and Why Fat Doesn't Make You Fat

A t my practice in Oregon, clients quite often say to me, "Don't bother explaining why I should change; just tell me what to do." They are motivated—or desperate—for change, which is understandable. But for any significant change to succeed and stick, you really need to understand what you are doing and *why*. A basic understanding of the science behind the changes you make provides a rope to hold on to—one that will help you find your way onto the path to change and steer you back on track when you falter or lose your way. In Part Two, we'll take a closer look at the science of energy metabolism, the foundations of a well-adapted fat-burning or ketogenic state, its impacts on your overall health and longevity, and its potential for achieving weight loss, reversing disease states, and optimizing athletic performance.

CHAPTER 4

You Can Choose Your Fuel (Just Please Don't Choose Glucose)

Some years back, a Canadian physician by the name of Dr. Jay Wortman arranged for a yearlong experiment with one hundred members of a Native Canadian fishing village community in Alert Bay, off the coast of Vancouver Island in British Columbia. The Namgis First Nation people living there had been suffering from increased rates of metabolic diseases, such as diabetes and heart disease, at a rate three to five times higher than in the general Canadian population, and it was devastating their community.

A member of the Métis First Nation, Wortman himself had at one time been diagnosed with type 2 diabetes with all the classic symptoms: he was overweight, was always thirsty and fatigued, had blurred vision, and urinated too frequently. Unwilling to be dependent on medications for the rest of his life, Wortman changed his diet by simply following his intuition—at that point he was not aware of the metabolic effects of food or ancestral diets. He eliminated sugary and starchy foods and instead ate higher amounts of natural fats and a small amount of protein.

Even he was surprised by the results. His blood sugar dramatically improved almost instantly, followed by a dramatic and steady loss of weight at the rate of about a pound a day. His other symptoms began to resolve themselves as well: his eyesight returned to normal, his excessive urination and thirst disappeared, and he had enough energy to start riding an exercise bike daily. Within four weeks he had normalized his blood sugar and blood pressure—he had completely reversed his condition.

Wortman felt called to bring this kind of dietary resolution to the First Nation people, for their advanced metabolic diseases were closely tied to their shift from traditional fare to the modern Western diet of high-carb, low-fat, processed foods. These diseases were devastating aboriginal communities, causing huge costs for health care services—from the costs of testing supplies, drugs, and insulin to the costs of treating and transporting patients living in the far northern reaches of the country for serious complications such as kidney failure and amputations. Despite the money being thrown at the problem, the tide was not turning; things were getting worse. In Wortman's own words, "Travelling into the affected communities, there was almost a sense of fatalism, a feeling that it was hopeless. Even in communities where extra resources were being applied and research was being done to see what would work, we weren't able to reverse the terrible trend. The problem was confounding everyone involved."[1]

To find a suitable community to work with, Wortman had to submit proposals for approval to multiple medical and governmental authorities. The resistance he faced was monumental. No medical authority was willing to consider that such a nutritional experiment was safe, let alone that it could offer any promise of success. But one medical authority in the small village of Alert Bay was open-minded enough to say yes. For a year Wortman guided and oversaw his participants to follow a diet high in fats and minimal in carbohydrates, one that mimicked their traditional one. They ate only meat, fish, non-starchy fibrous plant foods, and healthy fats, mostly from a native fish called oolichan and from animal-source foods, along with some plant fats such as olive oil.

The results were striking: as the year progressed, they lost weight, improved their healthy blood chemistries, got off medications, and made an inroad into reversing type 2 diabetes, a disease that is directly tied to the shift to starch- and sugar-based eating. Furthermore, their community spirit was reignited as they collectively felt better and got stronger. (A documentary team from the Canadian Broadcasting Corporation captured the experience in a poignant documentary called *My Big Fat Diet*.)

Wortman's approach in this social experiment powerfully illustrates that when the dominant modern Western macronutrients (sugar- and starch-based foods) are removed from the diet and traditional dominant macronutrients (fat with a little protein) are put back in their place, the body can restore order where there was metabolic dysfunction. It also illustrates a key concept that is central to the Primal Fat Burner Plan: when it comes to weight loss, long-lasting success comes from adjusting your food groups and, most important, your food quality. It does not come from obsessively counting your calories. (The bumper stickers for this would read "It's the carbs, not the calories!" or "Fat is where it's at!") The moral of the Alert Bay story is that no one has to be stuck relying on sugar as a primary source of fuel, and everybody has a remarkable and little-understood capacity for change when the right foundations are in place.

The Metabolic Secret: You Have Two Fuels

It's universally accepted and rarely questioned that glucose is the body's primary fuel and is required by all tissues, including the brain, for everyday energy. Or as the education website dummies.com puts it, "Carbohydrates are an essential part of a healthy diet because your body converts them to glucose and your body runs on glucose."[3] Some variation of that concept is standard issue in almost any quick Internet search you do on "carbs."

But look deeper and you discover that this "truth" is misleading and only conditional: *glucose is the body's primary fuel only if your diet is full of starches and sugars.* If your caloric intake is skewed toward healthy fats instead, with minimal starches and sugars, a different outcome results: the body primarily uses the energy from fat (including the fat on your body you want to get rid of) for the vast majority of its needs. It's certainly *possible* for us to run on sugar, but we have another, better choice. Your "primary fuel" is, it turns out, dependent on what food source you've conditioned your body to use. And the fuel source you choose to exploit has major ramifications for influencing how you feel, think, and function. To better understand this concept, let's take a look at how energy in the body is made.

Energy 101

The science behind cellular energy—what it is and how we make it—can get infinitely complex. To simplify things, first understand that human beings use something called adenosine triphosphate (ATP) for energy. ATP is manufactured by the mitochondria, tiny energy-producing organelles that exist within the majority of your cells. Your health and freedom from disease are intimately tied to the health and efficient function of these tiny cellular powerhouses. After you breathe in oxygen, the mitochondria combine oxygen that is dissolved in the bloodstream with the available fuel source, creating cellular energy through the process of cellular respiration. This is an astonishingly unrelenting process: a typical human cell may contain nearly one billion molecules of ATP at any one moment, and those may be used and resupplied every three minutes.[3] Suffice it to say that we have a massive, obligate dependence upon ATP; it must be supplied with raw materials in every single instant.

To meet this demand, we evolved to have a couple of supply chains for this raw material. We can utilize carbohydrates from food, and to a lesser extent protein from food, to create glucose, and/or we can use fats—both fats in the diet *and* fats stored on the body—to create free fatty acids and ketone bodies for fuel. (There are other contributors to ATP generation, but these two by far produce the largest amount.) Just as nature designed us with two ways to take in oxygen, a nose and a mouth, in case one gets blocked by a cold or a foreign object, we also have two ways to create energy. Nature is smart. Having more than one way to meet any needs essential for life equals higher survival odds. Or, in my less-PC version: when it comes to sugar, Nature would never be so shortsighted as to automatically enslave us all to such an unstable, damaging, and unreliable form of fuel as sugar!

The average person typically stores a relatively small amount of glucose, maybe 2,000 calories' worth, in the form of glycogen in the muscles and liver. The level of glucose in the blood is controlled—somewhat by default by a hormone called insulin, together with other hormones including glucagon, cortisol, adrenaline, and growth hormone. You may be familiar with what happens when you run low on blood sugar and suddenly feel cranky and even light-headed. Fat has a more natural and primary role as an abundant, stable, and reliably slow-burning energy source. The average person stores a good 150,000 calories' worth of fat on the body at any given time (even the thinnest person reading this probably has close to 100,000 calories' worth of fat). And burning fat confers all kinds of "clean energy" benefits: it delivers significantly higher energy compared with glucose and leaves less damaging free radical activity in its wake.

In fact, our mitochondria actually evolved as fat-burning structures. (If you are especially science-minded, you can google "eukaryotic cells" to discover the exciting way this evolutionary development occurred; otherwise, just take my word for it.) *Mitochondria like to burn fat!* And since they supply us with at least 95 percent of all the energy required for every one of our physiological processes—they keep the lights and heat on, as it were—and they also determine the overall health and resilience of our physiology, we want to keep them happy. By burning fat, we get a payout in the form of greater resistance to disease and anti-aging effects. (See "Defending Your Mitochondria" on page 60.)

Your body chooses its primary fuel based on what you habitually eat. And your dietary choices condition your metabolism. On a carbohydrate-rich diet, the body will burn mainly sugar; on a fat-rich, low-carb diet, it will burn primarily fat. My friend Dr. Ron Rosedale, a brilliant, respected metabolic expert and medical pioneer and author of *The Rosedale Diet*, was the first to state it this simply: we are all primarily "sugar burners" or "fat burners."

How We Burn Sugar (and Why It Is Perilous)

The term "carbohydrate" refers to the sugars, starches, and cellulose (fiber) found in fruits, vegetables (including root vegetables), grains, rice, legumes, seeds, nuts, and milk products. All starchy forms of carbohydrate and other sources of sugars (grains, rice, legumes, root vegetables, and milk) turn to mostly sugar, in the form of glucose, the minute they hit your bloodstream. Starch is basically highly concentrated sugar. In the case of sugars from fruit, the sugar is fructose, which gets used a little differently (glucose stimulates insulin, while fructose mostly doesn't and is directly metabolized by the liver) but still has a major metabolic impact.

Glucose burns hot and fast. It plays an important evolutionary role as our version of rocket fuel—a short-term, quick-burning fuel that is meant to exist as an auxiliary to fat energy. It exists as a reserve fuel that can kick in during an emergency (such as a fight-or-flight situation) or in a situation where brief but pronounced exertion is needed (sprinting, lifting heavy weights, heroic moments, etc.). After it enters your bloodstream, whatever is not burned immediately gets stored in your liver and muscles as glycogen, serving as a backup so that when you really need it you don't fall short. Strange as it may sound, the amount of glucose your body truly needs is actually minute—and as you'll see in Chapter 5, your body can readily make it on its own, without consuming carbs!

At any given time the average healthy adult human has some-

NICE CARB, MEAN CARB?

While it's appealing to think that some carbs are "good," such as the complex carbohydrates in starchy vegetables and fruit, while others are "bad," such as refined carbs and table sugar, the truth is that to your body and brain, there's really no such distinction; it's all sugar in the blood. A regular potato can spike your blood sugar even faster than a candy bar! Often overlooked is alcohol: it, too, has its metabolic and blood sugar dysregulating effects. And since less than 1 percent of the human pancreas is devoted to producing insulin, which by default is the only hormone we have to help us rid ourselves of serum excesses of glucose, we are all demonstrably ill equipped to handle such surges. Where the truly "good carbs" come in is with the fibrous vegetables and greens that grow aboveground, such as broccoli, asparagus, kale, spinach, and many others. Their actual sugar/starch content is minimal, and fiber (cellulose) dominates their makeup, along with water, minerals, certain vitamins, and valuable phytonutrients.

where up to about 5 grams (just under a teaspoon) of glucose circulating in the 9 liters or so of blood in the body. For your primal body,
this is normal; any more than that is something your body treats like
an emergency overload to be immediately burned or stored. Every
utilizable carbohydrate you eat raises that blood sugar level. Imagine
that you put a teaspoon of sugar (about 5 grams) into your coffee
and drink that. You have almost instantly doubled your blood sugar!
What if you eat a chain-restaurant chicken sub sandwich—17 grams
of sugar—and then wash it down with a soda containing 36 grams
of sugar? You've suddenly ingested more than *seven times* what your
body wants to allow at any given time. And sorry, but that whole
wheat burrito wrap doesn't do much better: there could be close to 30
grams of starch and sugar in an eight-inch whole wheat burrito wrap
alone, not including the carb content of all the starchy beans or rice
you may have in it. That's one heck of a carb bomb! Finish lunch with
a vanilla yogurt for dessert, and you might then add 30 more grams
to the mix—closer to 50 grams if it's a fruity flavor!

The Insulin Effect

When you consume dietary sugars (be they from sweets, sodas, and
juices or from wholesome-seeming grains, legumes, or starchy vegetables such as potatoes—or from processed foods that have a combination of starches and sugars), your body will increase the production
of the hormone insulin in order to remove the damaging sugar from
your bloodstream and attempt to convert it as immediate energy for
your cells. Insulin's job is not really to manage your blood sugar per
se. Instead it tries to take certain excess nutrients from your bloodstream and put them into storage for later, in case of a famine. Since
sugar offers exceedingly little structural value for the body or brain,
virtually all the sugar you eat is considered pure caloric "excess," and
it automatically evokes a strong insulin response. Now, you need a
little insulin for different things, but too much damages your arteries
and tissues, and shortens your life. The level of insulin in the bloodstream surges in order to swiftly transport this excess sugar to the

liver, where it is converted to hepatic glycogen (long strings of tightly packed glucose molecules stored in the liver for later use, as long as there's room) and also into glycogen for storage in your skeletal muscles. Once those storage sites are full (and it doesn't take a whole lot to fill them), the rest gets converted by your liver into triglycerides (blood fats), which are transported to fat cells throughout your body for later storage in places you would probably rather not have it.

If this scenario takes place only intermittently, it isn't too much for your body to handle. But when you consume significant amounts of carbohydrate on a routine basis (i.e., daily), your cells start to noticeably lose their sensitivity to insulin's constant message—sort of like tuning out a nagging spouse. After a while, instead of giving you energy, your body starts working harder at turning more and more of the sugar and starch that you eat into stored fat. You might find yourself getting drowsy after a meal as your body undergoes the energy-intensive process of making more and more body fat in an effort to get the sugar out of your bloodstream, which also helps temporarily keep you from becoming diabetic. Instead of feeling full after a big meal, you might find yourself craving a nap. You might also find yourself craving dessert—in other words, you want more sugar because your body feels starved for energy. Your cells have trouble hearing insulin's message after a while and your body has to work hard to make more body fat instead, which can make you feel tired after eating. This tends to become a self-perpetuating and relentless cycle. Only in modern times have humans created this constant emergency need to lower our blood sugar through insulin stimulated by chronically unnatural dietary choices.

Over time, your body becomes less sensitive to insulin, and it becomes easier and easier to gain weight, while also becoming harder and harder to lose it. This dysregulated state is called insulin resistance, and it disrupts the normal signaling process, ultimately creating a state of chaos. As your blood sugar creeps up over time, glucose commingles with your vulnerable tissues, doing more and more damage to your arteries, organs, and nervous system. If this continues unchecked, sooner or later the result is type 2 diabetes, which comes with multiple other problems and risk factors, including neuropathy, visual problems, poor circulation to peripheral tissues leading to gangrene and the need for amputations, renal damage (the number one condition leading to a need for dialysis is diabetes), not to mention an increased risk for cardiovascular disease, Alzheimer's and other dementias, and cancer.

The Plight of the Carbovore

If you have high serum triglycerides, then dimes to donuts you are a rampant (and dysregulated) "sugar burner."[4] I affectionately refer to such people as carbovores. Their elevated serum triglycerides are not the product of eating fat; they are the product of dietary sugar and starch. With high triglyceride levels, it is very hard to lose weight. Your body will seek to utilize sugar preferentially as fuel. With the emphasis on sugar burning, fat burning is effectively shut down.

Furthermore, when you eat sugar and fat at the same time, your body generates insulin (the fat-storage hormone), then stores that fat for later and tries to burn the sugar first, which is *not* a good combination. According to metabolic biochemist Dr. Richard David Feinman, it's like dietary carbs are a lit fuse and fat becomes a powder keg. Fat on its own is not problematic, but in the presence of carbohydrates, it creates a totally explosive minefield of metabolic dysregulation.

A Wild Ride—and Not the Fun Kind

The life of a carbovore is a constant roller coaster. Carbohydrate-laden meals, even healthful-seeming ones like a hearty bowl of oatmeal or a fresh focaccia sandwich with a locally microbrewed beer on the side, send blood sugar on a destructive series of swoops up and down. The insulin level rises to clumsily remove the excess sugar from the bloodstream, drastically lowering the blood glucose. When the blood sugar goes too low, the body essentially panics, triggering the release of the stress hormone cortisol (or even adrenaline), which causes anxiety and/or cravings for carbs (to refuel and to help soothe that stress response). The presence of cortisol causes your adrenals to send the blood sugar rocketing back up yet again, as fuel for a potential fight-or-flight scenario. This stimulates the release of insulin again, which then activates cortisol once more, and . . . you see where this is going. It becomes a vicious cycle, which gets the carb-dependent eater in its grip. You get set up to crave sugar anytime glucose starts to run low, always looking for that source of fuel—baked potatoes, pretzels, fruit, even alcohol—to replenish your supplies. Sugar surges also trigger

SUGAR STATS

Humans did not evolve to rely on foods so volatile, damaging, addictive, and unreliable as sugar and starch to fuel our bodies. But unless you blaze your own path in the opposite direction from the standard American diet, you are setting yourself up for suffering.

- Roughly a fourth of the calories we consume in Western society today comes from added sugar in some form—and this does not even include starchy grains, legumes, or root vegetables, which ultimately become sugar by the time they hit your bloodstream.[5]
- At least 80 percent of all processed foods contain some added sugar.
- Fructose consumption alone has increased over fivefold compared to a hundred years ago and has doubled in just the last thirty years.[6] Fructose is found in fruits and concentrated in dried fruit and fruit juices, as well as in table sugar (which is half fructose), honey, processed foods and sodas containing high fructose corn syrup, and anything-but-healthy agave syrup. Fructose is many times (anywhere from ten to thirty times) *more damaging* than glucose and is by far the sugar most responsible for burgeoning and rapidly accelerating rates of diabetes and obesity.
- Whole grain cereals, as well as potatoes, can spike your blood sugar faster than a candy bar. In fact, grains spike your blood sugar faster and higher than just about anything else (they are also used to fatten cattle—something that gives us one hint of what they do to us).

powerful opiate centers in your brain, adding to its addictive potential. By contrast, fat, which we can learn to depend on, is pleasurable to eat, and not addicting.

With carbs always offered as the go-to plate fillers for breakfast, lunch, and dinner wherever you go, it becomes all too easy to spiral down into metabolic disorder. This is a state that is the root cause of obesity and its commonly associated conditions, including heart disease, diabetes, PCOS, stroke, neurological problems, and cancer.

There's another major pitfall of this dependency. When you're a sugar burner, you inadvertently train the body to become more efficient at converting other things into sugar as well—primarily the protein reserves in your skeletal muscle and bone. During times when you are failing to supply enough carbohydrate to meet your energy demands (such as at night, while you are sleeping and not eating) your body starts to tap into these reserves, turning them into sugar to feed your sugar habit. Scary as it sounds to say this, it is a type of cannibalism, potentially resulting in reduced lean tissue mass and damaged heart muscle as well as osteoporosis. Don't panic, though: an effective state of ketosis retrains your body to burn fat and not sugar, thereby *protecting* your muscles, tissues, and bones.

The Damaging Effects of Glycation

All forms of utilizable sugar add to insulin resistance over time and also damage your body through *glycation*, a process by which sugars combine with proteins and fats in your tissues and cause them to become sticky and misshapen. The resulting combination is referred to as an advanced glycation end product, or AGE—an appropriate acronym, since sugar is a major factor in how the human body adversely ages over time and begins to lose function. Know anyone with chronic pain or inflammation? Glycation is in part to blame for that, as well as for many of the uncomfortable symptoms people associate with aging. Just because aches and pains are common as you age does not make them normal or inevitable!

A certain amount of natural and necessary glycation regularly takes place in the human body as a part of normal metabolism. But the kind of uncontrolled, non-enzymatic glycation I'm discussing here, the kind that is the result of consuming sugars and starches, is anything but beneficial. In a similar vein, a certain amount and type of free radical activity (unpaired electrons that cause oxidative damage to your tissues and mutate DNA) are also necessary for proper human metabolism. But, much as with glycation, the excessive generation of free radicals that is the result of consuming sugars and starches is not healthy, necessary, or beneficial. It's important to make this distinction.

Sorry, There's No Safe Threshold for Sugar

Ample research has tried to determine whether there is a safe threshold for glucose, one that would avoid the adverse aging, endocrine, metabolic, and glycating effects. In other words, as long as I keep the oatmeal, pasta, sandwiches, and potatoes within reasonable ranges each day, won't I be fine? The data is convincing that no safe threshold exists, as the damaging effects occur across the *normal* ranges of glucose. It is key to note that this research does not distinguish whether the sugar originates from a bowl of rice, a potato, a can of soda, or a candy bar. The inescapable conclusion: sugar is sugar, and all sugar is damaging, no matter what the source.

TESTING YOUR BLOOD SUGAR

Long-term glycation of your red blood cells (one of many susceptible tissues) may be assessed through a simple blood test measuring something called *hemoglobin A1C* (Hgb A1C, also known as glycated hemoglobin). This blood test offers a window of approximately three months into the damaging effects of sugar in your body as focused on your red blood cells. Keeping levels at 5.4 percent or below is optimal. Even as some inflammatory agents are produced through acetone (a form of ketone), a quality, low-carbohydrate, ketogenic diet does *not* result in the same damaging increases in Hgb A1C.

The studies also show that humans are becoming increasingly metabolically vulnerable to the effects of chronic sugar burning. Once metabolically deranged (as most of us are today to one degree or another), we are less able to effectively compensate for occasional indulgences and less able to tolerate even supposedly "healthier" or more natural sources of carbs. This is one of many reasons why the foods that recent generations ate—daily bowls of pasta or French baguettes—might have more of a negative impact on us today, and why a contemporary reevaluation of what we eat is so very essential.

From this abbreviated look at a very complex subject, you might now have a good idea of why relying on dietary fat and the abundant fat stored inside our bodies as a primary fuel source, and avoiding the negative consequences of sugar, has the power to transform your health.

THE STORY OF A GRATEFUL GENTLEMAN

Some time ago, I received a note from a medical doctor who is a fan of my work and my book *Primal Body, Primal Mind*. He forwarded a letter from a patient who had experienced dramatic changes in his health entirely by following my fat-burning, primal diet. This gentleman, at seventy-four years of age, had been sixty-five pounds overweight, was prediabetic (fasting glucose 140 mg/dL), had elevated cholesterol, was on medication for high blood pressure, had ghosting vision, suffered from an enlarged prostate (and was on medication for this), and also had knee and hip pain, asthma, pain in both his thumbs, and allergies. Within the first two weeks of adopting this ketogenic dietary approach he began seeing positive changes: he felt stronger, had more energy, experienced fewer food cravings, and felt less pain. After three weeks, his hip and morning pain had totally disappeared, 95 percent of his thumb pain was gone, his allergies had completely abated, his nails and hair started getting stronger, and his urine flow increased significantly. After four and a half months, he had lost fifty pounds and was off his blood pressure and prostate medication, his glucose and cholesterol levels had normalized, his asthma symptoms had significantly improved, and his ghosting vision had greatly improved. The man's letter to me was signed "Forever Grateful."

Defending Your Mitochondria

Mitochondria are more than simply tireless microscopic energy-producing factories operating in and fueling most of your cells. They are also central players in maintaining your healthy physiological makeup. Mitochondria enable us to adapt to a range of environments, climates, and conditions; they helped us evolve into human beings. Mitochondria have their own DNA, separate from the nuclear DNA in your cells at large. Known as mitochondrial DNA or mtDNA, it is very vulnerable; it has far fewer defenses against free radical damage and mutation, which cause inherited diseases, than the relatively protected nuclear DNA has.[7] Mitochondrial dysfunction is a key biomarker of aging, sapping our organs, tissues, and brain cells of energetic capacity as we grow old. Research shows that there is 50 percent more mitochondrial damage in the brain cells of people over seventy years of age compared with middle-aged individuals.[8] This vulnerability is of special concern, since mitochondrial damage increases the risk of Alzheimer's disease (5.4 million new cases in 2015, and rates are skyrocketing) and of cancer (also a product of severe mitochondrial dysfunction).

Ketones exert their magic within what is called the Krebs cycle—the biochemical cellular process of respiration and basic energy production within the mitochondria. Many people who are overweight have an impaired Krebs cycle. Resistant weight loss and many diseases such as Alzheimer's have what is called a block of mitochondrial pyruvate dehydrogenase (PDH). Ketones bypass this block. They also help protect your cells by blocking a certain class of enzymes (called *histone deacetylases,* or HDACs) that contribute to the aging process. Normally, these enzymes serve to suppress the expression of two types of genes (FoxO3a and Mt2). But increasing BOHB (ketones) instead *activates* their expression, which leads to numerous health benefits, not the least of which is a pronounced resistance to oxidative stress (the root of most disease). Scientists speculate that this mechanism could also represent a way to slow the detrimental effects of aging in all cells of the body![9]

Burning fat instead of sugar is one of the most proactive steps you can take to protect your mitochondria. Here's how.

- The free radicals and glycation incurred by chronically burning sugar for energy result in damage to mtDNA. It is certainly true that uncontrolled, non-enzymatic glycation occurs in everyone, with cumulative, deleterious effects as we age. But it becomes more rapid and aggressive if blood sugar levels are high. Minimizing chronic exposure to sugars and insulin and improving the function of antioxidants within the body is key to minimizing mitochondrial damage and the degenerative effects of aging.[10]

• Fat-burning improves mitochondrial efficiency, plain and simple. Many people, in an effort to lose weight, desperately try to speed up their metabolism—say, by exercising constantly to burn more calories as fast as possible, plunging their bodies into freezing water to achieve a thermogenic fat-burning effect, or even taking caffeinated supplements. This is unwise, if not dangerous, because the mtDNA lives totally exposed in the inner mitochondrial membrane, where the mitochondria's perpetual heat-generating factory blazes continuously. It's like a sweltering boiler room in there, oxidizing away, and when you intentionally turn up the burn, you generate an enormous volume of toxic reactive oxygen species (also known as free radicals) that can damage mtDNA—directly counter to your workout goals of improving health and longevity. A slow-and-steady, fat-burning ketogenic diet will help protect your cells from the excesses of oxidative stress and establish a healthy metabolism and healthy weight.

• Eating red meat, especially lamb, can help supply nutrients that better facilitate fatty acids actually reaching the inside of your mitochondria, where they can be burned for energy. One of the compounds derived from breaking down red meat is called L-carnitine (found in greatest abundance in red meat and especially lamb). It is the substance responsible for shuttling fatty acids across the mitochondrial membranes. Without it, your mitochondria find it very hard to burn much fat or fuel your muscles. It also helps to powerfully fuel your heart! It's one more example of how meat and quality fat burning are designed to go together.

Fire-Starting the Right Way: With Fat (or, How to Stop the Carb Roller Coaster and Get Off)

As someone who grew up in Minnesota, I am pretty handy when it comes to stoking a fire. Many of us had wood-burning stoves in our homes, and building a good fire was paramount for keeping home and hearth heated by day and by night. I always picture the stove I used to have in my northern Minnesota wilderness cabin when I explain how sugar and fat differ in the ways they affect our health, weight, and energy. Remember how all other forms of carbohydrate—sugars and starch—are ultimately reduced to sugar by the time they reach your bloodstream? (The exception is pure fiber, which we cannot digest or use for energy.) Think of carbs as the equivalent of kindling: small twigs, crumpled-up pieces of paper, or even lighter fluid that you might use to start a fire. Brown rice, beans, whole grains, potatoes, and pasta are the metabolic equivalent of twigs, while white potatoes, cereals, white rice, bread, pasta, and so on are the crumpled up paper—the former add a little more fire-building heat, the latter mainly hot flame. Sweetened beverages, juices, sports drinks, and most alcoholic beverages are like lighter fluid or gasoline on that metabolic fire. All of them supply a quick burst of energy, and while kindling burns fast and hot, it won't keep a fire (or your metabolism) going for very long.

If you try to maintain any fire with nothing but kindling, you effectively become a slave to that fire. You will be constantly preoccupied with where the next handful of kindling is coming from. You would have to wake up several times during the night to add more kindling to keep the fire going. You would also probably end up spending a lot of time and energy, money, and storage space keeping a lot of kindling handy so your fire wouldn't go out and you wouldn't freeze to death. Is that any way to live? Well, when it comes to human metabolism, the majority of people everywhere are metaphorically doing exactly that.

The same problem arises when the human body depends on sugar and starch as its primary source of fuel. You will constantly crave sugary and starchy carbohydrates and need to eat them frequently to keep your fire burning and your energy levels up. At night while sleeping, you might slip into a state of hypoglycemia, or low blood sugar; your sugar-dependent body will consider this to be an emergency and will stimulate either cortisol or adrenaline to raise your blood sugar back up again. This can wake you up or make your sleep restless. At the same time your body may also tap into your protein stores in muscle and bone to make more sugar to feed that metabolic fire. People who have trouble maintaining and balancing their blood sugar during the day are also more likely to feel irritable and reactive. They tend to seem a bit harsh, neurotic, angry, reactive, hypersensitive, negative, or edgy by nature. Know anyone like that? Yet often it's actually their diet, not their innate temperament, making them that way.

What if, instead of kindling, you placed a nice big log (of fat) on that metabolic fire? Now you'll have the freedom to do more important and productive things with your time and energy, while the fire burns steadily. Heck, chances are good that you'll even sleep through the night! Come morning, if you notice that the fire has died down a bit, all you need to do is toss on another log by eating a breakfast of a small amount of protein that's rich in fat, or a rich cup of bone broth with a spoonful of Pure Indian Foods Cultured Ghee or Turmeric Superghee (wonderful products you'll discover in Part Four). It's unbelievably liberating—suddenly there's a lot more time and attention available to actually live your life!

But sitting by the fire, twigs in hand, endlessly feeding the flame lest it go out, is actually what conventional wisdom and mainstream nutrition, with its emphasis on carbohydrate-based eating, advises us to do.

The American Paradox

You've likely heard of the "French paradox"—that, despite the French people's high consumption of saturated fat, their rates of heart disease are lower than ours in the United States. Here in our country we're stuck in an unfortunate situation that I call the American paradox: the more closely you follow official dietary government guidelines, the worse your health is likely to be![11] The USDA is busy telling Americans to base their daily diets upon low-fat, starchy carbohydrates and get more exercise; meanwhile, the obesity epidemic and related health challenges continue to grow. (This paradox is global, by the way—countries such as India are seeing skyrocketing rates of diabetes, and the vegetarians of southern India have literally the world's shortest life span.)

Trying to make sense of all this is a bit like Alice falling down a rabbit hole; everything seems upside down and nonsensical. Let's take a brief look at the stats. According to the Food Research and Action

Center (FRAC), after decades of being subjected to government guidelines promoting a low-fat and high-carbohydrate diet, Americans show the following problems:[12]

- 68.5 percent of adults are overweight or obese; 34.9 percent are obese. (Compare this to the 1971 overweight statistic of 42 percent.)
- 31.8 percent of children and adolescents are overweight or obese; 16.9 percent are obese.
- 30.4 percent of low-income preschoolers are overweight or obese.

Yet another study published in May 2015 examining the impact of dietary guidelines on the health of US citizens yielded some shocking but undeniable conclusions: rates of obesity and diabetes have increased dramatically.[13] The official government dietary recommendations were intended to prevent weight problems and obesity, along with diabetes, cancer, and other chronic diseases. The fact that this has not happened—and that the reverse is true—is officially rationalized in a number of ways.[14] But the underlying message is that we are dumb and lazy. That's right—the party line about why official dietary recommendations (such as from the American Heart Association and the US Departments of Agriculture and Health and Human Services) have failed is that Americans are to blame because we don't follow the guidelines and we don't work out enough.[15] In other words, if we're sick, it's our own fat, stupid fault.

This is such a persistent, morale-killing, and completely misleading message that I want to address it directly before we move on.

First, we *have* collectively and diligently followed the guidelines. Here's what official guidelines recommend for our daily diets versus what we are currently doing in reality (RDA stands for Recommended Daily Allowance):

Total fat consumption. RDA says a maximum of 35 percent of calories; reality says about 34 percent. (Let's not pat ourselves on the back, though—the number one source of those fat calories is partially hydrogenated oil from genetically modified soybeans, one of the worst things for the body!)

Saturated fats. RDA says a maximum of 10 percent saturated fat; reality says just under 11 percent (not terribly naughty or rebellious relative to established government recommendations).

Carbs. RDA says 55 to 65 percent, with 45 percent the smallest amount necessary to meet the (unfounded) "optimal dietary requirements"; reality says over 50 percent. This is more than enough to create a health-compromising, sugar-burning metabolism.

Protein. RDA says between 10 and 35 percent; reality says 15 percent.

As you can see, Americans *are* meeting the established dietary requirements, and we have largely eschewed our national interest in protein in favor of far more addictive carbohydrates. Isn't it strange, then, that the predominant health messages we hear are that we eat too much animal protein and saturated fat for our own good, and that those are the things that make us overweight and cause heart-related and other health problems?

Meanwhile, FRAC looked at historical shifts and found that the consumption of fats dropped from 45 to 34 percent of total caloric intake between 1971 and 2011, while carbohydrate consumption jumped from 39 to 51 percent. In the same time, obesity has surged by over 25 percent. We have diligently increased our consumption of carbohydrates and reduced our intake of animal fat and cholesterol for over five decades, according to the rules—and we have gotten fatter. Processed foods that contain chemicals such as MSG, Frankenfoods that contain genetically modified organisms (GMOs), hydrogenated and interesterified vegetable oils, and other damaging ingredients such as high fructose corn syrup are to thank for a good part of this disaster. But the promotion of higher-carb, low-fat diets has also undeniably served to push everyone in the wrong direction. (FRAC concluded, as many scientists have, that the increased consumption of carbohydrates is what has caused the huge increase in overweight and obesity.)

"If You Worked Out More, You Wouldn't Be Fat"

Let's burst another morale-killing myth: the idea that we are a super-sized nation because we simply don't exercise enough (that is, we are lazy, ignorant, or both). A study of a remote people still living in ways similar to some of our primitive Neolithic ancestors was performed to investigate the persistent (and judgmental) idea that, to para-phrase, "if you worked out more, you wouldn't be fat."[16] Researchers wanted to investigate if this primitive people—the Hadza, a group living in northern Tanzania—were lean and healthy because their hunter-gatherer lifestyle had them walking and moving vastly more than industrialized Western people. They measured the two groups' daily energy expenditures, took variables between the two groups into account, and came up with the surprising result that energy expenditures for both hunter-gatherers and those living in modern Western society were *essentially the same*. The researchers concluded that the Hadza's hunter-gatherer diet was the primary reason for the significant differences in health and lean tissue mass. This finding correlates with what is now more current thought—even among pro-fessional personal trainers—that *diet accounts for at least 70 percent of the health-and-weight loss equation*. Movement and regular exercise are important for many reasons, but they don't mean much if the foundation of your nutrition is full of holes.

The convergence of flawed science and profit-driven agendas has got us in a real pickle, to put it lightly. It's time to point the finger where it needs to be pointed. Since the very beginning of govern-ment efforts to guide the health habits of the nation, the officially sanctioned dietary guidelines have targeted dietary fat (especially dietary animal fat) as public enemy number one. These policies have relentlessly focused on the *hypothesis* that limiting fat intake would decrease obesity and promote better health. The lipid hypothesis launched an obsession with vilifying fat consumption (especially animal fat) that has persisted despite the recent, immense body of evidence countering it. We now can conclusively demonstrate that the lipid hypothesis was based upon numerous flawed assumptions and has had nothing short of catastrophic results.

Why is the truth dawning only now, fifty-plus years after this hypothesis was born? Big Agribusiness lobbyists and political appointees, seeking to maintain the profitable status quo and save bureaucratic face, have done their best to block the implementation of updated science. The renewed effort by the World Health Organization—based on weak, epidemiological evidence—to place red meat on a list of "probable carcinogens" (right up there with plutonium), is grossly misleading. (It haphazardly lumps in processed, chemically laden, and inflammatory bologna, hot dogs, and feedlot meats in with exclusively grass-fed liver or steak.)

As long as the USDA's Center for Nutrition Policy and Promotion can effectively sell us the illusion that we are suffering ill health and obesity because we aren't following their rules (which is a lie), we will continue to accept blame for our own struggles—and, worse yet, continue to rely on those rules for guidance. It seems we are mostly playing by the official rules, but the embarrassing proof of the catastrophic failure of these official guidelines is in the high-carb pudding—a dish that most definitely does not agree with us and is making us sick.

What If . . . We Started by Just Ditching the Carbohydrates?

Maybe you can see where I'm going with this. You've learned that the body can, and likes to, burn fat as fuel. You're about to learn more about how it can manufacture its own glucose as needed. So the next step in this seemingly logical (or radical, depending on your viewpoint) proposition is this: *we don't actually need carbohydrates in our diet at all.* Notice how this doesn't exactly jibe with the contemporary paradigm of six to eleven servings of carbs per day? Exactly.

Here's the unvarnished reality: The concept that humans need a certain amount of dietary carbs for proper function of the body is not grounded in actual science. It's a popular belief—otherwise known as a myth—that has persisted thanks to the interplay of agricultural and food industry interests, the dietetic establishment and government policy, combined with perhaps our own very "civil" modern tendency to obediently follow the experts, along with (frankly) wishful thinking. That is how myth often becomes accepted truth.

Except that when you look closely at the scientific literature, you find a wealth of information that challenges the status quo around carbohydrate consumption. The National Research Council has not established an RDA for carbohydrates, probably because the human body can adapt to a carbohydrate-free diet and manufacture the glucose it needs.[17] The 2010 Dietary Guidelines for Americans stated that "the lower limit of the dietary carbohydrate compatible with life apparently is zero, provided that adequate amounts of protein and fat are consumed."[18]

Maybe you're wondering, "Aren't we all different in our needs? Maybe a few unusual types can get by with no carbs, but surely most people need some dietary sugars and starches to survive." Again, the answer is no. We are all forged from the same human blueprint; there isn't a different textbook of human physiology for every person reading this. There is essentially only one. Beyond our most basic foundations and foundational needs lies mere nuance. Yes, there is a certain degree of biological individuality to consider, but to argue that everyone's foundations are different has no basis in science. It's a subject clouded in misinformation, misunderstanding, and quite a bit of nutritional politics (with an occasional pinch of wishful thinking). I like the way that diabetes and blood sugar expert Richard K. Bernstein, MD, puts it: "It is possible to suffer an amino acid deficiency. It is possible to have an essential fatty acid deficiency. But there is no such thing as a carbohydrate deficiency."

Seen through the lens of this scientifically supported approach, the fact that carbohydrates from starches form the massive base of the food pyramid—the foundation on which everything is supposed to stand—is utterly confounding. There is a functional and much safer workaround, one that is available for anyone to use: maximize your fat-burning ability and minimize your need for sugar.

CHAPTER 5

Harnessing Your Superfuel:
Flipping on the Fat-Burning Switch

Energy from fat is produced only when blood sugar and insulin levels are low. This happens during fasting conditions (or starvation) or when dietary carbohydrate levels are kept consistently low and protein levels are not excessive. This opens the door for the body to gain access to fat for fuel, which it does by breaking down first dietary fat and then stored body fat (triglycerides) to release free fatty acids.[1] These free fatty acids can be burned through a process known as beta-oxidation, or they may instead move to the liver where they are then converted into ketone bodies, which are more commonly referred to simply as ketones.

The Making of a Superfuel: Ketones

There are three different types of ketones: beta-hydroxybutyrate (BOHB for short), acetoacetate, and acetone (which is basically a degradation product of acetoacetate, but some evidence shows it also has the potential to help your body make some glucose when it needs it).[2,3] BOHB, considered the principal ketone, is not just a fuel but a "superfuel," more efficient at producing energy than glucose or fatty acid.[4] Once the ketones in your bloodstream reach your tissues and organs, the mitochondria within the cells use these unique energy units of fat to produce ATP. After somewhere between twenty-four and seventy-two hours of no carbs, the body begins to produce ketones in significant amounts. As ketones begin to circulate, the cells of the heart, brain, and muscles begin to use them. Within about 3 days your brain is already getting about 25 percent of its energy from ketone bodies. After just four days this goes up to about 70 percent![5] Soon your body begins to generate ketones and free fatty acids from your body fat for fuel as well.[6] When this happens, your body has shifted from a glucocentric (sugar-focused) metabolism to an adipocentric (fat-based) one. The basic definition of being ketogenically adapted in this way is that you are essentially burning your own body fat for fuel. Who in their right mind does not want this?

If you maintain the correct conditions for a few weeks—and now I'm talking about following a healthy diet low in carbohydrates and moderate in protein with sufficient dietary fat, not fasting or starvation—your body finds its groove and gets into a well-adapted, fat-burning state in which it makes regular efficient use of ketones and free fatty acids for energy. During a full state of EKA your BOHB ketone levels can healthfully vary from 0.5 to 7 mmol (though 1 to 3 is typical). This confers on you a very valuable asset: you are able to readily maintain a constant access to this energy supply by accessing your body's abundant fat stores when you need them. In other words, as long as enough fat is coming in to reassure your body that "hunting is good," your body will freely turn to the reserves you already have stored on your body and burn *them*. It's like getting the key to a well-stocked pantry, and that is why you can safely and very comfortably go longer without eating when you are burning fat—whether out of preference (for example, doing safe, short-term "intermittent" fasting for its added therapeutic benefits or if medically necessary) or out of sheer everyday necessity, such as a hectic schedule forcing you to skip lunch. It's liberating! Maintaining your energy and full mental clarity, even if hours go by between meals, and taking the power back from cravings can be life-changing!

This benefit applies even if you are slim, as you still have fat reserves that can be freed up for energy. (Don't worry; if you are healthfully slim and follow the Primal Fat Burner Plan, you will be eating well enough to maintain your healthy weight.) And if you typically have excess fat stored in places such as your belly, love handles, hips, and thighs, this excess begins to get burned as fuel. This is a state of effective ketogenic adaptation (EKA)—or, to put it another way, a healthy and well-adapted fat-burning state. Barring some underlying condition that might interfere with effective ketone utilization (such as undiagnosed adrenal insufficiency/autoimmunity, undiagnosed infections, or certain sources of inflammation that may depress cortisol availability, which I'll discuss in Chapter 8, or the ability to produce sufficient cortisol when needed), your body can happily run on fat. In fact, it is likely to run far better—not to mention longer, a topic we'll get to later.

In addition to securing a stable, long-lasting fuel source, you also avoid more of the invisible harm caused by chronic sugar and starch consumption: metabolic confusion and dysregulation, rampant inflammation and disease-causing free radical activity, and the glycation that causes malfunction and aging across all your organs and systems. You support your best mitochondrial health and protect yourself against the mitochondrial damage that causes disease and dysfunction, which makes you more vulnerable to cancer. An effective ketogenic state also helps to correct cellular metabolic dysfunction—hence Dr. Wortman's success with diabetes reversal, described at the start of this chapter.

The Benefits of Fat Burning

The many possible benefits of being in a healthy, well-adapted ketogenic state include:

- Easier weight loss, without hunger or cravings
- Stabilized neurological functioning in the brain, which makes you less susceptible to migraines, panic attacks, mood swings, and seizures
- Long-lasting stable energy that your body and brain can use all day long—even in the absence of regular meals
- An anti-inflammatory effect and a dampening of free radical activity, which causes tissue damage
- Protection of the brain from hypoxia (low oxygen flow)

- Increased blood flow to the brain and improved overall brain function, cognition, and memory; reduction of the risk of Alzheimer's disease
- Protection of lean tissue mass
- Improved sleep
- Increased mitochondrial efficiency
- Reduced blood pressure
- Improved immune function
- Healthier skin
- Reduced blood sugar issues; lower hemoglobin A1C and other metabolic markers associated with metabolic diseases such as obesity and diabetes
- Improved thyroid efficiency
- Improved cardiovascular markers: a rise in quality HDL, a reduction in small-particle LDL, lower triglycerides
- Possible reduction of cancer risk
- Anti-aging effects, with improved cellular regeneration and DNA repair

On top of this, as research and clinical experience have shown, a moderate ketogenic state, implemented correctly, can benefit a variety of disease states, which we'll look at more closely in the chapters to come. And moderate ketosis is physiologically safe to continue indefinitely.

Being *primarily* a fat burner or a sugar burner does not mean you are *exclusively* one or the other, mind you. We always make some use of both fuels. Once your body adapts to a primary reliance on ketones and free fatty acids, your overall requirement for glucose is greatly reduced—but you still need some. For the most part, the tissues and organs of the body prefer to use ketones and will selectively consume the types of ketone bodies they need. The exception is the liver, where ketones are actually made. But your liver can use fatty acids instead. The heart and brain, which are especially mitochondria-dense, are the most avid users of BOHB ketones, which are a clean, steady, and non-damaging fuel, even conferring protective properties. Your skeletal muscles love burning fat, too!

But some cells contain very few mitochondria, such as the renal medulla (inner part of the kidneys), white blood cells, and testes. And a very few others contain no mitochondria at all (red blood cells and the retinas, corneas, and lenses of the eyes). These mitochondrially devoid cells depend on glucose as their sole source of fuel, though they require extremely small amounts. Your body can easily make the small amount of glucose required by these tissues without ingesting any sugar or starch. This glycolytic energy demand is met by *gluconeogenesis*, the process of making glucose as you need it, which can come from dietary proteins and dietary or stored fats (triglycerides) inside the body. Needed glucose can also come from *glycogenolysis*, the process of drawing from glycogen that is either already stored in the liver or stored in the muscle for specific, short-spurt muscular demands. But unlike a glucose-based metabolism, ketones actually spare that precious emergency glycogen (and your lean tissue mass) for the times you really need it; they don't squander it on everyday activities, which simply feeds your unnecessary sugar habit.

Gluconeogenesis occurs only in the absence of dietary carbohydrate, and it is very efficient: the body makes the right (read: minimal) amounts of necessary sugar on demand, instead of depending on it to come from starch- and sugar-filled foods, with the consequent burdens on your metabolic, oxidative, and endocrine-related systems. Your brain may continue to draw upon very small amounts of glucose, but in a state of fully effective ketogenic adaptation, glucose will not supply much more than 10 to 15 percent of your brain's total energy needs. Meanwhile, your muscles have access to a small supply of auxiliary glucose to serve as a sort of "rocket fuel" in the event of either a sudden emergency or a need for pronounced (anaerobic) exertion.

It's quite a paradigm shift to accept that glucose isn't the indispensable resource you thought it was. It will make you look back and question everything you were taught about how to eat and who—or what interests—directed your dietary norms. This can be unsettling, to say the least. I invite you to consider this quote by Dr. Rosedale: "Your health and lifespan will mostly be determined by the proportion of fat versus sugar you burn over a lifetime. I've said that for 20 years. I've not found anything to contradict it. All the evidence that has occurred in the last 20 years has supported that one statement. Everything there is to know about health, and aging, can be summarized right there."

Won't Eating Fat Make Me Fat?

Despite the fact that for the majority of people diets don't work and weight lost is very soon weight gained back, I often find resistance to the idea that eating dietary fat will not make you gain fat. In fact, if done correctly, eating fat will even help you burn more fat.

Let's quickly run the numbers to put this in perspective. The breakdown and utilization of fats create four times more energy than that of utilizable carbohydrates or protein on average, yet fat has only twice the caloric density of carbohydrate. So by doubling the caloric intake—something that sounds scary to calorie counters—fat actually delivers *four times* the energy. That's one reason why looking at calorie counts on foods is fairly useless when it comes to weight loss. It doesn't tell you what happens when that food is turned into utilizable energy.

Furthermore, how we make use of the food we eat is dependent not upon its caloric content but upon the complex interaction of our hormones and enzymes in response to that food. The human body is not a heat engine, but rather a complex biochemical factory where structural and complex biochemical needs are given the highest priority; whatever is left over is used for immediate energy or stored energy. Dietary fat actually fulfills a host of structural and functional needs before it is used to fill energetic needs—or before getting stored as excess energy on your thighs.

Relying on fat as your primary source of fuel also affects your appetite through several different mechanisms. First, eating enough fat creates healthy leptin levels, which help keep your appetite in check. A hormone that acts as a fat sensor, leptin is found in fat tissue and helps your brain decide whether to make you hungry or not, and whether to store or burn fat. It is arguably your body's single most important hormone, regulating all others. When you aren't eating enough fat, leptin makes you hungrier; it prompts you to make more fat from other foods in your diet (namely, carbs), which then keeps you hungry.

Eating fat while eliminating sugar and starch also helps dampen ghrelin, the hunger hormone that acts as an appetite stimulant. The more quality fat your meal contains and the more nutrient-dense it is, the less ghrelin your body produces and the less hungry you feel. An effective ketogenic state can also lower the amount of ghrelin your body produces over time.[7] When you attempt weight loss the old way, by simply counting calories, ghrelin levels tend to creep up as the weight comes off, making it harder and harder to suppress cravings and the desire to eat. In a state of fully effective ketosis, though, instead of getting hungrier as you lose weight, you gain better appetite control.[8] And without needing and generating so much insulin, you will automatically store less fat. This can make weight loss virtually effortless. It's really the amount and quality of the energy you make that count, and eating enough fat to feel sated will always work best. It's almost impossible to overeat fat because of its inherent richness and satiating quality. After all, when was the last time you saw anyone bingeing on lard? A little fat really goes a long way to satisfy you!

It turns out that a high-fat, low-carbohydrate way of eating can flip a switch in the way your genes are expressed, helping to code for specific proteins that increase your metabolism of fats. This also helps your body burn even more fat than ever before during exercise —even during higher anaerobic intensity.

All of this helps to explain why some impressive studies have observed that a ketogenic diet can be used safely and effectively for weight reduction (and long-term weight loss) in obese patients.[9] Others have shown that it leads to a significant decrease in the level of triglycerides, total cholesterol, LDL, and glucose, and a significant increase in the level of HDL.[10]

Losing Weight . . . and Keeping It Off

When you restrict your fat intake and total calories, which is what decades of weight-loss programs have advised, you might notice some initial weight loss. But this tends to plateau quickly as your body adjusts to the minimal amount of fat coming in and becomes increasingly efficient at hanging on to the precious fat stores that you already have. You may find yourself struggling more with cravings. Your body senses a famine and struggles to compensate for the lack of fat-soluble nutrients coming in, slowing down your metabolism. This not only stalls additional weight loss but also speeds weight gain once you get off the diet and return to a more normal fat and caloric intake. It's inevitable.

But if you are able to consistently reassure your body and brain that enough fat is coming in, which you can do by eating enough of it, then your body has no reason to hang on to anything extra and will readily shift into that consistent fat-burning state without "worrying" about a famine. And because fat is so inherently satiating, hunger and cravings tend to be a thing of the past—allowing you to make consistently better food choices, automatically helping to ensure your longer-term success. Whatever small amounts of carbs that come in are more likely to be stored as reserve carbs (glycogen) in your muscles and liver, just in case you might need them later in an emergency.

Only one in six overweight or obese adults reports having maintained weight loss of at least 10 percent for one year.[11] Other studies suggest that long-term weight loss success rates from conventional dieting may be even lower.[12] Conversely, numerous studies have demonstrated both the safety and efficacy of ketogenic approaches, also demonstrating the ability of subjects to *maintain healthy weight loss for over a year* (something other dietary approaches clearly tend to fail at).[13] The researchers concluded: "Ketogenic Enteral Nutrition treatment of over 19,000 patients induced a rapid 10 percent weight loss, 57 percent of which was Fat Mass. No significant adverse effects were found. The treatment is safe, fast, inexpensive and has good one-year results for weight maintenance." Why wouldn't you try a more natural way of eating—eating fat to lose fat—and see what it holds for you? This approach is psychologically liberating, too, because *Primal Fat Burner* offers a foundational program for health and longevity. Effortless weight loss is a mere fringe benefit for those who need it. As a diet, it tends to feel more positive, more constructive, and less

WATCH FAT BURNING AT WORK

Maybe you still doubt that you could eat as much fat as you like and still get lean. Sometimes it helps to see this play out on the big screen. A terrific documentary called *Cereal Killers* follows one young man as he attempts to "hack his genes" and avoid his family legacy of heart disease by adopting a fat-based diet. For a month he ate a very low-carb diet, with 70 percent of his caloric intake from fat and consuming a total of around 4,000 calories a day, under the supervision of South African sports nutrition expert Tim Noakes. He worked out intensively for a mere eight minutes a week. Yet he saw impressive positive results in his physique, blood test markers, and more.

filled with self-doubt, self-criticism, struggles with cravings, and all those other negative aspects of fad diets. The approach is inspiring: give your body what it truly needs, avoid the things that interfere with it, and nature tends to take care of the rest! Nothing could be more self-empowering!

Oh, the Places It Goes! The Body's Many Uses for Fat

Next to water, the single most abundant nutrient in any human body is fat. Our bodies contain from 55 to 65 percent water. According to the American Council on Exercise, body fat percentages in average, non-obese men are up to 24 percent and in women up to 31 percent. But that doesn't count all the fat in your cell membranes, essential fatty acids in your organs and tissues, the fats functioning as part of your immune and endocrine systems, or all the fat and cholesterol in your brain. The first priority for dietary fats is to support your body's structural and functional needs; only then whatever is left over is stored or burned for energy. (This is in strong contrast to carbohydrates, which serve little structural function at all—less than 2 percent or so.) Fat provides a *lot* of these structural and functional needs, which is another reason why consuming ample fat doesn't equate with you getting bigger.

What follows is just a rough sketch of where they go and what they do. Pay attention— these are all the things your body needs fat for before ever extracting a single calorie!

- Your nervous system and the myelin sheath that protects neurons are made up of what are called *sphingolipids*, an important class of fat without which your nervous system simply could not function.

- Saturated fat, cholesterol, phospholipids, and omega-3 fatty acids together with omega-6 fatty acids are critical components of every cell membrane in your body.

- Fat plays a critical role in the functioning of your immune system (as do the many fat-soluble nutrients). Most fats are immediately absorbed into your lymphatic system once you've eaten them, rather than into your bloodstream. Certain short- and medium-chained saturated fats tend to bypass digestion and get absorbed more directly into the blood, where they have potent antimicrobial properties and can supply nearly instant energy as free fatty acids and ketones. Saturated fats also prime white blood cells to destroy invading bacteria, viruses, and fungi, and tumor growth itself tends to be suppressed during an effective state of ketosis, essentially by depriving cancer cells of what they crave most: sugar.

- The body's endocannabinoid system, responsible for maintaining the homeostasis of every single hormone and neurotransmitter, neurological stability, and bodily systems, is *lipophilic* (fat-loving). After all, endocannabinoids are fatty acids! This system helps to maintain homeostatic balance and works to keep away disease and inflammation. Omega-6 and omega-3 essential fatty acids form its foundation, as they are required for the production of endocannabinoids and cannabinoid receptors. Excessive plant-based omega-6s are pro-inflammatory and block the action of anti-inflammatory omega-3s.

- Your heart prefers saturated long-chain fats, such as stearic acid, with eighteen carbon atoms, and palmitic acid, with sixteen carbon atoms, as its primary source of fuel. (The heart also uses ketones, which may improve its efficiency up to 28 percent.) Your bones need dietary saturated fat and fat-soluble nutrients to assimilate and utilize calcium and other minerals effectively. Your hormones use cholesterol as a substrate and use certain saturated fats as signaling messengers for their production. Your lungs use an oxidation-resistant saturated fat (palmitic acid) to make lung surfactant (a disaturate molecule), which forms a protective barrier for your vulnerable pulmonary tissue.

Flipping on the Fat-Burning Switch

So here's the million-dollar question: what does it take to switch from being a sugar burner to being a fat burner?

There is a threshold of dietary carbohydrate intake at which the changeover from glucose burning to fat and ketone burning takes place. This threshold is measured in the amount of utilizable carbohydrates you consume per day. This is the amount of actual sugars in a food. To calculate it, you subtract the fiber from the total carbohydrate value. For instance, a medium apple contains about 25 grams of total carbs; when you subtract the fiber, about 6 grams, you see that there are about 19 grams of utilizable sugars. While some clinicians and researchers have suggested the threshold for sugar burning can vary, being somewhere between 65 and 180 grams of carbs per day, the famed ketogenic researcher George F. Cahill Jr., MD, was clear that 100 grams of utilizable carbohydrates per day was more than enough to kick you unceremoniously out of ketosis. Most ketogenic experts recommend no more than 50 grams of utilizable carbs a day to maintain the most effective state of ketosis. When it comes to eating carbs, a lot depends on how insulin sensitive you are to begin with; some individuals can get away with eating slightly more carbohydrates than others. But this kind of personal tweaking is advanced-level stuff. That's why the Primal Fat Burner Plan sets a universal target threshold that is low enough for everybody to benefit. In my experience the modern human metabolism is too vulnerable—and the compromising stresses of our modern lifestyle and environment too strong—to risk playing around or pushing that carb threshold envelope.

I have found that most people achieve optimal, maximally effective states of ketosis, and consequently the most successful weight loss and good health results, by limiting their daily utilizable carbohydrate consumption to roughly 50 grams (obtained from the small amounts of carbs in veggies, nuts, and maybe a few berries) and allowing relatively unlimited consumption of non-utilizable carbohydrate from fibrous vegetables and greens. (Fear not: on the

Primal Fat Burner Plan you won't need to measure out precise portions of vegetables to hit this target. When non-starchy vegetables are the carbohydrates in your diet, it's almost impossible to exceed that limit.) According to Dr. Cahill, "If a diet contains over 100 grams of carbohydrate [i.e., sugar/starch per day], there is no ketosis (<0.1 mM)." And "high protein, as well as carbohydrate, has to be avoided."[14]

Once you have achieved a state of effective ketogenic adaptation (EKA), a blood test will likely show BOHB ketone levels between 1 and 3 mmol/L (later in the book I will show you how to measure this at home). Some therapeutic protocols even shoot for slightly higher levels (up to about 7 mmol/L), though such refinements are beyond the scope of this book. Dreaded states such as ketoacidosis (typically with ketones measuring in excess of 15 to 25 mmol/L) occur in the rarest of instances and only in those with poorly managed type 1 diabetes. (See the important note on type 1 diabetes on page 137.) For the average person, monitoring ketone levels isn't necessary unless you feel you are running into sticking points . . . or you have a geeky disposition.

The Twenty-First-Century Ketogenic Phenomenon: Where Primal Fat Burning Fits In

From my vantage point on the podium at many a paleo conference, I've seen more definitions of a "paleo" diet than Baskin-Robbins has flavors. Similarly, "ketosis" has multiple identities—experts will offer contrasting approaches and definitions according to the priorities they feel are important. Some approaches to ketosis are more effective and healthier than others, and if you go too far down the wrong road you will actually put yourself at risk. All ketogenic diets are *not* the same. So let's take a closer look.

First and foremost, the point of the Primal Fat Burner Plan is not to fanatically pursue the production of ketones. Yes, these simple organic compounds can be measured and tracked easily if you are so inclined, letting you see if you are successfully and safely burning fat instead of sugar—I'll explain this in Part Four. But it's not the ketones that make the approach in this book so valid; in part it is the fact that you are effectively burning ketones for fuel as part of a fat-based (rather than carbohydrate-based) metabolism. Ketones are just a *part* of the energy you generate from fat—don't get obsessed with them or assume that making more is always better. For example, you can produce some ketones by eating a high-protein, very low-carb diet, and you might lose weight with that, but you wouldn't be in a fully effective ketogenic state. For that matter, you can also produce ketones by starving yourself or by chugging shots of canola oil on a low-carb diet, but you would not be anywhere near optimally healthy! Also, today there is no shortage of racemic (synthetic) ketone powders and supplements promising instant ketosis. Remember: more is not at all necessarily better, and creating more ketones in your body by taking large amounts of MCT (medium-chain triglyceride) oil or some expensive racemic ketone powder does not necessarily mean your body is efficient at using them, much less that you are healthier for it. Strategic use of some of these supplements may have their place, but cannot take the place of a fully natural, safe, and effective fat-burning metabolism.

One of the motivating forces behind writing *Primal Fat Burner* is to help people avoid the problems and issues associated with other ketogenic diets. Most are strictly focused on macronutrient ratios (in other words, the amount and ratios of fats, protein, and carbohydrates in the diet) and pay little attention to the quality or sourcing of these macronutrients or their nutrient content. In some circles, a ketogenic metabolism is associated with a state of starvation. Primal Fat Burner does not starve you. It nourishes you as never before. Other fat-based ketogenic approaches also fail to take into account the rapidly growing epidemic of autoimmune disease and the possibility of immune reactivity to certain commonly antigenic/potentially compromising (but otherwise seemingly keto-friendly) fat sources such as butter, canola or soybean oil, sugar and carb substitutes (including artificial sweeteners), and even commonly antigenic or immune-compromising inclusions such as soy, dairy, or genetically modified foods. Inflammation-provoking food sensitivities often matter at least as much as the actual macronutrient ratios in what you eat. This is why the Primal Fat Burner Plan insists upon whole, uncontaminated, unprocessed organic/exclusively pastured foods, those most in alignment with our human genetic makeup.

Medically prescribed ketogenic diets for conditions such as epilepsy, Parkinson's, and amyotrophic lateral sclerosis (ALS, or Lou Gehrig's disease), which have been used for years, can help to resolve some serious symptoms very quickly, but patients may miss out on the opportunity to build optimal health. These old-school medical protocols frequently involve the consumption of meal replacement beverages that contain partially hydrogenated/interesterified oils, corn syrup solids, artificial flavors, powdered milk, and even high fructose corn syrup. Sources of protein in these beverages often include commonly antigenic and highly processed milk, corn, and soy products (also likely containing GMOs and/or trans/interesterified fats, in the case of corn, canola, and soy). The recommended menus for these medically sanctioned diets also often feature undressed feedlot-sourced hamburger patties and bland, highly processed "carb substitutes" (read: artificial sweeteners). No wonder many medical doctors claim ketogenic diets are "unpalatable" and "difficult to sustain." (If you suffer from neurodegenerative disease, Chapter 8 will show you the benefits of becoming a primal fat burner.)

And then there's the issue of how much protein to eat. In the late 1960s, Dr. Robert Atkins proclaimed his now famous Atkins diet to be ketogenic, but he actually recommended excessive amounts of protein as its means of establishing positive ketosis—which may have inadvertently prevented many of its adherents from adopting a fully efficient ketogenic state. This would have allowed for the ongoing (albeit less inefficient) production and metabolism of sugars from protein. This may have been the reason so many Atkins dieters wound up succumbing to growing carbohydrate cravings—in effect, they never fully ceased to be fundamentally sugar burners. Also, little attention was given to the quality of food that followers were to eat. Canola oil and rancid bacon grease were on the same level as fresh tallow from grass-fed animals or organic virgin coconut oil. Highly processed and refined carbohydrate and sugar substitutes were marketed alongside his dietary recommendations.

A high-protein, high-fat diet such as Atkins will generate a lot of ketones in the absence of sugar and starch, but you may never become fully efficient at using them—especially if you happen to be coming off a high-carbohydrate diet. Remember, when you have been relying on carbohydrates as a primary source of fuel for a long time, your body becomes *really efficient* at converting other things, namely proteins from your diet, into sugars. It also saps protein from your muscles, bones, and organs to make more sugar. When you suddenly switch from a high-carbohydrate diet to a high-protein diet, your body will try to create as much sugar from the excess protein as possible in order to compensate for the lack of incoming dietary sugar; this is equally undesirable and frequently unsustainable.

If your diet is high in protein and low in carbohydrate, chances are good that you're still making significant use of glucose throughout the day and may never quite lose that craving for dietary sugars and starches. This is also one of the reasons that weight loss efforts can plateau for many individuals. You're also putting yourself at considerable risk with all that protein (see "Running on Protein" on page 85).

On another note, it can be limiting to go too far down into the low-carb wormhole—a dietary niche that obviously intersects with primal fat burning. But the low-carb movement tends to focus on one small piece of the puzzle while overlooking the more complex picture: by putting an emphasis on weight loss alone, it too often assumes that good health necessarily goes along with it. It doesn't necessarily! Being at a healthy weight can be a very welcome by-product of achieving optimal health—but simply being slender does not in any way mean that you will have healthy blood sugar, triglyceride levels, DHA levels, inflammatory markers, gut health, and nutrient absorption. Foundational health requires high-quality, nutrient-dense, and uncontaminated food. We must connect the dots to see the bigger picture of how our bodies and brains function as whole, complex systems. This is the very heart of functional medicine/functional nutrition and the *Primal Fat Burner* philosophy.

You achieve a state of effective ketogenic adaptation by eliminating the carbs and moderating your protein intake to just what you need each day, then adding as much fat as necessary to satisfy your appetite and calm leptin production (thereby signaling to your metabolism that "hunting is good" and that there is enough fat available to be able to let some go for energy). This gives the brightest green light to your full-time, full-speed-ahead fat-burning metabolism. The magic does *not* lie in producing lots and lots of ketones; the magic lies in being a primal fat burner, first and foremost.

NEWS FLASH: BOOSTING KETONES, BY HOOK OR BY CROOK

Any dietary approach that gets popular inevitably generates a market for hot new products that will make it work "even better!" Not surprisingly, a stream of ketone-based supplements is trickling onto shelves. I'm not exactly a fan. Ketone esters made in a laboratory have been used for medical therapies—potentially miraculous if you have epilepsy, but not appropriate, affordable, or even available for the average person. Now we're seeing approaches that use high quantities of MCT oil and/or supplemental "racemic" ketone salts (which are synthetic) to mimic the effect. Although it could be argued that they have the potential to ease the transition to fat burning, they are not optimally health-promoting on their own and may even complicate your health. I am highly skeptical of supposed "shortcuts"—potions and methods that seek a way around natural adaptation. It is also difficult to accurately measure the blood levels of racemic ketone salts found in popular supplements, which are quite different from the ones your body naturally makes itself. They actually do not fully register on conventional blood ketone meters (only the biologically active "D" fraction shows up), leading to potential problematic errors in accuracy. In Part Four I'll show you how small amounts of a certain kind of MCT oil may help you if you hit a plateau, but I advise skepticism when it comes to any supplement or product that purports to be a ketogenic magic bullet. Slow and steady wins the race: focus on optimizing your diet, day in and day out, and use my suggested MCT supplementation if your particular weight loss or performance goals call for it and it feels right to you. But remember, nature doesn't like shortcuts.

Running on Protein: Why It's a Bad Idea

If you cut back on carbohydrates, can't you just fill the gap with more protein instead of fat? A reasonable question, but the answer is no—and the reasons are important, because the term "low-carb" has become mistakenly linked with "high protein" in the cultural conversation.

Low-carb, high-protein weight-loss diets allow abundant muscle meats, dairy, fish, and protein powders, minimal carbs, and varying amounts and types of allowable fat, often from highly questionable sources. A lot of protein-rich regimens are marked "paleo," but using protein for energy is anything but healthy for the long term, and actually quite dangerous. This is why the Primal Fat Burner Plan includes modest to moderate protein portions along with ample fat. It is quality fat (with quite a bit from animal sources) that delivers the bulk of the caloric intake on this plan.

Consider what protein delivers. It is necessary for hormone and neurotransmitter production and basic structural maintenance and repair. Anything we consume in excess of those needs (roughly 36 percent worth, according to diabetes expert Richard Bernstein, MD) eventually gets converted to glucose and gets used the same way.[15] The reason that eating a high-protein diet adds significant stress and burden to the body has to do with its chemistry. Carbohydrates and fats are made up of mainly three elements: carbon, oxygen, and hydrogen. Proteins contain these elements as well but also contain nitrogen and other components that have to be disposed of through a process called *deamination*. The liver and kidneys handle this, but it is taxing work to break down nitrogen into ammonia and urea (which are toxic to the body) and then excrete them, and there are limits to what these important organs can handle. As a result, the body has a limited capacity to healthfully process protein in large amounts—particularly in the absence of fat, because fat dilutes the protein while helping facilitate its absorption and utilization. When more than 50 percent of calories consumed come from strictly lean protein, you hit and then surpass your physiological "protein ceiling" and must start paying the price of the excess digestive and metabolic burden. You also put yourself at increased risk for cancer and accelerated aging. If your fully grass-fed meat is quite fatty, or if you combine small amounts of lean meat with plenty of animal fat, you offset this ceiling and allow for a far less toxic metabolic burden while improving your utilization of the protein.

That's why the lean protein protocol that was de rigueur in the paleo movement in the early days (about twenty years ago) and still persists in some circles is seriously flawed. Early enthusiasts of ancestral eating heaped their plates with lean cuts of meat (and sometimes used plant seed oils to cook them—a *really* bad idea due to the dangers of instantly oxidizing those delicate and unstable oils through the application of heat). This approach probably took hold because of our cultural fear of fat (especially animal fat), but our ancestors would have never willingly elected to eat that way. As we saw in Part One, prehistoric humans selected for the fattiest meat possible to survive the harsh Paleolithic extremes and feed their (then still) sizable brains. If you go down this road and eat lean protein and other low-fat foods to excess, you are in trouble, because this makes you vulnerable to hyperammonemia—a buildup of ammonia in the bloodstream. This can lead to weakness, diarrhea, severe debilitation, heart abnormalities, and even death in a matter of just a few weeks.[16] The Native peoples of the Arctic had a term for this: "rabbit starvation," the unfortunate consequence of being forced by hunting hardship to subsist on animals with no fat stores.[17] (It illuminates why Vilhjálmur Stefánsson, the Arctic explorer, made the comment that meat is a complete meal only in the presence of fat.) The liquid protein diet fad of the 1970s led to "rabbit starvation"–type problems,[18] and the more recent explosion of protein powders has created a worrying new predicament, by providing unnaturally easy ways to load up on protein throughout the day with just a scoop and a blender. I'm not a fan: excess protein not only generates unnecessary glucose (the least of its problems) but burdens the body with its excess metabolites, speeds up aging, and also facilitates the expression of the mTOR pathway, which strongly promotes cellular proliferation of all kinds, potentially including tumor growth. For optimal health, healthy protein moderation (so that you meet but do not exceed requirements) is every bit as important as limiting carbohydrates.

Don't let this seriousness scare you, however. It's fairly easy to get your protein right, and the Primal Fat Burner Plan will help you do it with minimal angst and ample common sense. Here is what you need to know.

1. *What kind of protein.* We need to eat a certain amount of complete, animal-source protein with its naturally occurring fats in order to be optimally healthy. Significant protein value from plant sources (grains, legumes, or soy—or, say, combining beans and rice) generally comes with higher amounts of starch, almost no useful essential fats, and a plethora of potentially immune-compromising lectins and foreign proteins, even when the food is grown organically. It's preferable and most natural for your body to get your protein from animal-source foods.

2. *Quality.* When it comes to animal proteins, it is essential to eat high-quality, *fully pastured* meats, which means meat from an animal that lives its entire life eating grass

and other natural forage, not one that is fed grains and legumes (and God knows what else) in crowded, inhumane (and environmentally polluting) feedlots before slaughter.

3. *Combining it.* You need to eat a good amount of quality natural fat with that protein for your body to make the best use of it. This is achieved by eating naturally fatty meats as well as cooking leaner cuts in healthy fats such as lard, tallow, or coconut oil, and ensuring your accompanying vegetables are topped with quality fats as well. If you cook fish, which is naturally full of omega-3s that are prone to dangerous oxidation when overheated, it is helpful to use these same saturated fats to cook it— they confer protective benefits that help mitigate that risk and improve your body's utilization of the omega-3s.

4. *How much.* Eat just enough protein, but not more than you need; this amounts to about 0.8 gram of protein per kilogram of your estimated ideal body weight. This typically reflects an amount in the range of the currently accepted RDA for protein. You do, however, need to tweak this according to specific variables such as age, life stage, health status, or elite sports and fitness needs.

5. *Digestion.* When you're eating less protein than you might be used to, it's important to help your system digest and utilize the protein you do eat. It's not about eating more—It is about optimizing digestion of animal-source foods, by chewing well and by using hydrochloric acid and pancreatic enzyme support when needed.

In the pages that follow, I'll show you how to address all these points to get the most out of moderate protein. It is possible to mindfully restrict your protein intake while still meeting your body's essential amino acid needs for repair and regeneration and—maybe best of all—enjoying delicious, satiating meals. In so doing, you can help your body become the healthiest and most effective fat-burning machine.

Fasting, Restricting, and Burning: How Three Powerful Approaches Intersect

Caloric restriction and intermittent fasting were inspired by anti-aging research and popular nutrition advocates. These approaches stimulate the body to burn fat by mimicking conditions we would have faced between hunts. Here's how they intersect with primal fat burning.

Caloric Restriction

Safe caloric restriction protocols have proven effects in enhancing longevity, improving brain function, and avoiding disease. (One interesting longevity study on elderly people showed how it helped protect the brain and memory function.)[19] But more recent research has shown that the actual documented benefits of this approach come from restricting insulin-provoking carbohydrates and excess protein. It turns out that you don't need to restrict your fat calories at all to get all of the brain-boosting, longevity-enhancing, and anti-disease benefits![20]

The primary mechanism driving caloric restriction's benefits is *a decreased need for insulin (and the inhibition of mTOR)*. Insulin is the single most powerful driver of rapid aging, metabolic diseases such as diabetes and obesity, and cognitive degeneration. By moderating your dietary protein intake to a level that meets but does not exceed your daily needs, and by avoiding sugars and starches, you mostly eliminate the need and impetus for constant insulin (and mTOR) production. The subsequent effective state of well-nourished ketogenic adaptation (EKA) lets your body shift to maximizing its maintenance and repair, as well as maximizing its NAD+ production (the linchpin substrate of mitochondrial function and cellular metabolism), improving NADH to NAD+ ratios (which protects against free radicals, ionizing radiation, and inflammation), and maximizing mitochondrial health and efficiency. By not exceeding your protein requirements, you are less likely to trigger sugar production from the excess protein intake or your own tissues—as long as you eat sufficient dietary fat. Your body becomes focused on repairing what's broken instead of proliferating new cells you may not need (and that may also create a vector for cancer cell growth). In other words, caloric restriction really just means restricting only your carbohydrate and protein intake: quality dietary fat is (with credit to Ron Rosedale) a "free fuel" in this equation! You can eat as much of it as you need to satisfy your hunger—and because fat is so satisfying, you actually wind up eating less overall, while feeling even more satisfied, without cravings. It's a win-win for your health—and your pocketbook!

Intermittent Fasting

Popularized especially in fitness and CrossFit circles, intermittent fasting has many varied interpretations. Basically, it alternates periods of eating solid foods with not eating, with the longest fasting period generally lasting about fourteen hours at a time. It mimics *some* of the beneficial effects of caloric restriction. Some form of intermittent fasting can be helpful for some people, but it stops well short of making you a full-time fat burner or fully optimizing your diet for health and longevity. But used as a stand-alone approach, conventional intermittent fasting basically yields intermittent results. It generally does help increase the production of ketones, but by no means is the production of ketones the same as the body using them as effectively as it does in a state of effective ketogenic adaptation (EKA). It takes consistent effort over at least three weeks, and sometimes even up to a couple of months, to arrive at fully efficient ketone utilization. Furthermore, if your intermittent fasting program includes eating foods with sugars and starches when you are not fasting, or foods to which your genetic makeup may not be suitably adapted, then you are constantly taking one small step forward and two significant steps back.

Intermittent fasting used as a stand-alone approach puts you in a state of metabolic limbo—you are not quite a full-time fat burner and not quite a full-time sugar burner. Though it mimics short periods of famine or compromised nutrient availability typical in more primitive times, that doesn't mean it is fully optimal for us today. A primal fat-based ketogenic plan largely eliminates any need for intermittent fasting, though this technique can potentially be employed as an auxiliary tactic in special circumstances, especially for those who need to lose a lot of weight.

———

The Primal Fat Burner Plan employs the same longevity- and health-building mechanisms behind caloric restriction and intermittent fasting, while enhancing the focus on food quality, but it also avoids the downsides. The result is a combination of the best of all these approaches. Fusing ancestral approaches with longevity research is the smartest possible approach to health today, with the least potential for health compromise if done correctly.

CHAPTER 6

Becoming a Lifelong Fat Burner

Kerry, a legal professional, was postmenopausal and suffered from mood swings and brain fog, along with chronic joint pain. Kerry came my way for help with her persistent weight issues. She was clinically obese, and her blood chemistry profile showed signs of her metabolic disorder: elevated fasting glucose, elevated triglycerides, borderline high Hgb A1C, and higher cholesterol. She also showed depressed serum levels of vitamin D_3. Luckily, in her case, she showed no signs of thyroid issues or thyroid antibodies and was not yet diabetic. I suspected the presence of possible autoimmune issues, particularly since her son had been diagnosed with one (and these things tend to run in families), and because her symptoms were so doggedly persistent. Unfortunately, Cyrex Labs, which offers a number of highly accurate tests for identifying autoimmunity in its earliest stages, as well as food sensitivities, wasn't available then. We had to make do and proceed as best we could. She was a little on the functionally anemic side from a lack of iron, and as a result she struggled with fatigue, as well.

Kerry was an enthusiastic client out of the gate, eager to get started. Right away, she eliminated all grains and dairy, all processed foods, and all dietary sources of sugar and starch. She dialed back on her protein intake to just what she needed and made sure she was getting enough healthy fats and essential fatty acids (the supplemental EFAs were mainly from Antarctic krill oil—a pure and concentrated source of important omega-3s, EPA, and DHA). She committed to the primal fat-burning dietary approach and began sourcing a lot of food at her local farmers' markets. She also started culturing her own vegetables as well as making bone broths at home—which she discovered she really enjoyed doing. Fortunately for Kerry, her family was supportive and everyone began to eat the same way. This always makes a big difference.

Kerry's enthusiastic attitude was a great asset in resolving her long-standing issues. She never complained about the rather large lifestyle adjustments she had to make—she made it an adventure (an attitude I highly recommend, by the way), finding new places to procure her food, meeting farmers face-to-face at the farmers' markets and their actual farms, and reveling in the delicious dishes she was cooking. (In fact, she would mischievously comment how her fat-rich meals felt so wonderfully indulgent, almost like she was really getting away with something.) I could tell that it was a pure delight for her to turn her own life around. Kerry steadily lost more than forty pounds over the next six months or so and turned her obsession about weight into a focus on health and making healthy choices. Her metabolic lab test results and ferritin (iron) levels normalized, and she was able to bring her vitamin D_3 levels back up into a healthy range. She was also far less emotionally reactive to sources of stress that had previously driven her to snack—she was seeing her world through a clearer lens and knew that she could deal with things as she had to.

Kerry has happily maintained this new level of health in the years since we first met. Her remaining excess weight has gradually melted away, and she has become even more passionate about the power and pleasure of truly *good* food.

———

Becoming a primal fat burner is not a program for dietary dilettantes. It is really for the person seriously committed to restoring or maximizing their health for the long haul, and someone who isn't afraid of challenging the status quo. As such, you do have to be prepared to work at it a little. This isn't an 80/20 approach, where you follow a recommended plan 80 percent of the time and the other 20 percent of the time eat whatever you like. This is a 100 percent approach—a high goal that promises and achieves high results.

How Much Fat Do I Eat?

The healthiest and most effective state of ketogenic metabolism is achieved through getting 70 to 80 percent of your calories from dietary fat, while strictly moderating your protein consumption so you meet but don't exceed your daily requirements of no more than 6 to 7 ounces of meat, fish, or eggs per day, or about 50 to 70 grams of protein (that's about 0.8 gram of protein per kilogram of estimated ideal body weight per day). I'll walk you through how to do this—rest assured, it does not mean eating coconut oil out of a jar all day or drinking lard, nor does it mean doing percentage calculations over the breakfast table!

In addition, you will be essentially eliminating sugar and starch and instead eating as many *non-starchy* fibrous vegetables and greens as you want: broccoli, cauliflower, asparagus, kale, spinach, field greens, lettuce, cabbage, Brussels sprouts . . . the list goes on. (See complete lists of foods to eat and foods to avoid in Chapter 11.) These vegetables provide additional potassium, magnesium, phy-tonutrients, and antioxidant activity–promoting substances, which help to protect you from numerous cancers while helping to detoxify you. Include some naturally fermented, probiotic-rich foods, too (all cheaply made at home), such as sauerkraut, coconut kefir, other cul-tured (not simply brined) vegetables, and kvass, and you will be vastly improving the nutrient density and health value of those plant foods. The fermentation process allows the healthy bacteria to produce en-zymes and additional nutrients that make them more digestible and provides even more nutrition than you would have gotten from the raw vegetables.

To cultivate and maintain a state of effective ketogenic adaptation—where you produce and actively use ketones as your primary source of fuel—you need to avoid the "cheats," like the occasional donut, daiquiri, hunk of bread, handful of snack chips, or slice of pizza. One single slip-up can knock you out of effective ketosis for a day or two, not to mention that cheating with foods containing gluten (and quite possibly also dairy) has the potential to severely adversely affect autoimmunity and damage your gut and brain. Not worth it, *ever*. Also, even if you happen to be ketogenically well adapted when you decide to have that sugary dessert or a bag of corn chips, it may take a couple of days or longer to return to a full state of efficient ketone *utilization* again, while firing up your previously conquered cravings all over again.

No More Carbs? *Ever?* (Are You Completely Nuts?)

It is impossible to avoid all carbs forever (there will always be some in the vegetables and nuts you eat), plus there will be occasions where you might want to have a bowl of berries, some dark chocolate (really not the worst thing in tiny amounts), or even a glass of champagne to celebrate something special. There are times when things like this are decidedly worth it (though read the label on that dark chocolate carefully first for signs of gluten). But if you do make such infrequent exceptions, it becomes easier for some to rationalize more serious indulgences or "cheats," so you need to consider these occasions carefully. Things like sugary desserts, a pitcher of margaritas or a daiquiri at girls' night out, a bowl of popcorn while watching Netflix, or stopping on the way out of town on vacation for crappy fast food may result in a noticeable and frustrating backslide where you gain a couple of pounds overnight, feel the return of certain symptoms (and old cravings), or stop losing weight for a few days or more. Those having diagnosed or undiagnosed autoimmune issues tend to experience a lot more backlash from such slips. Others for whom this is not so forgiving include migraine sufferers, seizure sufferers, and those with mood instabilities or bipolar disorder. One indulgence tends to trigger more, and cravings often rush right back in to torture you. This is especially a danger if you have been heavily addicted to sugar in the past. You need to know that it can take a few days and some extra discipline to get back on track again. The best policy is generally to keep these rationalized indulgences to a minimum.

How many carbs you may personally be able to tolerate depends in part on how insulin sensitive or metabolically dysregulated you are to begin with. People who are not overweight or who are especially athletic might be able to get away with eating slightly more carbohydrates than others while maintaining a state of EKA, but once your body has fully adapted to the primal fat burner metabolism, ketones in particular become even more efficient at producing energy than either glucose or free fatty acids and are far better for you. The more adapted to making efficient use of fat you are at any weight, the better off you will be! And the less you stray, the less you will rock the boat.

The Lost Art of Digestion

It's not just the nutrients in the food you eat, or even their quality, that determines whether your cells get the substances they need for life; it's also the *proper digestion* of these nutrients that can make or break your health. There are two aspects of the digestive process that bear looking at to ensure you safely and optimally become a primal fat burner and achieve its full promise.

Hydrochloric Acid

A considerable segment of the population is deficient in the stomach acids required to fully break down proteins (and absorb vitamin B_{12} and minerals). This can be because of age (those over forty have less of it), stress, thyroid issues, certain nutrient deficiencies (B vitamins, zinc), and other problems. This is problematic in general—and becomes even more important when following a moderate-protein primal fat burner diet, where you want to get as much as you can from each meal. Digestion is a north-to-south process: everything begins in the stomach (following signaling from the brain), and having a properly acidic pH in your stomach sets the tone and initiates the subsequent signaling for all that follows. But this part works well only if you have the right conditions: a calm, relaxed autonomic state of parasympathetic functioning and the presence of about seventeen different nutrients.

Without enough hydrochloric acid production, you simply cannot properly digest protein into its component amino acids and peptides needed for proper protein synthesis in the body (and poorly digested proteins are more likely to eventually result in triggering food sensitivities). You also can't properly digest and absorb dietary minerals from any source, much less digest and absorb the critical vitamin B_{12} (even if you are eating lots of animal-source foods) without sufficient stomach acid. If you also happen to have a "leaky gut" (small intestinal gut barrier compromise), you run a greater risk of mounting an inappropriate immune response to the foods you eat, which can lead to rampant food sensitivity issues, systemic inflammation, and autoimmune conditions. Poor protein digestion also readily results in things such as muscle loss, the inability to form collagen, and hair loss. It can also lead to an increased risk for *H. pylori* infection and ulcers, gastric reflux symptoms, dysbiosis (unhealthy composition of bacteria in your gut), and parasitic infections.

As just noted, any inhibition of normal hydrochloric acid (HCl) production also affects your ability to digest and absorb vitamin B_{12}— an animal-source nutrient essential for healthy cognitive function and healthy blood cells. Deficiencies of this critical substance have been widely associated with B_{12}-based and/or pernicious anemia, poor sleep, cognitive decline, brain shrinkage, memory problems, Alzheimer's, and other dementias.

A compromised thyroid almost always compromises the digestive process, as the thyroid gland partly controls the release of the hormone gastrin, which signals for additional production of HCl when the presence of complete protein is detected in the meal. HCl production is a precise orchestration, without which no other digestive processes in the body can properly take place.

If you have any of the signs and symptoms of poor digestion, you may likely benefit from hydrochloric acid supplementation taken with meals, as long as your stomach and esophagus aren't inflamed. If they are, then you will need to heal the inflammation first. (Medications for acid reflux, by the way, are almost never the answer and only deepen the problem. They are also linked to numerous additional problems, including neurological problems such as dementia.)[1] HCl tablets and capsules can be readily purchased over the counter, but finding

COMMON SYMPTOMS OF LOW STOMACH ACID (HYPOCHLORHYDRIA)

Belching, bloating, burning, or "acid reflux" shortly after meals

A sense of excessive and/or prolonged fullness after eating

Indigestion and/or constipation (because food is not being digested properly)

Anemia (a result of poor iron and vitamin B_{12} absorption)

And many more: memory issues, fatigue, hair loss, leg and foot cramps, restless leg syndrome, slow healing, skin problems, weak/ridged fingernails, gallbladder (biliary) issues, low bone density, and multiple food sensitivities

the right amount for your needs can be tricky. Work with a qualified health care provider (holistic or functionally oriented practitioners should be particularly familiar with these issues) to walk you through the process of determining the dosage that is right for you, as it can vary widely from person to person. Over time, when or if your HCl production improves, you may find you can take fewer capsules, though some people do need to supplement with HCl on an ongoing basis. People in their seventies and beyond particular may require supplemental HCl and pancreatic enzyme digestive support in order to make the best use of protein, vitamin B_{12}, minerals, and other nutrients in their diets; these supplements may also indirectly help improve biliary health. On the Primal Fat Burner Plan, you'll be encouraged to pay attention to your digestion. Poor production of hydrochloric acid and pancreatic enzymes, as well as thyroid-related issues, can also predispose you to have biliary issues—and you need a healthy gallbladder to optimally digest your fats and fat-soluble nutrients.

Gallbladder

Though it's small and underappreciated, a healthy gallbladder confers the considerable capacity to digest fat and is absolutely key to long-term mental and physical health. Many people, especially in the medical establishment, believe that eating animal fat or adopting a fat-based, ketogenic diet leads to the creation of gallstones. This is not supported by the research available. It *is* true that gallbladder attacks tend to occur following fat-containing meals, but *only if you already have preexisting gallstones in your gallbladder.* The actual dietary causes seem to be associated with low-calorie, low-fat, higher-carbohydrate diets as well as the low levels of intracellular magnesium that are common with high-carbohydrate diets.

A quick primer: Located beneath the liver under the right side of your rib cage, the gallbladder's main purpose is to collect, hold, and dispense the bile from the liver, which allows for the proper emulsification, digestion, and absorption of dietary fats and fat-soluble nutrients. Bile also works to emulsify, or make water soluble, spent hormones and other substances so they readily move safely out of the body with bowel movements. We were all born with a gallbladder for good reason: to be able to consume natural dietary fat in considerable amounts. We can get into trouble, however, when unaddressed digestive and nutritional problems—as well as other issues such as diabetes, excess belly fat, excess estrogen, or cirrhosis—conspire to thicken and slow down the bile, which can ultimately precipitate gallstone formation.

There can be serious ramifications to having gallstones. The consumption of a fatty meal naturally causes your gallbladder to contract, and this may inadvertently force one or more of these stones into your bile duct, where they can become stuck, causing tremendous pain, inflammation, and a dangerous blockage that may require surgical intervention. The passing of small stones or sluggish bile following fatty meals can also result in painful gallbladder attacks. Note whether you feel aching or pain under the right side of your rib cage following meals. This could be a problematic sign that should be checked out by a qualified health care professional. If left unchecked and unaddressed for too long, the gallbladder itself can become infected or the bile duct blocked to the point where immediate surgery becomes necessary.

But all that needs to be put into proper context: the gallstones did not form *because* of a high-fat diet, and in fact, it's often just the opposite. (On a carb-heavy diet, if you don't "use it"—your gallbladder—you can "lose it.") And for people with normally functioning gallbladders, a high-fat diet is not only okay, it is optimal. Furthermore, a weight-loss study on obese people found that a higher-fat diet *prevented* gall-stone formation in comparison to a low-fat diet.[2] High-carb, low-fat diets consistently lead to a higher risk of gallstones.[3,4] One study in 2014 summed it up neatly by stating that "Diets high in fat content reduced gallstones, compared with those with low fat content."[5]

WHAT TO DO IF YOUR GALLBLADDER HAS BEEN REMOVED (OR IF YOU HAVE ONE AND IT ACTS UP)

Yes, you can still become a primal fat burner without a gallblad-der! But please go about this systematically and intelligently.

- Try to find out what underlying issue led to your gallbladder removal in the first place. The long-term ramifications of that issue, whether it's a thyroid condition, excess estrogen, an autoimmune disease, food sensitivities, or something else, may still be working against your long-term health in spite of whatever symptom relief you may feel.

- Without a gallbladder, you will have a compromised capacity for fat digestion, leading to the potential for weight gain and deficiencies in critical essential fatty acids and fat-soluble nutrients. You will likely have to take supplemental bile salts (frequently sold as "ox bile") with every meal that contains fat. The addition of lecithin from non-GMO sources to the diet can also help a little with proper fat emulsification. Don't be intimidated; a fat-burning regimen with these aids is completely within reach.

- If you have gallbladder issues—and many people don't know they have them; a clue would be problems after eating fatty meals (a digestive intolerance to dietary fats), or regularly getting achiness or pain on your right side after eating—find a qualified functional medicine specialist to help you get to the bottom of your biliary issues first, so you can then take carefully directed steps to restore your biliary health and be ready to embrace the Primal Fat Burner Plan.

The Primal Fat Burner Plan includes foods with gallbladder-supportive properties: foods rich in EPA/DHA, along with beet kvass, which contains betaine (also known as trimethylglycine or TMG, an important methyl donor capable of promoting the regeneration of liver cells and the flow of bile, as well as promoting fat metabolism). I heartily encourage you to make beet kvass from the recipe in this book and enjoy it regularly. In addition, including things like garlic and onions, turmeric, and daikon in your everyday fare will help support your biliary function.

If you have a known gallbladder issue or no gallbladder at all, please see the box on page 99 before proceeding.

Making the Switch: How Your Body Converts from Sugar Burning to Fat Burning

Just like converting your home to run on solar power or your car to run on biodiesel, there are adjustments that need to happen when you convert from sugar burning to fat burning. Numerous metabolic pathways are involved in this process, and it pays to understand them, because for almost everyone, the shift away from carb-based foods is a big deal—it's quite frankly the change of a lifetime. This gets slightly technical, but stay with me (unless you would rather skip the science class and jump ahead).

One particular enzyme, called hormone-sensitive lipase, is key to this process. It is normally inhibited by insulin, but once you stop consuming sugar and starch, insulin tends to get out of the way and allows hormone-sensitive lipase to begin to work its magic. Hormone-sensitive lipase allows for the breakdown of triglycerides and the formation of free fatty acids to be used as an energy source. Your body then makes use of free fatty acids for energy by moving them from the periphery of your circulation into your liver, where they undergo something called beta-oxidation in the hepatic mito-chondria. This converts the free fatty acids into acetyl-coenzyme A (acetyl-CoA).

Now, as long as you are a carbovore (i.e., a sugar burner), this acetyl-CoA enters something called the tricarboxylic cycle. To do this, acetyl-CoA first needs to pair with something called oxaloacetate, which is derived from pyruvate during regular sugar burning (glycolysis). But when sugar is not available for this oxaloacetate, activity gets shifted instead toward the gluconeogenesis pathway, allowing you to make your own glucose. The buildup of acetyl-CoA then gets diverted instead toward ketone body formation. Voilà! You now have the energy units from fat beginning to form! Unfortunately, your body is not so quick to give up its dependence on sugar and initially treats most of the ketones you are making as waste products.

Once your body begins producing ketones in earnest, it is also desperately trying to create sugar by stimulating your body's blood sugar hormones (glucagon, adrenaline, and cortisol). These initially serve to raise your blood sugar back up by using the glycogen in your liver (breaking it down through the process called glycogenolysis), which makes more glucose available to your cells. All this transpires quite rapidly and takes far less time to happen than it has taken you to read this. The more you restrict sugar and starch intake in the beginning, the more your glucagon (blood-sugar-raising hormone) output becomes amplified. During this time, you may notice a temporary increase in your blood sugar level measurements as your blood sugar hormones attempt to overcompensate for the lack of dietary glucose by creating more of it internally. Glucagon, seeing the writing on the wall and looking for help, also begins stimulating hormone-sensitive lipase as an indirect means of increasing the release of free fatty acids from your triglycerides. Glucagon then stimulates the uptake of these free fatty acids by the liver and its mitochondria so they can begin to be burned for energy.

Once the demand for energy overwhelms this process, it further promotes the more efficient production and eventually utilization of ketones. The entire adaptation process takes roughly three to six weeks for most people. Even though glucagon—normally the key hormone that upregulates blood sugar—is also an important part of generating ketones, it can play this fat-burning role only in the absence of insulin.[6] This complex metabolic dance is regulated and carefully orchestrated by two master hormones, leptin and insulin.

———

Before you flip your own fat-burning switch, read on to discover the often overlooked critical importance of fat-soluble nutrients and how the Primal Fat Burner Plan can help protect you against the vast range of diseases of modern civilization—and support you in maximizing your sports and fitness goals.

PART THREE

The Unrivaled Power of Primal Fat Burning

Optimizing Your Health, Preventing and Resolving
Disease, and Achieving Peak Performance

CHAPTER 7

A Field Guide to Fat-Soluble Nutrients

One reason that so many people begin to feel and function better when they become primal fat burners is that a mainstream diet has left their body depleted and desperate to replenish its stores of critical nutrients. By optimizing the diet with nutrient-dense high-quality foods, the cells, tissues, and organs finally receive the amount of fat-soluble nutrients they need to function best—sometimes for the first time in years (or ever).

To my mind, fat-soluble nutrients are the true unsung heroes of the fat milieu. While ketones are the hot new celebrity getting the glory, and debates about macronutrient ratios grab the headlines (in the niche environment of the paleosphere, that is), the *micro*nutrients made available by eating animal-sourced foods might deserve our respect even more. They let us claim the gift of our primal birthright— *if* we eat enough dietary fat from the right sources.

If you're confused about what fat-soluble nutrients are, you're not alone. Most people have only a vague notion of what vitamins, minerals, and other micronutrients do, and are unaware that almost all the ones required to fund a healthy metabolism, healthy heart, and optimally functioning brain are *only* or *primarily* found in or best gotten from healthy, pasture-fed animals. The conventional "five a day" servings of fruits and vegetables simply cannot cut it.

We need the abundance of critical nutrients found in fat-rich, animal-source food—some of which may also be found in plants but are ultimately *dependent* on dietary fat (and hydrochloric acid produced through the consumption of complete, animal-source proteins) to be most properly absorbed and used. The fat-soluble nutrients do everything from supporting immunity to building our bones, and they even directly affect the way the human genetic blueprint gets transcribed and activated. The steady supply of fat-soluble nutrients was a major factor in our early ancestors' robust physiology, rapidly evolving brain, resilience, and resistance to disease; conversely, recent low-fat diets and taboos against consuming healthful organ meats have led to widespread suboptimal levels of these nutrients today, a factor that has contributed to cardiovascular disease, cancer, osteoporosis, cognitive/neurological issues, and other chronic diseases.[1]

This is why committing to upgrading your food sources to fully pastured animal sources, while removing the grains that block proper micronutrient utilization, delivers health payoffs. Regularly consume the meat, organs, and fat of 100% grass-fed and grass-finished animals, and you get most of the fat-soluble nutrients your body critically needs. *Grain*-fed (aka feedlot) animals—even if they're eating organic grain, I'm afraid—exhibit a minute fraction, if any, of the benefits. Make sure the meat you eat didn't spend time in a feedlot!

Will following a primal eating plan mean you don't ever need to supplement your intake of vitamins and minerals, among other essential micronutrients? Unfortunately, probably not. A fair amount of available evidence suggests that our soils are too depleted and our environment too polluted for foods to deliver enough of the nutrients we need, so we likely all need extra help. And if you have a preexisting health condition or immune compromise (such as cancer, autoimmune disease, Alzheimer's/dementia, or depression), I would certainly want you to work toward putting a smart and strategic supplementation program in place.

But being a primal fat burner ensures a very solid start and foundation upon which to build the rest. By eating meals that are rich in highly bioavailable and especially critical nutrients—and that also contain the fat that helps you make use of the nutrients right away—you take more of the guesswork out of how much of which fat-soluble nutrients to take every day. Then you can do some tweaking if and when you need it, assessing your unique needs for extra supplementation—a project that usually requires expert support, since random supplementation can be at best very expensive and at worst counterproductive.

The Perils of Modern Diets: How the Wrong Foods Deplete Your Nutritional Stores

If you have been eating/drinking significant quantities of modern processed/factory farmed foods, you are likely to be prone to the following deficiencies, which you can begin to resolve as a primal fat burner:[2]

Sugar: deficiencies in B vitamins, magnesium, and chromium

Sodas: deficiencies in all of the above, plus more mineral deficiencies

Feedlot meat or farmed fish: deficiencies in omega-3s

Factory-farmed chicken and eggs: deficiencies in omega-3s, vitamin A, beta-carotene, vitamin D, and vitamin E complex

Grains and legumes: deficiencies in minerals (especially zinc), omega-3s, and the amino acid L-tryptophan

Also, if you have a history of any of the following, you are prone to other deficiencies:

Vegetarianism: deficiencies in vitamins B_{12}, A (retinol), D_3, and K_2; coenzyme Q10 (CoQ10); many minerals, especially zinc, magnesium, and iron; protein and several amino acids, including L-tryptophan; L-carnitine (found mainly in red meat and needed for efficient fat burning); and elongated forms of omega-3 essential fatty acids (EPA and DHA)

Low-fat eating: critical fat soluble nutrients, such as carotenoids and vitamins A, E complex, D_3, K_1, and K_2; essential fatty acids, such as omega-3s and gamma-linolenic acid (GLA); CoQ10; minerals

Stress: magnesium, zinc, electrolytes, and water-soluble nutrients such as B vitamins and vitamin C complex

Low stomach acid or acid reflux: amino acids and protein; minerals, especially zinc, iron, magnesium, calcium, and phosphorus; and vitamin B_{12}

Drinking distilled water: minerals

Eating conventional (nonorganic) produce: minerals, vitamins, antioxidants, and phytonutrients

We Are Family: How Fat-Soluble Vitamins Team Up

Micronutrients don't exist as isolated entities. Nature designed them to exist in synergy with one another and with other compounds that help them get absorbed and used, and put them together into our food, including fat-rich food. Fat-soluble nutrients function like a family in the body—they rely on one another to optimize their beneficial effects for healthy DNA expression, immune function, and longevity. And all families work better with some order and balance.

Here's just one example of this. For every receptor for vitamin D on a human cell, there are two receptors for animal-source vitamin A (retinol, that is, not beta-carotene, which is a precursor to vitamin A);[3] therefore, you *need* ample vitamin A in order to be able to properly use your vitamin D, and you need the two vitamins in relatively healthy ratios to each other, because an excess of one can create a relative deficiency of the other.[4] On top of that, you also need vitamin K_2 from animal-source foods to properly utilize Vitamin D_3. Vitamin K_2 is actually the substance that makes the vitamin A– and vitamin D_3–dependent proteins come to life—it is the activator in the equation.[5] While vitamin D_3 (the activated form of vitamin D in your body) helps your body absorb minerals such as calcium, vitamin K_2 decides how and where that mineral is going to be used. Without vitamin K_2's balancing effect upon vitamin D_3, the calcium you consume can end up in the wrong places—your arteries, your heart, your joints, and your brain. Vitamin K_2 also protects the body from potential vitamin D overload, particularly if you oversupplement.[6]

Take it one step further, and you discover that vitamins A, D, and K also need certain minerals to fully realize their benefits. Vitamins A and D_3 require sufficient zinc and magnesium to do their job. And to absorb many of these minerals from our food in the first place, we need fats *and* the presence of these three fat-soluble vitamins, and we need hydrochloric acid in our stomachs, which we produce the most of when eating animal-source foods. It's a full and synergistic circle—one that nature helps you with by packaging all these elements together automatically in certain high-quality primal foods. (It's important to note that in today's era of depleted soils, relying on plant-based foods for minerals such as magnesium probably won't cut it. Pastured meat and seafood—to the extent you feel seafood is safe—thus become even more important sources of this nutrient.)

Vitamins A, D, and K are the three amigos in this story; they like to hang out together and resolve all kinds of sticky situations. Vitamin E complex is their sidekick, with an especially important role to play in higher-fat diets. Let's take a closer look at all of them.

Vitamin A: The Rodney Dangerfield of Fat-Soluble Nutrients

The astounding benefits of vitamin A, also known as retinol, are almost endless. It regulates your gene expression, functions as an important antioxidant, primes your thyroid receptors, and supports cell growth and differentiation (absolutely critical when it comes to preventing or treating cancers). As if that's not enough, it helps direct the normal formation and maintenance of your heart, lungs, kidneys, and other organs[7] and is essential for healthy vision, reproduction, immune function, skin health, and cellular communication.

Ever wonder why grandmothers of yore insisted that kids take a spoonful of cod liver oil (rich in vitamin A) every day? Prior to the development (and lucrative patenting) of antibiotics after World War II, vitamin A was the primary focus of anti-infective therapy and immune system enhancement.[8] In the 1930s scientists discovered that cod liver oil supplementation reduced the incidence of colds by fully a third. Today we have a better picture of how vitamin A builds strength and resilience into your immune cells and offers potent resilience against a full spectrum of serious infectious and immune-related diseases.

On top of all this, the abundant benefits that come from optimized vitamin A include healthy hormone and thyroid levels, stable mood, good skin, optimized fertility, proper digestion and absorption of nutrients, appropriate cortisol response, and stress management. Run low on this vitamin, and it can be tough to stay well.

If you're hoping to meet this need by crunching on carrots, you can't. This is where things get confusing and true vitamin A fails to get the respect it deserves. Beta-carotene, which is abundant in yellow, orange, and red vegetables, is *not* vitamin A, even though the industry allows it to be misleadingly labeled as such. Call it a pet peeve of mine. Beta-carotene can at times and under certain optimal circumstances eventually be converted to small amounts of vitamin A after an extensive, complex biochemical process, albeit at a highly ineffective rate. But it would require massive amounts of carrots to make minute amounts of vitamin A—more than you could consume! And if you have thyroid issues, celiac disease, or diabetes (which, unfortunately, many people do), you can't do this conversion at all and *must* get vitamin A from the sources below. The same applies to kids under about age six—which is why I urge you to help your kid fall in love with eating tasty dishes such as Liver and Bacon or Primal Pâté (the recipes are in Chapter 12).

With a nod to one of my heroes, the world-renowned biochemist Dr. Mary Enig,[9] be highly skeptical about the can of tomatoes or other processed foods labeled "high in vitamin A." They're actually hyping up the beta-carotene inside (and the FDA permits this deceptive verbiage). Only animal-food sources deliver true vitamin A—with liver being the king of sources—and when they are from organic, fully pastured sources, the vitamin comes along with its critical cofactors and fellow fat-soluble nutrients, including vitamin D_3, vitamin E complex, vitamin K_2, zinc, and cholesterol.

Best Sources of Vitamin A

Vitamin A is found in greatest abundance in liver, fully pastured meats, fatty fish such as sardines and fatty salmon, fish roe, egg yolks, shellfish, emu oil, cultured ghee, and butter from grass-fed cows (if you are not sensitive to dairy). Cod liver oil, with its pre-formed vitamin A along with some omega-3s, can be helpful if you truly can't

THE TRUTH ABOUT LIVER

Some people fear that liver is a compromised food source because they assume it stores toxins. Not true. Animal livers don't store toxic waste; they function as a clearinghouse for the detoxification and biotransformation of various food elements and environmental substances. Of course, it is clearly always important to make sure that any food you consume comes from the healthiest, most naturally raised and grown sources. And if you've heard that eating too much liver will make you overaccumulate vitamin A and suffer toxicity, fear not: there's no documented basis for this anxiety. The diets of healthy primitive and traditional peoples had ten times more fat-soluble nutrient content than those of modern Westerners, according to Weston Price's research—and his nutrient-deprived Westerners lived in the 1930s, when lard and butter from grass-fed cattle were the norm. It's hard to imagine even a diligent primal eater today getting anything near toxic levels, especially if consumed from natural sources in balance with the vitamin's other fat-soluble brethren.

stomach eating liver, but it's not at all the same thing nutritionally as eating whole liver with all the other synergistic nutrients contained in it. Vitamin A supplementation needs to be balanced by a sufficient intake of vitamins D_3 and K_2, zinc, and other nutrients for its optimal utilization. If you use cod liver oil supplements, I recommend avoiding the popular "fermented" form, because of the overwhelming likelihood that they are severely rancid.

Though official dietary recommendations for vitamin A are extremely (if not ridiculously) low—only 2,000 IU per day for women, for example—careful research has demonstrated safety and positive health benefits with doses of between 30,000 and 50,000 IU per day. Just one 3-ounce serving of beef liver can yield more than 20,000 IU, so eating it just once a week can significantly improve levels in adults and kids—and you can eat it safely several times a week. Two eggs from fully pastured (not simply "organic") chickens can even yield as much as 5,200 IU.

SAFE SUPPLEMENTATION

A little-known fact: close to 70 percent of supplement brands are owned by big pharmaceutical companies, which unfortunately tend to use the cheapest ingredients they can and often include additives, toxic compounds, coatings, and fillers that not only compromise effectiveness but often can affect safety as well. If you decide to supplement, it's wise to steer clear of the cheap drugstore and mass-market brands. I offer a list of recommended supplement sources in "Nourishing Resources" on page 285 and through affiliate links on my website at www.primal body-primalmind.com/store.

Note: When it comes to how much anyone should supplement with, it is literally impossible to generalize. This section of the book is designed to underscore the critical importance of these nutrients in your diet. If you are consuming animal-based and other fats from 100 percent exclusively pastured and organic sources and you are already healthy and asymptomatic, then for the most part this diet should be able to supply most of what you need on its own. Much will depend upon whether you happen to have symptoms of insufficiency (the symptoms are outlined in the section on each nutrient) or, in the case of vitamin D_3, whether you have tested as functionally low or not (anything below 40–60 ng/mL). With respect to vitamin D_3, it is extremely important to test, then retest regularly to be sure you are getting as much as you need and not too much. The circumstances under which supplementation may be necessary are discussed here in general and are not meant as any sort of prescription for specific supplementation. Please consult with your qualified health care provider for further information regarding your specific needs.

Vitamin D: The Rock Star (with Multi-Platinum Status)

Call it the "sunshine vitamin" or call it the "rock star vitamin": D is the household name of fat-soluble nutrients. More a hormone than a vitamin, it is essential to the proper function of every cell and tissue in your body. It supports bone health, can modulate autoimmune conditions, and confers immune support and probable anti-cancer bene-fits. It is known to be protective to the brain, have anti-inflammatory benefits, and protect the delicate and vital fatty acids EPA and DHA in your body. It helps the gut lining and heart work properly, helps protect against seizures and migraines, and even helps prevent cavi-ties and tooth disease (in close partnership with its pal vitamin K_2). Its reach is almost endless.

What the cereal and milk makers who "fortify" their foods with added vitamin D don't want you to know is that the numerous ben-efits associated with vitamin D are connected to its activated form, vitamin D_3 (cholecalciferol), and not to plant-based or synthetic vitamin D_2 added to foods.[10]

So what's the best way to get your fill of it? Humans can synthesize D_3 from a combination of cholesterol, its precursor analog D_2 (which comes from certain plant-based foods and mushrooms), and ample exposure to UVB rays in sunlight. That said, you need to expose a lot of skin to the sun by getting nearly naked at noon for at least several minutes to an hour or two on a fairly consistent basis—the amount of time depends on your geographic latitude, how many receptors for vitamin D you inherently have, your ethnicity, what time of year it is, and relative cloudiness. For most, this would be possible only if you live in a sunbelt state and can get outside during the day . . . and it wouldn't hurt if you live in a nudist camp! I jest a bit about the nudity—I live in Oregon, where aging hippies and virtual public nudity aren't that unusual—but a fairly lengthy period of broad skin exposure is typically required (i.e., more than just your face and hands, and no sunscreen lotion) for meaningful vitamin D_3 produc-tion from sunlight.

For everyone else, get sun when you can, but be sure to follow the example of your ancient primal brethren who lived and hunted at northern latitudes. They got their activated D_3 from the ample con-sumption of animal fat from large grazing and foraging animals. In the Americas, northern Native peoples got it from marine mammals (seal, walrus, and whale fat) and oily fish (especially their heads), while in Australia, Aboriginal peoples ate insects, grubs, and emu meat and fat. Interestingly, monogastric animals such as bears, emus, and pigs seem to carry the most readily utilizable vitamin D_3 in their fatty tissue. In our modern-day food supply, animal fats and fatty organs such as tallow, suet, brains, tongue, marrow, and organ meats offer the richest supply you can get. Start improving your levels by cooking with lard from a pastured pig: it's the richest food source of all!

Best Sources of Vitamin D_3

The best sources of vitamin D_3 are fully pastured pork fat (lard), tallow, marrow, organ meats, sardines, salmon, fish roe, and egg yolks. Poultry fat, especially from large birds such as the Australian emu (and emu oil), is also a good source. Contrary to contemporary popular belief, cod liver oil is actually a relatively poor source of vitamin D.

If you are consuming vitamin D_3 from natural sources or getting plenty of sun and getting enough dietary vitamin A (retinol) and K_2, there is little reason to be concerned about getting too much. The current RDA is only about 600 IU per day, but current research suggests that this number might need to be as much as ten times greater.[11]

Vitamin D_3: To Supplement or Not to Supplement?

If you live in a seasonal, northern climate and/or work inside all day, some supplemental D_3 tends to become necessary at various times of the year. Liquid, emulsified forms of supplemental vitamin D are some of the best, as they make it easier for the body to rid itself of unwanted excess and are readily absorbed even by those with impaired fat digestion. If you have a chronic inflammatory condition, such as an autoimmune disease, you may need to take vitamin D_3 every day throughout the year, testing your levels regularly and adjusting your dosage accordingly. (There are testing kits you can order yourself, such as from Direct Labs and ZRT Labs.)

If you supplement at all, it's wise to check D_3 levels with a simple blood test (the technical name is serum levels of 25, hydroxyvitamin D_3) a couple of times a year, or more if you have a chronic immune challenge, to ensure you have enough and are not using too much, as supplemental vitamin D *can* accumulate to levels that are too high.

As for what levels are optimal, newer research seems to suggest that a good range is 40 to 60 ng/dL, but absolutely *no lower than 35 ng/dL*. Below this level, there are many issues with bone health, mood- and cognition-related disorders, cardiovascular disease, cancer, and most forms of autoimmune disease.[12] Going above 60 ng/dL, meanwhile, may also cause problems, the latest science shows, so don't think that more is necessarily better.[13] If you are struggling with a chronic infection, autoimmune condition, or cancer, vitamin D gets used up fairly quickly, so know that more supplementation might be needed. Remember, vitamin D_3 requires the presence of the animal-source fat-soluble vitamins A (retinol) and K_2 in balanced amounts to give you its benefits, preferably through using the foods in this plan.

This is especially key if you have a diagonal earlobe crease, which may be a sign of progressive heart disease or arterial calcification, and vitamin D supplementation without added supplemental vitamin K_2 is ill advised. If this is true for you, avoid calcium supplements at all costs. Be smart and seek expert counsel in this case. Remember, the three amigos must ride together!

Vitamin K_2: The New Rock Star

Mark my words: vitamin K_2 is hot on the tail of vitamin D, about to steal the limelight. Weston Price was the first to reveal this mysterious nutrient—he called it "Activator X"—which appeared to be a powerful key to the robust health conferred by traditional diets. Latter-day science now knows it as vitamin K_2, a key fat-soluble vitamin and the better half of the vitamin K family (its other sibling being vitamin K_1). In the hip and happening paleosphere, it is the trendy subject of many a blog and podcast.

You may be familiar with K_1, the plant-derived form of vitamin K, found in leafy green vegetables such as kale, lettuce, broccoli, and spinach. It makes up roughly 90 percent of the vitamin K in a typical Western diet, and its action is associated mostly with increasing the capacity for blood clotting (which is a mixed blessing—essentially beneficial after injury, but more blood clotting also means more potential for certain kinds of stroke or infarction in vulnerable individuals). The benefits of K_1, as it turns out, pale in comparison to those of its newly celebrated sibling, K_2.

Vitamin K_2 is the animal-source version of vitamin K (MK-4) and the one our ancestors would primarily have gotten from their diet rich in fats and organ meats, and some from fermented or rotting foods (MK-7). (There are a few versions of vitamin K_2; see page 118.) Today, however, animal-source vitamin K_2 accounts for only about 10 percent of the vitamin K in the Western diet, meaning most people are quite deficient in it. This is a big problem. For one thing, there are dozens of proteins in the body that are reliant upon K_2 for their activation. One of the most important is osteocalcin,[14] a protein responsible for organizing the deposition of calcium and phosphorus salts in bones and teeth. Osteocalcin is produced only in the presence of vitamins A (retinol) and D_3; K_2 is the principal activator of this important protein secreted by osteoblasts, the body's bone-building cells. When osteocalcin is activated, it draws calcium into the bones, where osteoblasts then are able incorporate it into the bone matrix. In addition, vitamin K_2, when combined with vitamin D_3, helps inhibit osteoclasts, which are the cells responsible for bone resorption.[15] Without it in your diet, calcium fails to incorporate into your bones and is far more likely to calcify things that were never meant to be calcified, such as your heart, arteries, and joints. The same osteocalcin that vitamin K_2 activates also triggers the activation of another protein called matrix GLA protein (MGP). This unique protein is responsible for removing excess calcium that can accumulate in soft tissues such as your arteries and veins. And as you likely know, arteries that become brittle and inflexible—a condition called arteriosclerosis—make you much more vulnerable to stroke. Meanwhile, similar calcium deposits in the heart are making it weaker. In other words, you are risking a possible death sentence simply because your diet is lacking in dietary animal fat and K_2. Vitamin K_2–activated MGP may well be the strongest factor in preventing, and possibly even reversing, tissue calcification involved in atherosclerosis and is required to prevent vascular calcification.[16]

A lack of vitamin K_2 may be what actually killed my father. He had lost his gallbladder years prior (after years of dutiful low-fat eating) and doggedly persisted in his low-fat dietary approach to his dying day. He also confirmed and discussed his diagnosis of advanced coronary calcification with me and confided that he believed this would likely be the cause of his death. He had been avoiding fat, and for years following his cholecystectomy he had a compromised capacity to digest fat. He had the earlobe crease that indicates susceptibility to arterial calcification. And he would have been undoubtedly quite resistant to the idea that eating more foods rich in saturated fat and taking extra steps to digest it better with necessary supplementation following the loss of his gallbladder could have saved his life.

The takeaway? Boosting your intake of this critical nutrient through an optimized diet can literally change your life—arterial calcification is shockingly pervasive in industrialized populations and it is nearly universal by the age of sixty-five to some degree.[17] (As an aside, it is the vitamin K_2, in combination with vitamins A and D_3, that gives primal diets their potential for reversing tooth decay.)[18]

And there's more. Your brain contains one of the highest concentrations of vitamin K_2 in your body in the form of MK-4 (one of its variants; see page 118). It is involved with the formation of myelin in your nerve cells, which is partly responsible for your capacity to learn. There are also strong benefits associated with vitamin K_2 for conditions such as multiple sclerosis, cerebral palsy, epilepsy, and some forms of mental retardation associated with both glutamate toxicity and cysteine depletion. Research into the applications of vitamin K for brain health is still in its infancy, but early studies are extremely exciting.

Given all this, the fact that conventional dietary guidelines for vitamin K supplementation are still based solely upon plant-based vitamin K_1 and the levels required to ensure adequate blood coagulation—as if K_2 doesn't even exist—is a really big deal. It leaves countless millions deficient in vitamin K's most important and bioactive form, and thus vulnerable to bone loss and osteoporosis, cardiovascular disease, organ and tissue calcification, and quite possibly even cancer.[19] The lesson here is to infuse your daily diet with this health-giving nutrient.

Vitamin K₂: Its Mysteries Explained (And Why Emus Deserve Your Awe)

There are a few types of vitamin K_2. The MK-4 version comes from pastured eggs, butter from 100% grass-fed cows, and foods from animals that are exclusively grass-fed. Duck and goose liver and fat are essentially the richest sources. MK-4 is well absorbed by the body[20] and is primarily responsible for K_2's benefits for bone health.

The MK-7 version (as well as the MK-8 and MK-9 types) comes from bacterial fermentation and dairy fats (luckily for the dairy-sensitive, these variants are found in Pure Indian Foods Cultured Ghee; see "Nourishing Resources" on page 285). Cultured vegetables can also potentially contain these versions, but only if the culture used was specifically designed to do that. For my Beet Kvass recipe (see Chapter 12), I recommend a starter culture called Kinetic Culture that is designed to infuse K_2 into your food through specialized bacteria. One kind of bacteria-derived MK-7 is made from a fermented soy product called natto. You likely won't want to eat natto—it has a slimy and putrid texture and taste—but it is made into MK-7 supplements (these are fine to take if the soy is certified non-GMO and you don't have an immune reactivity to soy, which many people do). But there is no MK-4 in natto. Note, too, that taking K_2 as a supplement on its own in part negates the importance of its essential synergy with its other fat-soluble amigos, vitamins A and D_3. It's far better to eat the natural fats containing these three fat-soluble nutrient compadres that naturally work together optimally.

Finally, the MK-3 version, also called menadione, is synthetic, is poorly recognized by the body, may contribute to excessive clot formation, and is *not* recommended. If you choose to use supplements, please read all labels carefully! Most commercial vitamin K supplements feature this cheaper, synthetic, and less effective form of the vitamin.

My personal go-to for a comprehensive supplemental source of vitamin K_2 (in its natural MK-4 form), along with its natural A and D_3 companions, is emu oil—yes, you read that right! The emu is a large ostrich-like bird indigenous to Australia, venerated among Aboriginal peoples there for tens of thousands of years because of its superior fat quality. It contains as much natural MK-4 K_2 (all other MK-4 supplements are synthetic) as goose liver pâté and comes with every one of K_2's essential cofactors. It also is unique in naturally containing highly beneficial, particularly biologically active, non-synthetic conjugated linoleic acid (CLA), which is nearly impossible to come by in a supplement (virtually all CLA supplements sold are synthetic and ineffective). But not all sources of emu oil are of equal quality. The oil I personally recommend is a humanely sourced, meticulously researched product from a highly specific genotype of emu and is sold exclusively through Walkabout Health Products in the United States and Baramul Processing in Australia (where it is sold as Baramul 100). See "Nourishing Resources" on page 285 for more information. In addition, emu oil has been shown to have profoundly anti-inflammatory effects, inside and out.[21] And it is a potentially potent inhibitor of angiogenesis, thanks to its high CLA[22] and vitamin K_2 content.

Finally, although there are potential concerns with excessive intake of vitamin K_1, there are no such concerns about overdosing on vitamin K_2 in almost any amount, even over time.

Vitamin K_2 and Metabolic Diseases

There's a special reason that vitamin K_2 ties into the goals of the Primal Fat Burner Plan. Vitamin K_2 plays an important role in preventing metabolic diseases, because when osteocalcin is activated, it goes beyond its primary job of calcium ion homeostasis: it also helps to regulate insulin and enhance insulin sensitivity by signaling the fat cells to release something called *adiponectin*. Adiponectin is powerful: in addition to its insulin-sensitizing qualities, it has strong anti-diabetic and anti-inflammatory activities.[28] One of its key effects is to lower the plasma levels of triglycerides and fat accumulation in the liver, muscle, and visceral adipose tissue. It also prevents pancreatic β-cell apoptosis (cell death) and it improves hepatic insulin action as well as mitochondrial function, ultimately improving glucose tolerance.[29] That's a pretty extraordinary range of benefits for something most people have never heard of! Interestingly, omega-3 fatty acids also have a strong adiponectin-enhancing effect.[30] It's ironic that after decades of propaganda about low-fat diets and heart health, a fat-soluble nutrient (from animal fats, no less) and an animal-source essential fatty acid can have such a powerful effect on metabolic dysregulation.

Best Sources of Vitamins K_2 and K_1

The best sources of vitamin K_2 are meats and organ meats from 100 percent fully pastured animals, fish roe, shellfish, insects, certain

SPINACH IS GOOD, BUT BEEF MIGHT BE BETTER

When it comes to preventing arterial calcification and resisting cancer, animal-sourced vitamin K_2 has proven superior to vitamin K_1.[23] A research report out of the Netherlands called the Rotterdam Study[24] tracked 4,600 men over fifty-five years of age. By far the lowest rates of heart disease were found in those having the highest levels of vitamin K_2: they exhibited a 41 percent lower risk of cardiovascular disease, plus a 51 percent reduced overall mortality from coronary heart disease. And the patients having the highest levels of K_2 had 52 percent less arterial calcification. A subsequent study called the Prospect Study followed 16,000 women for ten years and showed that vitamin K_2—but not vitamin K_1—was able to significantly reduce the risk of developing cardiovascular disease.

In addition to the abundance of research proving K_2's preventive impact on cardiovascular disease and related deaths, there is impressive research for its potency against cancer. One German research study showed a 52 percent reduction in prostate cancer in men who consumed larger amounts of vitamin K_2 (with, again, no similar effect from K_1).[25] In 2010 researchers from the Mayo Clinic found that the risk of developing non-Hodgkin's lymphoma was roughly 45 percent lower in people having a vitamin K intake of at least 108 μg a day, compared with people having an intake of less than 39 μg per day.[26] Vitamin K_2 has also proven itself in a number of studies to have a potentially stunning preventive role in liver cancer and death in patients with liver cirrhosis and hepatocellular carcinoma.[27]

types of cultured vegetables (depending on the culture used to make them), cultured ghee from grass-fed animals, emu oil, emu meat, and full-fat dairy products from pastured animals (for those who are not dairy sensitive).

The best sources of vitamin K_1 are green leafy vegetables and (to a lesser extent) animal sources similar to those for K_2.

The US RDA for vitamin K—they're talking primarily about K_1—is only 90 mcg. Current research shows we likely need about ten times as much and should focus instead on vitamin K_2, aiming for a daily intake of roughly 800 to 1,000 mcg of vitamin K_2 a day, especially to keep calcium where it's needed and away from where it's not.[31]

Vitamin E Complex and Tocotrienols: Primal Fat Protector Pals Extraordinaire

When we talk about vitamin E, we're really referring to a complex or group of at least eight fat-soluble antioxidant compounds, including several types of mixed tocopherols. Commonly found in nuts, seeds, and green leafy vegetables, vitamin E is also found in foods and fats from fully pastured animal sources. Vitamin E requires the trace mineral selenium to most actively function as an antioxidant—this is rich in pastured meat as well as Brazil nuts.

Researchers at the Centers for Disease Control back in 1999 looked at the vitamin E status of 16,000 American men and women. Twenty percent of white Americans, 41 percent of African Americans, and 28 percent of Mexican Americans back then were deficient in vitamin E. Vitamin E deficiencies have been linked with diabetes, immune disorders, AIDS, muscle damage in exercise, Parkinson's disease, eye diseases, and lung and liver diseases.[32] While this fat-soluble vitamin also exhibits important properties that help guard against cancer,[33] benefit cardiovascular health,[34] support vision,[35] prevent obesity-related fatty liver disease,[36] and help improve brain health and reduce the risk of Alzheimer's disease,[37] there are two things that make it especially relevant for the Primal Fat Burner Plan. One is that it is a precursor to the enzyme glutathione peroxidase, which is a critical antioxidant enzyme. Second, vitamin E complex protects the body from the presence of potentially peroxidized (rancid) fats—something that is quite important when consuming higher-fat diets, to protect against any spoiled fats you might happen to ingest (see "When Good Fats Go Bad" in Chapter 11). It's one fat-soluble vitamin supplement that many of my clients do add to their plan when they transition to fat burning, as it is a fairly simple extra insurance policy if you have the inclination and budget for it.

Quality is *everything* with vitamin E; I tend to recommend a product called Mixed Tocopherols Concentrate from Unique E. It sidesteps a pitfall of vitamin E supplementation, which is that most are synthetic, meaning less potent, frequently detrimental, and in fact even delivering the opposite effects of natural sources of E.[38] You can tell if a supplement uses synthetic vitamin E, as the label will say "dl-alpha tocopherol acetate" or "dl-alpha tocopherol succinate." If you use a quality source of supplementation, then safety is well established across a wide range of dosages.[39]

Best Sources of Vitamin E

Fats from fully pastured meats, nuts, and seeds are the best sources of natural vitamin E.

Key Supporting Players: The Other Fat-Soluble Micronutrients You Need to Know

Carotenoids

There are at least six hundred varieties of carotenoids, typically found in plants, pastured meats/eggs, pink/red salmon and related fish species, certain organisms (krill), and fungi around the world. The most important for humans include beta-carotene, lutein, lycopene, astaxanthin, and zeaxanthin. These are found in colorful yellow or reddish vegetables and some greens, and also in fats from fully pastured animals and in Antarctic krill oil. Also known as pro-vitamin A, these micronutrients require dietary fat for their proper assimilation and use.

CoQ10

Perhaps the single most important nutrient for your heart is coenzyme Q10, which is critical to the health of your mitochondria as well. CoQ10 is found mainly, if not exclusively, in animal-source fats, and it requires fat for its absorption and utilization. CoQ10 is also heavily used by all your other organs, including your brain.

PQQ

Pyrroloquinoline quinone, or PQQ, is a fat-soluble nutrient (found to originate in star dust!) that has recently come to notice. PQQ literally has the capacity to increase the number of healthy mitochondria you have. It is found in high concentrations in leafy greens such as parsley and spinach, green and oolong tea, and natto. There is also a small amount in egg yolks. Dietary fat is required to absorb it.

Genetics, Epigenetics, and the
Fat-Soluble Nutrient Connection

Nutrigenomics is the interdisciplinary study of hereditary factors that influence a person's response to diet—both how genes influence nutrient absorption and metabolism and how nutrients in our diets (or their absence) influence gene expression. Genes, both those with positive effects and those with negative effects, are expressed when the environment surrounding them is favorable for that expression. Many different stressors—both internal and external—affect how your genes behave and thereby influence the initiation and progression of chronic disease through certain non-modifiable risk factors associated with your genetic blueprint.

The magic here lies not in your particular genetics per se but rather in *epigenetics*, the study of these external or environmental factors that turn genes on and off and affect how cells "read" and interpret your genetic blueprint.[40] Getting enough vitamins A, D_3, and K_2 in your diet is the most amazingly simple way to promote healthy gene transcription and DNA expression. (For the science geeks, some of the processes most adversely affected by fat-soluble nutrient deficiency are DNA methylation, histone modification, small and non-encoding RNAs, chromatin architecture, and other transcriptional regulating events such as stem cell creation.)

GRASS-FED MEAT/ORGANS: YOUR HEALTHIEST ONE-STOP SHOP FOR FAT-SOLUBLE NUTRIENTS

Far from being cancer-causing, as some reports have proclaimed, the moderate intake of red meat/organ meats and a more unrestricted intake of animal fat from healthy animals that have been fed on nothing but fresh green grass and natural forage their entire lives supplies innumerable anti-inflammatory, anti-cancer compounds and may just be among your ultimate anti-cancer health foods—as long as you keep total amounts of meat at a moderate level, as I'll explain in Chapter 12.

Research comparing exclusively grass-fed beef to grain-fed has revealed that meat from fully pastured animals has:

- Much higher levels of key antioxidants vitamin C and vitamin E, ten times the levels of beta-carotene,[41] and enhanced amounts of total CLA and omega-3 fatty acids.[42] (Grain feeding rapidly depletes most of these things—sometimes in as little as seven days.)
- Higher levels of vitamins A and E as well as the cancer-fighting antioxidant glutathione (GSH) content, the last of these a result of the tremendous density of glutathione compounds found in fresh green grass. GSH is an absolutely critical enzyme that protects cells from oxidized proteins and helps prevent damage to DNA, among many other things.
- Greatly improved concentration of superoxide dismutase and catalase, which provides additional antioxidant support and also protects meat muscle lipids from peroxidation.[43]

All these things help to explain why cancer has been consistently reported to be extremely rare in red-meat-eating hunter-gatherer societies.[44,45]

CHAPTER 8

Primal Fat Burning May Help
Prevent and Alleviate Disease

Over my years of practicing and teaching primal nutrition, I've heard from thousands of people who have used the principles outlined in this book to improve, and sometimes resolve, some of today's most prevailing chronic health problems. Many have lost weight, having tried and failed at every other program out there. Others have reduced or eliminated depression and anxiety, lessened or stopped seizures and migraines, or reversed worrying mental decline and memory loss; some have even improved autistic symptoms. Many see improvements in gastrointestinal functioning, arthritis, polycystic ovarian syndrome (PCOS) symptoms, fibromyalgia, cardiovascular diseases, high blood pressure, and dysregulated sleep patterns. Diabetic symptoms are frequently greatly improved, with some diabetics even reporting they were able to transition off of insulin and other diabetic medications. I have also heard quite a bit from those who have struggled with various forms of autoimmune disease, and they report dramatically improved symptoms and quality of life, including many with type 1 and type 1.5 diabetes. I've even received stories from cancer patients, reporting how it has indispensably supported them as part of their recovery plans.

In the face of so much bad news about diseases that are mostly, in fact, preventable, these people had the conviction to take back control of their quality of life using a nontoxic metabolic support mechanism they created for themselves through the simple act of eating.

This potential is available to you, too. By harnessing the power of ketones, quality fats, and fat-soluble nutrients, you can benefit from their protective *and* therapeutic benefits. Augment this by using quality sources of food and nutrients and avoiding inflammatory and immune-triggering foods, and you can really start to maximize your resilience, optimize the functioning of your heart, brain, immune system, and metabolism, and feel confident that you are taking proactive steps toward staying healthier longer.

The scientific literature contains many studies that corroborate that a ketogenic state can by itself affect several major areas of health and disease—and remember, the Primal Fat Burner Plan goes well beyond mere ketosis. The brief survey that follows will give you an idea of the benefits of this dietary approach. No one will ever care more about your health and well-being or the health and well-being of your family than *you*, so please consider the healing potential that primal fat burning can confer.

Heart Disease: Overturning Decades of Misinformation

It goes against decades of anti-fat propaganda to say this, but the truth is that your heart loves fat. In fact, next to the human brain, there is no physical organ for which fat is more natural a fuel than the human heart. Your heart is actually a natural-born fat burner! Fatty acid oxidation— fat burning—accounts for up to 70 percent of the ATP that your heart produces, day in and day out,[1] and ketones (specifically natural R-beta hydroxybutyrate, or BOHB) can add to this in a way that can improve its efficiency by up to 28 percent (according to Dr. Richard Veech, a forty-seven-year ketone research expert and award-winning senior researcher and laboratory chief at the National Institutes of Health)![2]

In other words, nothing could possibly be healthier or better suited to the daily functioning of your beating heart than natural dietary fat. The less sugar and starch you eat, the more your heart automatically uses fat and ketones to fuel itself. As the carbs are replaced by natural fats, the side effects tend to be very good ones for your heart: your triglyceride levels,[3] a prime marker for cardiovascular disease,[4] drop, often significantly.[5] Your blood pressure is also likely to drop, and other problematic metabolic markers often return to a normal range.[6]

Yet this natural order got sidelined when the flawed "dietary heart hypothesis" of the early 1960s, positing that a high intake of fat and cholesterol causes heart disease, became generally accepted. Caught in a twisted net of profit, pride, and prejudice (to paraphrase lauded researcher George V. Mann, of the famed Framingham Heart Study), we humans were lured, disastrously, away from our natural evolutionary diet. The demonization of naturally occurring fats and the subsequent promotion and mainstream acceptance of artificial or highly processed fats such as margarine and commercially produced seed oils, as well as the invention of industrial trans and interesterified fats (which are artificially saturated fats), went hand in hand with the fanatical promotion of so-called heart-healthy carbohydrates. Result? An explosion of sickness and unprecedented pharmaceutical intervention. These unhealthful foods, along with the institutionalization of a host of misguided ideas about preventing heart disease, added up to "the greatest health scam of the [twentieth] century," to quote Mann again.[7] This took a devastating toll on millions of ordinary people. I recognize that my tone here may seem a bit harsh, but I have lost loved ones as a result of that lie. I imagine you have, too.

The hypothesis was wrong—dead wrong. Numerous studies and meta-analyses over the ensuing decades have come to similar conclusions, leading to the exoneration of fat and natural, nonoxidized cholesterol, which are not the culprits in heart disease.[8] More recently, in April 2016 the long-lost results of what was once dubbed the Minnesota Coronary Experiment were found hidden in the basement of a home belonging to Christopher Ramsden, the son of one of the former lead researchers associated with the study. Ramsden now works for the National Institutes of Health. The experiment was conducted from 1968 to 1973, and included 9,423 participants between the ages of twenty and ninety-seven, making it the largest heart health trial of its kind at the time. It turns out that one of the other lead researchers of the study was none other than Ancel Keyes—the father of the fallacious lipid hypothesis. Despite the important and rigorous nature of the trial, the results did not see the light of day until now, forty years later. In the study, participants were told to replace saturated fat and foods higher in cholesterol with vegetable oil; meals were even prepared for them. The data analysis showed that the vegetable oil did indeed lower cholesterol in the subjects by an average of 14 percent in a year. But the likely reason the results were buried came with what followed: the research data actually showed that the lower the cholesterol levels, the higher the mortality rate of the participants.

For every thirty-point drop in total cholesterol there was a 22 percent increased chance of death. In those sixty-five and older who received vegetable oil, there were 15 percent more deaths as compared to seniors in the saturated fat group.[9]

After nearly a century of misinformation, we can finally state with confidence that there is no significant association between saturated fat intake and cardiovascular risk. In fact, the old, outdated dietary heart hypothesis has been increasing that cardiovascular risk. Instead, saturated fat has been found in many cases to be *protective*.[10] You may not have heard that one from Dan Rather, but study after study now affirms this.[11]

Cholesterol, once dreaded, is (slowly) being recognized for performing a variety of critical and wholly natural structural roles in the body, while supplying the substrate for critical hormones and brain protection, even acting as an antioxidant and protecting tissues from inflammatory damage that can lead to further dysfunction.[12] The assertion that high blood cholesterol levels will give you a heart attack is demonstrably erroneous: up to 75 percent of all people who die of heart attacks have what is considered to be "normal" cholesterol levels.[13] In fact, higher cholesterol has even been identified as a longevity marker in women[14] and may actually protect against atherosclerosis.[15] In the Framingham Heart Study, which followed people for decades, lowering cholesterol levels led to *increased* mortality.[16] A new, robust, and thoroughly reviewed study published in June 2016 found that a whopping 92 percent of elderly people with a cholesterol level that was considered high lived longer![17]

The surprising reality is that for many people, *low* cholesterol (below @180 mg/dl) confers more serious risks.[18] Research shows a shockingly wide range of consequences: hormonal imbalances, anxiety, depression, suicide, heart failure, stroke, kidney disease, violent behavior, dementia, Alzheimer's disease, Parkinson's disease, higher infection rates, birth defects, and cancer.[19]

So if naturally saturated fat (providing it is not oxidized or rancid) and cholesterol are not the problem when it comes to heart disease, what is? It turns out that 80 percent of what clogs your arteries isn't even saturated fat or cholesterol but rancid unsaturated fats, which come from refined and/or overheated vegetable oils.[20]

And these are just one part of a cocktail of artery-damaging modern foods contributing to the soaring rates of heart disease. The other parts are, not surprisingly:

- Carbohydrate-based diets of primarily grains, starches, sugars, and high fructose corn syrup[21]
- "Fake" fats, including trans fats[22] and interesterified fats[23] (which, unfortunately, are coming to replace trans fats but which are no better for you)
- Excess inflammatory omega-6s from processed vegetable oils, grains, and feedlot meat[24]
- Processed foods[25]
- GMOs and glyphosate (the pesticide most used in commercial agriculture)[26]
- Gluten (through immune reactivity and/or associated gut compromise)[27]

Remove these offenders from your diet for life, and you give your heart the basic conditions it needs. Then take it up a level by igniting your fat-burning metabolism, and you give it what it really *wants:* effectively usable ketone bodies, which research shows confer protective benefits in a safe and effective way, as long as you follow the plan correctly. Ketones may well be beneficial for those who have had cardiovascular disease or are recovering from a heart event of some kind.[28] (If that's you, please approach effective fat burning with the guidance of a qualified health care provider and use common sense by carefully monitoring your progress and the way you feel.)

"According to cardiologist Aseem Malhotra, studies do no not support any significant association between saturated fat intake and cardiovascular risk. Instead, saturated fat has been found to be protective."[29]

Brain Health: Protecting Your Brain for Life

Until now, the ketogenic approach has won its greatest renown for its profound impact upon neurological instabilities such as epilepsy. The extensive research[30] embracing its benefit on even intractable seizures is quite impressive and so conclusive that a ketogenic diet has become a standard treatment, recommended even by conventional neurologists.

But its neurological applications go far beyond seizures. Other disorders that are successfully addressed this way include (but are absolutely not limited to) autism,[31] attention disorders,[32] bipolar disorder, traumatic brain injury,[33] Parkinson's disease,[34] amyotrophic lateral sclerosis (ALS, or Lou Gehrig's disease),[35] mitochondrial disorders, and cancerous brain tumors.[36] The fuller the state of effective ketosis in these (and almost any) instances, the better!

In particular, a well-adapted ketogenic diet is proving effective in preventing and treating Alzheimer's and other forms of dementia.[37] When I share this with clients, it resonates: almost everyone knows somebody who is helping an aging parent struck with dementia of some kind.

Alzheimer's is now being called type 3 diabetes because one of its major drivers is blood sugar dysfunction and glycation, just as with diabetes. In this case, as with all dementias, the impact is upon the brain—the part of the body that is most vulnerable of all to the damaging effects of sugars. The advanced glycation end products (AGEs) generated when a high-carb diet floods the body with glucose and, even worse, fructose initiate a slow and steady neurodegenerative process that has important implications for memory function, mood instability, and cognitive decline. Furthermore, as chronic blood sugar surges cause a depletion of magnesium, binding sites in the brain become more vulnerable to accumulations of aluminum and other toxic metals. This can also result in electrochemical changes allowing more calcium into the cells, leading to subsequent cell death.

In addition, for your brain, just like your heart—and especially your *aging* brain—cholesterol is absolutely critical. Research is showing that people with low cholesterol levels are at increased risk of dementia in general, and that people with Alzheimer's disease generally are *lower* in cholesterol and other fats in the fluid that circulates in and around the brain and spinal column (the cerebrospinal fluid) than healthy individuals. (Cholesterol, as mentioned in Chapter 2, makes up 25 percent of the brain and is essential for optimal cognitive and neurological functioning.) The Framingham study showed that older people with low total cholesterol (under 200 mg/dL) were much more likely to perform poorly on tests of mental function than those having supposedly "high" cholesterol (over 240 mg/dL).[38]

For the record, I personally never like to see total cholesterol below 200 mg/dL, particularly in older women, for whom higher cholesterol is a longevity marker. When cholesterol uptake or availability by the brain gets impaired, Alzheimer's risk goes up. This impairment can be caused either by a certain gene defect or—and more commonly— by chronically elevated blood sugar levels from a carb-based diet, because glycation limits cholesterol uptake (as do statin drugs, by the way). This is why those with type 2 diabetes, who are struggling to control raised blood sugars, have a two- to fivefold greater risk of Alzheimer's disease. (Even so, currently sanctioned diets for diabetes tend to include a lot of "healthy carbs," which the diabetic is then forced to "manage" with insulin, an officially sanctioned scenario that tends to play out well for drug companies but poorly for the diabetic.)

It doesn't take massive doses of sugar to drive the development of dementia. Researchers see manifestations of these diseases even in the brains of those with supposedly normal, nondiabetic higher fasting blood sugar ranges—whether or not they happen to be genetically vulnerable to Alzheimer's.[39] Gluten consumption also adds to the risk.

Switch on a state of ketosis, however, and blood sugar tends to become a nonissue. Interestingly, ketones are profound memory-enhancing agents, and adherents to the ketogenic lifestyle frequently report clearer thinking, a better memory overall, and laser-like focus.

Even if such a devastating diagnosis as Alzheimer's does not touch you—yet—if your diet frequently contains starch and sugars (and remember, that includes whole grain bread, rice and beans, potatoes, fruit, honey, wine, and so forth), you are subjecting your brain to the detrimental effects of glucose/fructose metabolism, leading to higher oxidative stress and inflammation, two of the fundamental factors that contribute to neurodegeneration. Are your mood, concentration, focus, sleep, and energy levels stable, reliable, and unwavering? If not, take a look at your plate.

Using ketones to fuel your brain instead of glucose produces much lower oxidative stress on the cells and tissues and results in greater cellular energy output. Ketones as fuel also generate greater antioxidant capacity by increasing glutathione peroxidase in the cells of the hippocampus. Furthermore, cerebral ketones are associated with decreased apoptosis (cell death) and inflammation.[40] A genetic tendency toward Alzheimer's, scary as it may be, does not seal your fate. How your brain functions and how it ages is largely up to you. And the earlier you start optimizing your brain health, the better.

So to best protect your brain, add plenty of fat to your low-carb diet. On the Primal Fat Burner Plan, you'll enjoy medium-chain triglyceride fats, like those found in coconut oil, that help generate immediately helpful ketones. These have been found to improve cognitive impairment in memory-related disorders after just a single dose![41] So try a little Primal Keto-Coconut Pemmican (recipe in Chapter 12) the next time you feel your brain needs a boost!

Leaky Gut, Inflamed Brain

"Leaky gut" refers to a compromise in the gut barrier that allows unwelcome, potentially undigested foreign proteins, lectins, or environmental toxins to pass into your bloodstream, triggering an inflammatory immune response. The same mechanisms that contribute to leaky gut also control the integrity of your blood-brain barrier. This unique relationship between the brain and your gut has big implications. When brain tissue becomes inflamed or is compromised by exposure to too many modern-day toxins and antigens, it can lead to digestive problems and unfavorable changes in the makeup of the all-important gut flora (your microbiome). The gut-brain connection is very real and is a two-way street. The fermented vegetables, kvass, and coconut yogurt on the plan (along with the wide variety of delicious fibrous vegetables and greens) will help to ensure that your microbiome remains diverse and healthy, and in turn helps keep your brain healthy, too. One controversial study did show an increased risk of lipopolysaccharide (endotoxin) translocation from bacteria in the small intestine (resulting in more inflammation and leaky gut) in the presence of dietary fat in mice, but all the fats used in the study were vegetable fats.[42] Dietary cholesterol, conversely, shows a protective effect against these same endotoxins.[43]

Autoimmune Diseases: Relief for a Silent Crisis

Simply defined, an autoimmune condition is one in which your body's immune system becomes confused and starts to produce antibodies against its own tissue, leading to that tissue's gradual and progressive destruction. Some of the more familiar examples of this include celiac disease, thyroid autoimmune disease (Hashimoto's), type 1 diabetes, multiple sclerosis, asthma, psoriasis, Sjögren's disease, lupus, and rheumatoid arthritis. Even autism, often characterized by severe neuroinflammation, is now being classified under this umbrella. In the silent yet alarming explosion of autoimmune disorders today, many people are suffering from symptoms of several autoimmune conditions at once. In particular, women are at disproportionate risk for many autoimmune diseases, one reason for this having to do with hormonal issues. Mainstream medicine, with its very specialized, compartmentalized approach to the body, lacks the big-picture approach needed to tackle these system-wide imbalances.

Though there are many potential triggers for autoimmune diseases, you *can* minimize your odds of suffering and help manage your condition with a primal fat-burning approach to eating. This diet broadly addresses some of the key factors involved in the initiation and progression of immune dysregulation and systemic inflammation that is at the root of autoimmune diseases. (Research has demonstrated ketogenic diets' clear anti-inflammatory effects.)[44,45] It can help put out some of the fire; and for those suffering from autoimmune diseases, the difference can be like night and day. Primal fat burning can help to improve such conditions because it:

- Supports mitochondrial health like nothing else can. One of the prime hallmarks of all autoimmunity is mitochondrial compromise, because dysfunction in the mitochondria leads to an increase in oxidative stress, tissue damage at a molecular level, and free radical production, which in turn leads to antioxidant and NAD depletion. This all contributes to the progression of autoimmune disease. For those suffering from one of these disorders, supporting your intracellular fat burning and having healthy, ATP-generating mitochondria is absolutely critical.
- Supports stress response through the stabilization of the brain and nervous system and support of hippocampal integrity. The brain is a frequent inadvertent casualty of autoimmune conditions because rampant, chronic inflammation can have neurodegenerative effects. The stress of such illnesses alone tends to lead to chronically elevated cortisol levels, cortisol surges, and dysglycemia, all of which eat away at key memory structures in the brain.
- Lessens or helps resolve infections through improved immune response, increased fat-soluble nutrient availability, and natural anti-microbial factors in various fats. Both diagnosed and undiagnosed chronic infections can be an overlooked source of immune system overactivation—like a raging fire that has your emergency system dialing 911 all the time.
- Improves hormonal imbalance, in part at least, through improved insulin and leptin sensitivity, which builds overall foundational endocrine integrity. This helps because metabolic disorder (resulting in weight gain and other problems) is primarily an endocrine issue.
- Reduces the load of environmental chemicals, toxins, heavy metals, and haptens that trigger inflammation and immune response. This is accomplished through the plan's emphasis on uncontaminated, unprocessed, quality food sources,

and the inclusion of plenty of detoxification-supporting vegetables and greens.

- Helps to resolve dysbiosis, the overabundance of unhealthy gut bacteria caused by pesticides, chlorinated/fluoridated drinking water, and antibiotic use and/or residues (like glyphosate) in produce and this and others in factory-farmed meats. Dysbiosis can totally aggravate autoimmune illnesses because the relative balance of GI flora can have a profound influence upon inflammatory signaling and unhealthy cravings. The plan promotes a healthy fiber intake and cultured and fermented foods, all of which can help feed the "good guys" in the microbiome.

- Profoundly positively affects glutathione production. This all-important antioxidant enzyme plays a key role in the management of all autoimmune conditions, but people battling these conditions tend to have severely depleted levels of glutathione, because inflammation quickly wipes out glutathione stores. To anyone suffering from an autoimmune disorder, glutathione is your very best friend. It takes the hit from inflammation so that your tissues don't.

CAROL'S STORY

Carol initially came to me for help with her weight issues. She had tried and failed with the Atkins diet years ago, and so was skeptical that a primal, ketogenic approach could help her. Still, she was intrigued enough to try.

Her blood tests revealed that she was borderline diabetic, with significantly elevated fasting blood glucose, triglycerides, and Hgb A1C. Her total serum cholesterol levels were elevated, but her HDL level was depressed. Although she was taking prescription thyroid hormone for an underactive thyroid, her blood tests showed that her thyroid antibody levels were off the charts: she had Hashimoto's disease and didn't even know it. Hashimoto's is an autoimmune condition in which the immune system attacks and gradually destroys the thyroid gland. Often, autoimmune thyroid cases are poorly responsive to thyroid medications, as inflammatory cytokines can interfere with thyroid receptors, preventing them from responding properly to thyroid hormones. The symptoms persist, in spite of the healthier-looking blood TSH levels.

Since immune reactivity to gluten is implicated in nearly all cases of Hashimoto's, Carol cut gluten from her diet. Because of the advanced stage of her condition, she needed to continue taking Synthroid, but steps needed to be taken to slow or halt further tissue destruction. The Primal Fat Burner Plan, plus some additional supplementation uniquely designed to address her issues, helped her do just that.

Additional blood test results found that Carol had pernicious anemia (a vitamin B_{12} deficiency), very low vitamin D_3 levels, and other markers that were strongly suggestive of digestive problems and more than typical of her autoimmune condition. No wonder she couldn't lose weight!

Systemic inflammation—a flood of inflammatory compounds (known as *cytokines*) that continually circulate throughout the entire body—are typically found in sufferers of autoimmune disorders. Inflammation, eating sugary and starchy carbohydrates, and common dietary antigens such as grains, legumes, and dairy products are some often seen reasons why so many people are unsuccessful when it comes to their weight-loss efforts.

Carol, who happens to be a research chemist, began following my dietary recommendations despite her skepticism. She gave up bread, grains, starches, sugary foods, cereals, pasta, milk, and cheese. She learned to read labels carefully. She ate a diet in which most of her calories came from the omega-3-rich fats of pastured animals, and ate beef, calf, and poultry liver more frequently. She used coconut oil and tallow for cooking meats and vegetables and filled her plate with salad greens, broccoli, cauliflower, asparagus, and cabbage. She found local sources of fully pastured meats and organic vegetables. She started shopping at farmers' markets.

Within a month Carol reported back to me on her exciting progress. She no longer craved sugar or experienced low blood-sugar symptoms. Her sleep and moods were dramatically better. Her follow-up blood tests, run by her primary care doctor about two months later, showed dramatic improvements. Carol's fasting blood sugar was normal and her Hgb A1C had already begun to improve significantly. Her cholesterol was lower, thanks to less inflammation, while her HDL level was on the rise—a good sign.

Her energy levels were significantly improved. This didn't "cure" her thyroid condition, but she was clearly managing it better, and she felt greatly improved and more emotionally stable overall. Her own doctor was literally agog at the dramatic and rapid changes.

Although Carol admits to occasionally missing some of her old favorite indulgences, such as ice cream and bread, she continues to stick to the Primal Fat Burner Plan because she feels so great—a full ten years later. She lost thirty pounds (exactly what she needed to), has normal blood chemistry markers, and is managing her Hashimoto's much better, with less overall puffiness, fewer mood swings, and fewer bouts of the fatigue, nervousness, irritability, and agitation typically associated with the disease.

An Important Note on Type 1 Diabetes

Type 1 diabetics can also greatly benefit from a fat-based, ketogenic approach to eating, and many have—to positive life-changing effect. But the process *must* be carefully introduced and monitored. Eliminating carbohydrates from the diet greatly reduces the need for insulin, but if your condition is not being properly managed, your body may also begin producing ketones too rapidly, potentially resulting in a dangerous state unique to type 1 diabetics called *ketoacidosis*. In ketoacidosis, the body fails to adequately regulate ketone production, causing such a severe accumulation of ketoacids that the pH of the blood is substantially decreased. The result of this is potentially life-threatening for type 1 diabetics. This makes careful and conscientious self-monitoring of blood sugar (and typically ketone levels, too) crucial, and I recommend the supervision of a knowledgeable health care provider to get you started.

I have heard from numerous type 1 diabetics who successfully became fat burners and are thrilled by their dramatically reduced requirement for insulin and the improvements in their overall well-being. This includes young children, who have been guided through the process carefully by their parents and doctors. If you are willing to do the work, this kind of improvement is a definite possibility for you. Dr. Richard

Bernstein (himself a lifelong type 1 diabetic and author of *Dr. Bernstein's Diabetes Solution*), who advocates a similar dietary approach, has further resources available on his website, www.diabetes-book.com.

Cancer: A New Approach to a Uniquely Modern Problem

The modern cancer epidemic knows no precedent. The World Health Organization predicts that worldwide cancer rates will increase by 70 percent in the next two decades.[46] Cancer Research UK grimly predicts that the disease will soon hit one in two people.[47] Cancer is an infinitely complex subject, and what we don't know in many respects far outweighs what we do. Today's modern environment has myriad mutagenic and immune-compromising substances (and other stressors) potentially contributing to the initiation and development of cancer. Rather than get lost amid all the potential causes of cancer, I find that it's most helpful to look at how we can create conditions in our body that put any (potential or already developed) cancer cells at the biggest disadvantage possible, while strengthening our resistance against those cells' efforts to grow and spread. The truth is that at any given moment, there can be many mutated, cancerous cells in the body, but a healthy immune system is constantly working to identify and destroy them before they proliferate. The trick, in part, is to do everything possible to support that effort.

Today we are gaining ground in the understanding of the metabolic nature of cancer. This was first discovered by a pioneering 1930s researcher, Dr. Otto Warburg, who won a Nobel Prize for his work theorizing that cancer is foundationally a *mitochondrial, metabolic disease driven by the presence of sugar*. The CliffsNotes version of the Warburg effect[48] is that the fermentation of glucose and other sugars is what primarily fuels malignant tumors and other cancer cells. This creates lactic acid as a by-product, which generates a highly acidic pH in your tissues; this in turn encourages a cancer-friendly environment (and leads to extreme fatigue and weakness[49,50]—a state further exacerbated by the accelerated conversion of protein stores into sugar to feed ravenous cancer cells, with a tragic wasting effect for the sufferer, called cachexia). There are numerous peer-reviewed studies showing a close relationship between poor blood sugar control and significantly increased cancer risk.[51]

This vastly simplifies the concept, of course, but the validity of this metabolic mechanism for spreading cancer—and possibly even initiating it—has been the subject of mounting scientific study.[52] Cutting-edge research says that sugars play a central role in initiating cancer in healthy cells, not just spreading it.[53] (By contrast, the conventional view has always been that sugar metabolism by cancer cells is just a peripheral mechanism in the background of what is basically a genetic process.) Back in 2006, the Cancer Genome Atlas project boldly and confidently set out to sequence the genomes of cancer cells. This effort exceeded the scope of the massive Human Genome Project by ten thousand times, as researchers were intent on proving the genetic basis of cancer. But the results ended up proving something else entirely. In fact, some cancers weren't traceable to genetic mutations at all. The research of Dr. Thomas Seyfried (Boston College) later showed that the relationship between genetic defects and cancer was more one of association, not causation, and the core issues driving the defects were located elsewhere. One hypothesis is that it is mitochondrial damage that happens first, which then triggers genetic mutations that may then lead to cancer.

Actress Angelina Jolie opted for a preemptive double mastectomy following the discovery that she carried the breast cancer gene BRCA1. Medical authorities claim this genetic marker is a sign that women will likely develop aggressive and frequently fatal breast cancer, a scary prognosis for sure. Yet there is another side to the reports about the BRCA1 gene. A researcher by the name of Dr. Mary King published an article in the journal *Science* back in 2003 that gave a different view of this dreaded genetic maker: "The lifetime risk of breast cancer among female carriers [of BRCA1] is presently 82 percent. *Risks appear to be increasing with time* [emphasis added]. Before 1940 it was 24 percent. Lack of physical exercise and obesity in adolescents may be important modulating factors for risk in carriers."[54]

In other words, diet and lifestyle factors appear to be the key driving force when it comes to this particular gene's expression. The fact is, genes are mere blueprints contained within our DNA. As with any type of blueprint for building anything (including health), the quality of the outcome depends on the quality of materials used and further-more, genes are not destiny. Our ultimate salvation is anything *but* the medical/pharmaceutical industry. We are all far more in control of what our genes do than we might think!

The abbreviated takeaway is that there are three things that *all* cancer requires in order to survive, feed, and thrive: sugar,[55] lactic acid (a metabolic by-product of sugar),[56] and glutamine (a normally helpful amino acid that in excess can feed certain cancers).[57] The hor-mones insulin[58] and IGF-1[59] (similar to insulin) operate like fertilizer for cancer cell growth.

Given that sugar consumption feeds cancer and drives insulin lev-els, and the factor that most controls IGF-1 (a hormone similar in its structure to insulin) is the mTOR pathway, initiated by excess protein consumption (independent of total calories),[60] it stands to reason that one of the simplest and best strategies for creating anti-cancer condi-tions in your body is to greatly minimize starches and sugars and to restrict protein intake to meet but not exceed your basic nutritional requirements. (And *please* run away quickly from those high-protein weight-loss programs, with their excess of mTOR and IGF-1 triggers!)

In addition, sugars have a profoundly suppressing effect on what is referred to as your body's leukocytic index—the ability of white blood cells to keep developing cancer cells in check. This is crucially important for women with higher risks of breast cancer, especially estrogen-related types: insulin makes more estrogen circulate in the body, and both hormones accelerate cellular proliferation. A low-carb diet with low-glycemic foods offers powerful preventive help. According to the Harvard Health website, "The *glycemic index* is a value assigned to foods based on how slowly or how quickly those foods cause increases in blood glucose levels."[61] Bread, white pota-toes, white rice, and cereal have a high glycemic index and raise blood sugar very rapidly, while fibrous vegetables like asparagus, broccoli, and cabbage have a very low glycemic index and do not significantly impact blood sugar. High-glycemic foods also bring fat-burning and all the benefits of ketosis to a screeching halt!

When you successfully transition to a fat-burning metabolism, you have the advantage of ketones on your side. They efficiently produce energy *without* the excessive creation of reactive oxygen species (free radicals), as glucose or fructose does; they don't produce lactic acid as a by-product, and they support robust mitochondria, making your cellular respiration healthier and more disease resistant. Furthermore, cancer cells really can't use ketones as fuel.

The multimillion-dollar question is whether a state of EKA can help *treat* already existing cancer. A new wave of research suggests this diet's ability to improve cancer treatment outcomes, whether that treatment is conventional (surgery, radiation, and chemotherapy) or more holistic. It's been posited that particularly in hard-to-treat brain cancers the presence of cerebral ketones supports the healthy brain cells while reducing tumor growth and inflammation.[62] Anecdotal evidence also suggests that the utilization of EKA in tandem with existing therapies significantly improves outcomes. Ten years from now, we should have a deeper understanding of nutritional therapies for many different kinds of cancer, including, I predict, ways in which seemingly opposing healing approaches, such as EKA ketosis strategically combined/cycled with higher-carb juicing, may have a potential to more effectively deliver cancer-killing compounds to sugar-starved cancer cells, and could conceivably work in uniquely synergistic harmony.

Some successful holistic cancer treatment approaches utilize diets that seem to be higher in carbs, which I believe may function as a sort of "Trojan horse"—masking hidden anti-cancer compounds and nutrients within an irresistibly sweet matrix. No cancer can resist sugar. By preceding (and perhaps also following) this strategically placed "smart sugar bomb" by a period of strict ketogenic compliance, a weakened, starving cancer cell might find this lethal sweet cocktail irresistible and effect its own self-destruction. It's only a hypothesis, but I hope some researcher pursues it.

If you are currently living with cancer, the Primal Fat Burning Plan, with its emphasis on immune support, anti-inflammatory foods, avoidance of cancer-provoking sugar and insulin, and avoiding excess protein, provides an excellent foundation for your support and healing. Please discuss it with your trusted health care provider and ensure you get your nourishment through only the highest-quality foods and fats from organic and exclusively pastured sources. Two other important notes:

1. The most recent research suggests that with active cancer it may be advantageous to lower your protein intake further, to 0.5 gram per kilogram of estimated ideal body weight, instead of the plan's standard 0.8 gram.
2. If you want to include bone broth in your diet while addressing your own cancer, be sure to simmer it no longer than about four hours, to minimize the amount of glutamine you leach into it.

A nutrient-dense diet is your superhero tool for increasing your resilience to cancer. The fat in meat and organ meats from pasture-raised animals and ample bone marrow are rich in natural conjugated linoleic acid (CLA), one of the most broadly beneficial and potent natural cancer-fighting substances (as opposed to the comparatively ineffective synthetic supplemental sources).[63] Coconut oil's lauric acid is another anti-cancer powerhouse. Enhance this even further by keeping your stress in check and getting enough sleep: excess levels of cortisol and circadian rhythm dysregulation from chronic stress, antigenic exposures, steroidal medications, or hormonal/brain-based imbalances are also a potential problem, as cortisol freely generates blood sugar, helping to feed cancer cell growth (even in the absence of dietary sugars and starches).

Resistant Weight Loss, Resistant Insulin: Winning the Battle of the Bulge, and Type 2 Diabetes

Resistant Weight Loss

When George first came to see me, just retired from IT work at the age of fifty-four, he had been gaining weight steadily over the previous eight years. He had tried running and other forms of exercise to thwart the expansion of his girth and attempted to diet periodically using the old standard low-cal approach, to no avail. His less-than-flattering nickname was the "Bottomless Pit." At dinner, he would scan the table to see who might not finish their food and monitor the serving dishes to make sure he could get seconds of meat along with pasta, rice, potatoes, or bread. Nothing went in the fridge for later; he ate it all. He used to joke that he had a "broken full switch" and he knew that he was full only when it hurt—though the joke was definitely on him, and under the smiles, he knew it. He was considerably overweight, and his blood pressure had reached a borderline hypertensive state. He was tired a lot of the time, had trouble getting a good night's sleep, and often felt anxious or foggy, struggling to think clearly at work—a classic carbovore symptom. His complexion was bad, and he had digestive problems.

The nutritional approach I proposed was completely opposite his habits, but George was keen to put an end to the relentless battle with diets and find a better path forward. He agreed to stock his kitchen with pastured meats and eggs, bone-broth-based soups, and wild-caught fish. He cut out all grains, legumes, and starchy vegetables and made large salads full of dark green vegetables, with frequent additions of avocado, coconut, and extra-virgin olive oil. He cut out all fruit, save for a few tart berries, since weight loss was a goal. George even got into making his own homemade sauerkraut and kefir.

After about a week of this, he called me to recount "an incredible experience." One night, after eating a moderate-sized dinner, he noted a very new and foreign sensation: he felt comfortably full. He laughed out loud, surprised and awed. It had been a long time since he'd heard that message from within. As the days passed, that sensation continued: he'd note that he was satisfied after completing his meal, and he had no desire to overeat.

He also began to see improvements to his health. After five months, he had shed around forty pounds, reaching an optimal and stable weight. His blood pressure normalized, he slept better at night, and he felt calmer and steadier by day. His complexion cleared up and his brain fog lifted. He was thrilled. He reported another important shift: his perception of what constituted "food" had changed completely. He had been a self-proclaimed indiscriminate omnivore with a rather addictive personality—"if I see it, I eat it" had been his mantra. Now he was attracted only to the foods that worked for his body. The old foods simply lost their power over him. Even though he hadn't changed his exercise habits at all, he said, "I lost the weight anyway." And it stayed off. George became quite an advocate for this nutritional approach (remaining one to this very day, many years later), and even coached grateful friends, family, and colleagues to successfully make their own fat-burning switch.

Most of what you've read so far in this chapter applies to the two most common health problems of our era: resistant weight loss (where the pounds simply won't leave) and the insulin-resistant state of type 2 diabetes. When clients are following a well-balanced and properly implemented primal fat-burning diet, yet are frustrated they are not losing the weight they hoped for, there are commonly five starting areas we look at together. These are all the most common triggers for excess weight gain and common causes of plateauing and/or resistant weight loss:

- Consuming too much protein can stall your best weight loss efforts and interfere with ketogenic adaptation and efficiency. The mTOR metabolic pathway created by excess protein both triggers cellular proliferation and a partial conversion to sugar. Unless you need increased dietary protein for something important (if you are a youngster who's still growing, or if you are pregnant), mostly it derails your long-term weight loss efforts, your health, and your longevity. Get out the digital food scale and carefully measure out the directed (raw) protein amount for each meal; this can sometimes reveal that your protein portion sizes have expanded without your even realizing it.
- Hidden carbs are another oft-overlooked issue. Occasionally, nuts and nut butters (which often contain both fats and carbs) get overeaten as a "healthy snack." Some people get a bit lenient with fruit, migrating from occasional berries to more fruit, assuming it's "primal" because fruit's been around forever. However, fruit today is cultivated to be

bigger and sweeter than nature ever designed it to be, and our ancestors didn't typically have access to fruit all year round. Fruit sugars have a unique ability to trigger greater weight gain, but not because of their calories. It's about the activation of a specific enzyme, *fructokinase*, through the consumption of the predominant sugar in fruit, fructose. Fructokinase activates another enzyme that tells your body, "Hey, winter is coming—start putting on fat!" Nothing will make you fatter (and more metabolically dysregulated) faster than fructose and other purportedly "all-natural," "low-glycemic" sweeteners, which are typically high in fructose. Agave syrup—often added to prepackaged, so-called "health foods"—is among the worst of these.

- Chronic inflammation can be a result of many conditions: diagnosed or undiagnosed autoimmune disease, immune reactivity to certain foods and environmental compounds, infections, gut dysbiosis, or the excess consumption of pro-inflammatory omega-6 fatty acids in refined vegetable oils and feedlot meats. Inflammation can be measured with a simple blood test focused on specific inflammatory markers (CRPhs, homocysteine, uric acid, etc.).
- Excess cortisol output, frequently a result of chronic stress and/or a type-A lifestyle, can also readily dysregulate your metabolism, hike up your blood sugar, and cause your body to store more fat.[64] Cortisol can best be measured through a urinary lab test known as the DUTCH Test, or through a salivary ASI (adrenal stress index) test.
- Excess estrogen can be a result of certain medications (such as birth control pills or estrogen-based hormone replacement therapy), tainted feedlot meats, pesticides or herbicides, the use of plastics to drink/eat out of, other chemicals, and even personal care products (especially those containing parabens). Estrogen can also build up in your body as a result of poor biliary function and/or constipation, preventing you from properly eliminating excess or spent estrogen. If your gastrointestinal transit time is too sluggish, these excess

estrogens can get reabsorbed back into circulation again, adding to the unwelcome endocrine pool and resulting in unhealthy weight gain and increased cancer risk.

Adopting a high-fat, low-carbohydrate way of eating can flip a switch in your gene expression, helping to code for specific proteins that greatly increase your metabolism of fats.[65] In fact, this also helps your body burn *more* fat than ever before during exercise, even during high-intensity anaerobic exercise.[66]

While weight loss is often the biggest motivating factor for adopting a change in diet, the primary emphasis should always be first and foremost foundational health. This is the unabashed goal of *Primal Fat Burner*: to empower, educate, and inspire you to create optimal health for yourself. Weight loss is (and should be) a mere side effect of any quality health program. After all, it's entirely possible to be thin and diabetic, suffer from heart disease or high blood pressure, suffer from an autoimmune disease or Alzheimer's, or develop cancer. Being slender is not necessarily synonymous with being healthy.

That said, it is more than possible to have it all. The Primal Fat Burner Plan isn't just about burning fat to lose weight; it's about adopting a fat-burning metabolism in alignment with our ancestral and natural genetic heritage, as well as modern, scientifically validated human longevity principles. The idea is to go beyond conventional "paleo" or other popular ketogenic approaches to truly supercharge your health, brain, mood, and clarity, and to maximize your capacity for being your very best.

Type 2 Diabetes: The Effective Ketogenic Adaptation Solution

According to experts, the incidence of diabetes has increased by more than 700 percent in the last fifty years.[67] Type 2 diabetes is an advanced state of insulin resistance brought on by prolonged, excessive carbohydrate consumption. As such, it responds brilliantly when you switch to a fat-based metabolism. In type 2 diabetes, the body loses its ability to respond to insulin, causing even more of it to be produced while it

WILL THE TWO BIGGEST RESISTANT WEIGHT-LOSS CULPRITS PLEASE STAND UP?

By far the most common source of initially resistant weight loss in women involves the metabolic conversion of an enzyme produced in the ovaries, called *17,20 lyase*. In the presence of excessive insulin, this enzyme actually converts estrogen into the androgenic hormone *dihydrotestosterone* (DHT).[68] This often results in the condition referred to as polycystic ovarian syndrome. The symptoms of PCOS are actually almost identical to the symptoms of low thyroid function: weight gain that is unresponsive to exercise and even low-calorie diets, plus fatigue and hair loss. It is part and parcel of *metabolic syndrome* (endocrine dysfunction associated with insulin resistance) and can become self-perpetuating. Shutting down the need for insulin and addressing inflammation are key to helping reverse this process. Research done using low-carbohydrate, ketogenic dietary approaches have (according to one randomized, controlled study) "led to significant reductions in weight, percent free testosterone, LH/FSH ratio, and fasting insulin in women with obesity and PCOS over a six-month period."[69] Similarly, in men, the most common cause of resistant weight loss is the overconversion of *aromatase*, an enzyme produced in adipose (fat) tissue. Aromatase will combine with insulin to convert healthy testosterone into estrogen.[70] This is a major factor in today's epidemic of low male testosterone—for which testosterone supplementation is categorically *not* the answer, as over time it can greatly deepen the problem. The answer for both women and men lies in addressing the underlying metabolic issues and inflammation while working to *restore* healthy endocrine balance. A period of modified fasting, anti-inflammatory support, and careful food choices are essential to reversing both these forms of chronic weight-gain woes.

is progressively able to do less to remove damaging sugar from your bloodstream. The more insulin your body tries to produce to deal with the sugar, the more weight you begin to gain, as your body tries initially to prevent you from becoming diabetic. Unfortunately, this can work only to a point, and eventually blood sugar rises in a way that insulin cannot compensate for and the complications associated with type 2 diabetes begin to set in. Nothing is more consistently effective at reversing type 2 diabetes than an approach to eating that is low in carbohydrates, moderate in protein, and higher in dietary fat, because carbohydrate restriction automatically improves glycemic control, reduces insulin fluctuation and need, enhances insulin sensitivity, improves blood sugar levels, and subsequently improves states of stubborn insulin resistance, obesity, and inflammation. In essence, it improves and restores metabolic control.[71] Conventional treatments focus on lowering blood sugar by typically adding exogenous insulin-stimulating or insulin-enhancing substances; while on the surface this may appear to improve things, at least temporarily, it's not a wise long-term approach. Modern medicine tends to treat diabetes as though it were a disease of blood sugar. But diabetes is, in fact, a disease not of blood sugar but of *insulin resistance*, and it comes about because of repeated, excessive insulin production that stems from poor dietary choices. Elevated insulin levels, as diabetes expert Ron Rosedale, MD, has pointed out, are associated with and even causative of heart disease, peripheral vascular disease, stroke, high blood pressure, cancer, obesity, and many other conditions. As to why those with type 2 diabetes benefit so much when they achieve a successful state of EKA, I think Dr. Rosedale says it best: "Diabetes is a disease of nutrition, and it is the science of nutrition that must treat it!" If you are living with type 2 diabetes and about to engage in the Primal Fat Burner Plan, I strongly urge you to work with a knowledgeable and supportive qualified health care provider to help monitor your progress in the early stages and also carefully monitor your medications and need for possible rapid dosage changes. (See also "Ketone Meters" in Chapter 10.)

———

Becoming a Primal Fat Burner can do far more for you than help you fit into your skinny jeans; it has the potential to save your life.

CHAPTER 9

Carbovore No More

THE GAME-CHANGING EFFECTS OF FAT BURNING FOR PEAK PHYSICAL PERFORMANCE

Do a quick survey of the really passionate and engaged primal fat burners, and you'll find that a good number of them are athletes—both the everyday "workout warrior" looking to optimize workouts and recovery and the elite athlete seeking an edge in competition—from triathletes to basketball players, Australian football players to cricket players, strength competitors to surfers.

In fact, some of the most vocal (and visibly ripped) practitioners of a well-adapted fat-burning diet are top endurance athletes—people who push themselves to superhuman lengths on long runs, bikes, and swims. After they retire the pre-race pasta and ditch the post-game bagels, they report better performance, swifter recovery, better blood markers, and sharper mental acuity, as well as the leanest and most muscular physiques of their careers (along with fewer health/injury complications associated with endurance sports). It tells us that a fat-based metabolism can provide not just optimal support but performance- and health/physique-boosting benefits for the rest of us mere mortals, too, eager to stay fit, get lean, and enjoy sports and athletics even more.

Switching to fat burning for sports and fitness is a game changer. Consider that the world of physical performance has long placed its bets on carbohydrates: since the 1970s, athletes and coaches have been committed sugar burners, relying on carbohydrate-filled foods for much of their energy and practicing "carb loading" prior to events, to fuel them toward the finish line. This has become so ingrained as normal that we hardly question it. But after reading thus far, I hope you are questioning these practices, too. While the excess blood sugar and stored glycogen in the muscles is mostly used up in the long race that follows, the damage accrued from constantly loading up on and then metabolizing all that sugar cannot be undone. You can burn off the sugar, but you can't ever burn off the insulin, and any time you've instructed your body to repeatedly rely upon a lot of sugar—even in the name of athletic prowess—you invite some level of health and metabolic compromise.

Because of this, when carb-loading elite athletes retire from competition, diabetes can be the less-than-desirable prize. World-class rower Steve Redgrave was diagnosed with type 2 diabetes three years after earning his fifth Olympic gold medal at the age of thirty-eight.[1]

And it's not uncommon to see headline stories about long-distance runners dropping dead from heart failure. The newest thinking is that the overdependence upon carbs in conjunction with the body's efforts to reach for yet more sugar for fuel through the oxidation of the body's protein and muscle stores, coupled in some cases with excess cortisol from hard training, takes its toll on the heart—which is, of course, a large, very active, and vitally important muscle. By contrast, since a fat-burning metabolism is inherently sparing of the body's protein stores, it yields a net increase of lean tissue mass.[2] And, as you've read, the heart actually prefers and uses fat more efficiently than glucose.[3] If you're a marathoner, in other words, fat burning can do far more than improve your performance; it could literally save your life.

As for food quality in the world of sports nutrition—*ouch!* In recent decades even the occasional gym-goer has become familiar with the stacks of brightly wrapped "energy bars" (laced with high fructose corn syrup), tubs of protein powder (derived from soy or pasteurized milk), and Disney-colored energy, electrolyte, or recovery drinks for "powering up" before workouts or recovering afterward. In the sports mainstream, it's long been about chasing the perfect body and performance, while eating a pretty twisted diet with more than a shadow of the Frankenfood monster. Ironic? Tragic!

The Faces of Super-Powered Fat Burning

But it doesn't have to be that way, and a new wave of athletes is showing why. For fat-adapted ultramarathon runners such as twenty-eight-year-old Tim Olson, who shaved twenty minutes off the course record when he won the one-hundred-mile Western States Endurance Run from Squaw Valley to Auburn, California, his organic, grass-fed primal diet is key not just to success but to recovery. In an interview for *Runner's World*, he said, "My legs are less swollen after really long runs. I can go hard again sooner than I did before I went Paleo."[4] He still uses some carbohydrates (mainly non-endocrine disrupting energy gels during midrun), but in a strictly limited fashion in his daily life and while preparing for athletic performance—a tactic that applies mainly to competitive athletes, as I'll describe below.

Meanwhile, Ben Greenfield, Ironman athlete, author of the book *Beyond Training* and a friend of mine, successfully "bio-hacked" his way out of a prediabetic condition brought on by unusually excessive cortisol. Given his genetic predisposition to type 2 diabetes, had Ben not been savvy as he was about knowing how to be a smart fat burner, he might not have been so lucky. He now advises and coaches many others how to improve performance while protecting their bodies. (And he's particularly known for his willingness to participate in some extreme-sounding clinical trials to prove the safety and efficacy of fat-burning for hard-core athletes—quite the heroic effort!) Ben works hard at managing his personal tendency toward high cortisol levels—something that can get the best of *any* hard-core athlete, since the stress of training often jacks up cortisol levels, which in turn repeatedly spikes blood sugars. Transitioning from a sugar-burning metabolism therefore adds an important level of protection to people who give their bodies quite a beating and stress hormone blast in pursuit of their goals.

And it would be remiss not to call out world amateur Ironman champion Sami Inkinen, who also reversed a prediabetic condition brought on by (in his case) a carb-heavy, nearly zero-fat training diet. Sami began working with Steve Phinney, MD, PhD—physician, sports performance scientist, and coauthor of *The Art and Science of Low Carbohydrate Performance*—and reported a remarkable progressive change in his numbers, essentially reflecting much less inflammation and more stable, lower blood glucose levels. His capacity to burn fat literally tripled, going from a fat-burning capacity of only 200 kilocalories per hour to more than 700 kilocalories per hour. He had achieved an astonishing improvement in his athletic performance—so much so that he and his equally extraordinary (and keto-adapted) wife, Meredith Loring, then undertook and successfully completed a truly epic, 2,400-mile trans-Pacific crossing in a rowboat, powered (you guessed it) by a diet that was low in carbs, moderate in protein, and 75 percent fat from high-quality sources. The two-month trip was the performance equivalent of running two marathons a day *each*. (They not only made it, they stayed married! A testament to fat-burning's emotionally stabilizing effects if ever there was one. You can read about it at their website, fatchancerow.com.)

One of my personal favorite examples of the empowering effects of making the metabolic switch, however, is from a young woman named Maureen Quinn. After adopting my primal fat-burning dietary approach, she began strength training. She "entered her first competition in August of 2014, shocking everyone with a first place finish in the featherweight division."[5]

Then within six months, Maureen won sixth place in the featherweight division of the 2015 United States Strongwoman National Championships. Not only was her performance very impressive, but her ultra-strong body "became the leanest I'd ever been after eating all the fat I wanted." Maureen gets the majority of her calories from grass-fed animal fat and is no stranger to nutrient-dense beef cheeks, liverwurst, and bone marrow. Her diet (which she customizes with intermittent fasting) is the foundation of her training—fueling her to lift monstrously heavy things while ensuring she stays lean enough to stay under the 120-pound featherweight limit.

Uber hunky and insanely fit athletic superstar Adam Von Rothfelder of NBC television's hit reality show *Strong* is both a friend and a major fan. He says that "Utilizing a high-fat diet for competition brings an incredible sense of awareness and energy. I personally have been consciously living in a primal state with free-range meats and veggies for almost ten years and have seen not only incredible results in myself but also in my clients. While on *Strong* my partner and I stuck to a strict primal diet which she loved. Not only did she enjoy eating savory fats and rich meats but she lost weight, gained muscle, and even saw an improvement in her fibromyalgia."

After decades of carbohydrates being the undisputed title holder when it comes to sports, fat is now being recognized as a contender for the performance-enhancing crown—perfectly capable of making that knockout punch.

How EKA Supports Your Sports and Fitness Goals

Though the athletes I just mentioned were testing the merits of a healthy state of effective ketogenic adaptation at an intense and elite level of training, anyone who enjoys sports or fitness can hit his or her performance sweet spot as a primal fat burner, too, even with the lower levels of protein this approach involves. As dietary protein levels lessen to merely what is needed, efficiency improves, allowing for an enhanced recycling of available proteins and improved adaptation to fat burning. Sometimes a little less really is more.

A well-formulated ketogenic diet and well-adapted ketogenic state can:

- Spare your lean tissue mass by sparing protein from being converted to glucose and used for fuel in hypoglycemic states,[6] so you are less apt to use your muscle (including your heart) and bones for fuel while you sleep.
- Help spare your body's protein from oxidation,[7] so you get to keep all that muscle you've worked so hard for, instead of wastefully burning it for energy.[8]
- Improve your efficiency of protein utilization,[9] so you need less to gain and keep more muscle and recover faster.

- Reduce nitrogen excretion (provided you are eating sufficient fat),[10,11] to help further facilitate that positive nitrogen balance for better growth and tissue repair.
- Lower systemic inflammation,[12] so you are less prone to pain and excessive downtime or recovery time.
- Provide better maintenance of and even increase circulating levels of the branched-chain amino acids leucine, isoleucine, and valine, as there is less need to use them as fuel while operating in a ketogenic state; instead, your body is more able to rely upon them for driving muscle protein synthesis. Maintaining healthy ketogenic adaptation helps you build and maintain muscle.

Take note, however: these benefits do take some time to kick in. Athletes and workout warriors who train on a regular schedule often notice extra fatigue during the transition to a fat-burning metabolism. Where more sedentary folks might feel "off" for a few days—as I'll describe in Chapter 10—athletes can feel as if they are dragging for a week or two. If that's you, stay with the diet and take it a little easy; you are in the midst of changing over fuels, so it's natural that your engine may need to spend a little time "in the shop" as it gets the upgrade! Supplements such as L-glutamine, L-carnitine, and C8-type MCT oil (such as the Bulletproof brand Brain Octane) can help kick-start more efficient fat burning and stave off that low-sugar lag time. If you're a competitor, plan ahead and make your fat-burning switch during your off-season. (For the record, this is why some of the research comparing fat- to sugar-burning metabolism for performance previously failed to get encouraging results—the studies ended way too soon, before effective adaptation was able to take place.)

Who Might Need to Tweak the Plan?

For almost everyone working out and training at an amateur level, even if you are training fairly hard, the foods in the Primal Fat Burning Plan will most likely suffice, once you have fully adapted to the metabolic switch to a primary dependence on fats instead of sugar. This even includes those who do CrossFit-style workouts that include power lifting. There are a few special places where an elite athlete or someone with special requirements might need to slightly adapt things, however. But being a fat burner actually spares your glycogen stores so that in the moments you need it most, it's all there.

For high-intensity, short-duration activities such as sprinting, soccer (where an average player might run an average of 109 meters each minute in a seventy-minute game), and other anaerobic sports relying much more on glucose as an anaerobic rocket fuel, the primal fat-based approach can be tweaked with the strategic consumption of 50 to 100 grams of carbohydrate such as fruit (or a high-tech, non-insulin-provoking performance gel such as SuperStarch) immediately prior to, say, a professional game or sporting event in order to support the extreme anaerobic load for the duration of these events.

The "right before" part is key: the carbs can be burned off mostly by the intense physical demand of the event. It's a mistake to reload with carbs after the event, but the ingestion of sugars and starchy foods after exercise will largely bring your fat burning to a screeching halt. You will instantly lower the amount of fat being liberated from your fat stores for energy, and you will reduce the efficiency with which your body is able to use fat and ketones for fuel in your skeletal muscle.[13] It can even take a couple of days to restore your formerly healthy state of effective ketosis after that indulgence. You also unnecessarily, in some small way, increase your vulnerability to insulin resistance and metabolic dysregulation.[14] Also, adding carbs to your post-exercise regimen is simply not going to improve your muscular development.[15] On top of that, you run the risk of increasing your fat storage plus increasing your "rebound" cravings for carbohydrates.

For those endeavoring to engage in more superhuman feats such as Ironman events that draw mercilessly from pretty much every gas tank you've got, strategically adding some carbs or SuperStarch midrun can help add the extra rocket boost you may need to power through it. Even though Ironman champion Ben Greenfield may periodically use this type of extra help, his pre-race meal involves anything but carb loading. While detailing his pre-event diet on one of his podcasts, he said his breakfast the day of the event consisted of "half a stick of butter, two shots of MCT oil, and a cup of coffee."

Generally speaking, most elite-level athletes will need about 25 percent more protein each day than the average person on the Primal Fat Burner Plan. A small amount of extra protein can potentially help offset some glucose deficits, even as protein in excess of daily requirements for maintenance, rebuilding, and repair has its inherent risks and may compromise health and longevity—you have to choose your priorities.[16] As fat burning's first wave of elite passionate athletes is proving, it is absolutely possible to be an effective primal fat burner while achieving enhanced levels of peak performance unrivaled by professionally competitive carbovores. Whatever your current level of strength and fitness may be, let that inspire you to grab a spoonful of my Primal Keto-Coconut Pemmican, lace up your sneakers, and pick up that jump rope, kettlebell, or pair of swimming goggles!

PART FOUR

The Primal Fat Burner Plan

You're about to discover the transforming effects of transitioning to a fat-burning state: renewed energy, radiant health, and freedom from a compromising and potentially dangerous dependency on a sugar-burning metabolism. This three-week plan is designed to guide you through making the switch to a balanced and well-adapted fat-burning metabolism, and then support you to maintain it for the long term. It's not a program that you do periodically and then drop, like a cleanse or detox. It is a shift to a new way of eating for life and a new way of thinking about the link between your health and real food. For many it is a complete paradigm shift, opening the door onto a totally new way of prioritizing themselves and a healthy lifestyle.

As with making any significant change, some people move smoothly through it and others find it a little bumpier. To some extent, *all* change is at least potentially discombobulating. And how easy you find it may depend on how long you've been swimming against the current of good health—if you've gotten far out to sea with your eating habits and food sources, then turning around and getting back to shore will require slightly more effort. But rest assured that with steady strokes and by staying on course, you will find your way to terra firma!

Wherever you are starting from, know that the transition to a metabolic dependency on fat does not happen overnight. It tends to take about three to six weeks for your fat-burning metabolism to be fully up and running. During the first few days or even up to a couple of weeks of the transition, some people experience temporary symptoms of feeling a little off or uncomfortable as their bodies make the adjustment, though many do not. But by the end of three to six weeks, almost everyone I have worked with feels confidently established in this new mode. Many already experience significant improvement in energy and clarity, and often have shed stubborn pounds as well. By staying consistent with the Primal Fat Burner Plan for two months, most people will find themselves truly in their groove and notice significant changes in the way they feel, function, and look. With sixty delicious recipes to choose from, and tips and advice that have already helped thousands of others to successfully launch their fat-burning journey, you have everything you need to become a successful primal fat burner, too.

The meal plan and the recipes that follow will help you to achieve all this through balanced meals that deliver appropriate ratios of fat to protein. You will also find instructions for easily measuring protein intake.

THE PLAN AT A GLANCE

On the plan, you will:

- Essentially eliminate dietary sugar and starch.
- Moderate your protein intake to no more than 0.8 gram of protein (raw weight) per kilogram of estimated ideal body weight per day for average adults.
- Eat sufficient quality fat from a variety of animal and plant sources to satisfy your appetite and meet fat-soluble nutrient and essential fatty acid requirements. If you are eating animal fats from exclusively pastured sources, including some organ meats, you should be able to get most of what you need.
- Eat as many fibrous vegetables and greens (cooked, raw, or cultured) as desired. Unsweetened green drinks (or sweetened with a few drops of pure stevia) may also be used.
- Use the best-quality food you can find or afford, and fill your plate with nutrient-dense ingredients that supply your body and brain with what they might have been missing.

CHAPTER 10

Setting Up for Success

To successfully make a big change, it is important to capture the initial enthusiasm you feel and use it to generate valuable momentum for launch. This personal enthusiasm is like the jets strapped to a space shuttle for liftoff. It will give you the initial altitude to rise over the abyss of doubts, social pressure, addictions, and pitfalls that almost everyone faces around eating. Abyss avoided, you will soon find yourself afloat at cruising altitude, staying airborne without much effort. The best way to harness this power is to take a little time to plan your trajectory wisely using the following preparatory steps.

Getting Ready to Burn: The Prep Work

Physical Check-In

Almost anyone can make the transition to primal fat burning and get the benefits, with just a few exceptions that have been mentioned throughout Parts Two and Three. If you consult with your health care practitioner and you likely can consider yourself to be in relatively normal health with no issues you know of, you can get started right away. If you have the resources, doing a basic expanded blood chemistry panel can provide valuable information about where you are starting from. It's always nice—and recommended—to have that baseline of comparison, though it's not essential. If you suspect that you may be in something like a borderline diabetic state (with chronically high blood sugar), please undergo a basic health evaluation prior to embarking on the plan. It will be important for you to closely monitor your progress—preferably under the supervision of a qualified professional. If you are already diabetic, then you will want to notify your health care provider about the dietary changes you are making and carefully monitor your blood sugar and blood ketone levels throughout the day during this transition. You may also find the need to rapidly adjust (typically lower) exogenous insulin and other medication levels, which should be done only with a doctor's careful guidance.

If your health is compromised significantly in any other way, I recommend regular monitoring and supervision by a qualified health care provider during the process of implementation. If you are on medications, be advised that you will almost certainly require a change in those medications (and quite possibly sooner than you might expect) as your body adapts to the changes it will undergo. Be sure you have a licensed health care provider you can readily consult with about making those potentially needed adjustments.

And a note of support: If your doctor hassles or berates you over your proposed change in lifestyle, then consider getting another opinion or finding a different doctor willing to work with you, and to consider health choices outside an antiquated paradigm. There are plenty of MDs, DOs (doctors of osteopathy), naturopaths, nutritionally oriented chiropractors, functional neurologists, and functional medicine specialists who will be more than supportive of your health needs, choices, and journey. And they're not necessarily that hard to find nowadays.

BLOOD TESTS

A basic blood chemistry panel is a useful, albeit optional, tool for evaluating your current health baseline. You can then compare it with a second panel three months after you begin the Primal Fat Burning Plan, to chart your progress. (Three months is appropriate because the hemoglobin A1C test generally provides a window into the last three months' glycation damage.)

Below are the *functional* blood levels that I look for and help clients work toward achieving. (Functional levels show a more accurate normal and healthy range than the standard lab range on your printed lab paperwork, which compare you against other patients at your lab.)

If you are already at these levels when you start, that's great news; the Primal Fat Burning Plan will give you an extra buffer zone of health, an edge in sports and cognitive performance, healthier aging, and resilience from disease.

Fasting glucose: ideally between 70 and 85 mg/dL as long as you are not symptomatic (i.e., you have no issues with hypoglycemia or reactive hypoglycemia).

Triglycerides: below 100 mg/dL.

Fasting insulin: below 10 IU/mL (and ideally closer to 5 IU/mL or below).

Fasting leptin: ideally between 4 and 6 ng/dL.

Total cholesterol: roughly between 225 and 240 mg/dL. (The conventional medical standards are arbitrary and relative. Postmenopausal women, for instance, tend to do better with higher levels.) If your level is higher than this, it may be an indication that there is something else happening for which the extra cholesterol is necessary. Be happy that cholesterol is doing its job, then dig deeper with the help of a qualified health care provider well schooled in functional medicine to get to the bottom of what is generating your apparent increased cholesterol need.

HDL: Ideally between 55 and 75 mg/dL. Higher may imply either a genetic tendency or some hidden nonspecific source of inflammation.

Hgb A1C: between 4.7 and 5.4% is a good range.

Uric acid: between 3.2 and 5.5 for women and 3.7 and 6.0 for men.

TSH: between 1.8 and 3.0.

TPO antibodies: below upper reference threshold. (Elevated levels imply thyroid autoimmunity.)

Anti-thyroglobulin antibodies: below upper reference threshold. (Elevated levels imply thyroid autoimmunity.)

Homocysteine: below 6.0 μmol/L.

CRPhs: between 0 and 3 mg/L (and preferably not over 1.0 mg/L).

Fibrinogen: between 193 and 423 mg/dL.

BUN: between 13 and 18 mg/dL.

SGOT (AST): between 10 and 26 IU/L.
SGPT (ALT): between 10 and 26 IU/L.
GGTP: between 10 and 26 IU/L.

Preparing for Liftoff: Your Essential To-Do List

Here is where we maximize the aerodynamics of our soon-to-launch shuttle, by carefully plotting the trajectory. Sit down for half an hour and write out your best plan for accomplishing this change. Be brutally honest with yourself and actively anticipate your own vulnerabilities and adverse tendencies.

1. *Set a goal.* Choose one that's motivating to you, such as weight loss, improvements in certain symptoms, more energy, better moods and sleep. This will help focus you and keep you on track far more effectively. It's hard to reach a destination when you don't quite know where you specifically want to go. Setting a goal far better enhances your odds of getting there!
2. *Put the plan on your schedule.* Block out three weeks starting on a set date, factoring in a couple of days to shop, go through your pantry, and cook several meals, as this will help you start out on the right foot. Beginning on a Sunday can be helpful for this reason.
3. *Remove any obstacles.* Remove the "avoid" foods from your fridge and pantry to the extent you can. If others in your home are not on the plan, strike a deal to remove the obvious temptations, such as bread, crackers, tortilla chips, ice cream, and any junk food, if you can.
4. *Stock your home with better options right from the get-go.* Plan your meals ahead of time; write out a list for the first week by looking through the recipes and meal plans and deciding what you'd like to try. Use the food lists (see page 180) for reference, and shop accordingly. Look through the items listed in the "Supporting Players" section later in this chapter and add what you need to your list.
5. *Cook in batches.* Making soups and large portions that you can

freeze in small containers (glass ones are safest, by the way) will be invaluable in helping you stay on track. Not everything has to be from the recipes: a simple roast chicken can feed you for several lunches, for example. Though you will come to feel quite satiated between meals, it is good to have some primal, low-carb, higher-fat snacks on hand, especially at the start. Pick a few you'd like to make and add the ingredients to your list. And get some Brain Octane MCT oil or coconut oil—a teaspoon of oil here and there can take the edge off hunger.

6. *Consider your own areas of vulnerability.* Read through the sections below and think about what might trip you up. If you know you are likely to have issues with sugar cravings or symptoms of low blood sugar, then plan ahead for this and purchase a recommended supplement to take the edge off. If you often find reasons not to cook during the week, plan a cooking afternoon over the weekend. If you fall off track easily, try to find a friend or family member to do the plan with you. Do what it takes to minimize your own excuses and anticipate where you need more support.

Preparing Your Kitchen and Pantry

Shopping for a primal fat-burning diet can take a little getting used to. My clients sometimes tell me that this way of eating looks great on paper, but when they are walking down the aisle at the supermarket, they have trouble making the switch in their shopping lists at first. The truth is, when you commit to eating nutrient-rich foods from healthful and ethical sources, grocery shopping *will* become a bit more involved; you will likely not be able to do a one-stop shopping trip at your local store unless you have a market that is committed to quality meat and animal-sourced products. Look at this as part of the process: shifting to higher-quality foods involves discovering new sources and providers. It does *not* need to mean sky-high food budgets. Having read about fat-soluble nutrients, you now know I'm a passionate advocate for meat and eggs from fully pastured animals, as well as clean and safe sources of fish. You will be eating about one-third of the protein in the average American diet, using lots of cheaper cuts of meat (including bones), and saving considerably by cooking satisfying meals at home and minimizing snacks and packaged foods. Eating healthfully does not necessarily mean eating expensively. Some of the most budget-conscious people I know have maintained a primal fat-burning diet while accounting for every penny, and found they *saved* money over the typical American diet.[1] It can be done! The food lists in Chapter 11 and "Nourishing Resources" on page 285 will give you some guidance.

While you are on the plan, make it a point to familiarize yourself with all the available local sources of quality organic and grass-fed food. If you live in an area where these are difficult to obtain, use the websites I recommend to order some of the essential fat-burning items. Spend a little time looking up all the farmers' markets, co-ops, CSAs, and natural foods markets in your area—which often have screaming deals—and even venture out to local farms that have implemented quality crop-growing and livestock-raising practices (you can find a lot of these folks through www.eatwild.com). Develop first-hand knowledge of where your food comes from. Join a local chapter of the Hunt Gather Grow Foundation for even more resources and support (www.huntgathergrowfoundation.com), which lets you con-

---

I'M FINANCIALLY STRAPPED—WHAT DO I DO?

Ask questions, read labels. Bring some healthy skepticism to shopping. Don't give any store a free pass—even the "healthy" chain supermarkets. Read labels and look beyond the terms "organic" and "gluten-free" on the package; those words can be stuck on all kinds of non-supportive products. Remember, shopping healthfully involves asking questions. It's okay to ask butchers where the meat came from and how it was raised, or whatever else you need to know in order to make a purchasing choice. It also helps them better gauge what their patrons are looking for. Knowledge is power: without it, you can easily get caught in the tide of repeat-buying low-grade foods without realizing what you are getting—and missing out on the good stuff that might be right alongside!

nect with others already dialed in to the sources of the best-quality local foods. Check out the profusion of online sites about nourishing, traditional-style cooking and homesteading, often run by young and not-wealthy home cooks, which offer crafty and budget-conscious tips. My friend Marjory Wildcraft has an entire program showing you how to easily grow most of your own groceries at home, saving a fortune in food costs (www.growyourowngroceries.org).

Supporting Players: What You'll Need Alongside the Primal Fat Burner Plan

DIGITAL SCALE

An inexpensive digital scale that measures in ounces and grams will be very helpful for measuring protein portions until you can eyeball them.

MINERALS: Full-Spectrum (Himalayan and/or Celtic sea salt, potassium citrate supplements (just one 99 mg capsule/day is fine), and liquid ionic (preferably) magnesium (400 to 600 mg/day).

Adopting a low-carbohydrate and higher-fat ketogenic approach to eating will change the way your body uses certain minerals. You will tend to lose a lot more sodium (and stop retaining excess water) once you lose the carbs. This can sometimes result in temporary issues such as constipation. In fact, it's not uncommon to lose up to five pounds of water weight (plus fat) in the first week for this very reason. But if you don't replace the sodium, then you run the risk of your kidneys dumping potassium in an effort to keep a relative balance with sodium. Consequently, both these minerals become important during your transition. You don't need to eat sugary bananas to get your potassium: 4 ounces of meat in a day will give you a banana's worth, and you can get plenty of potassium from fibrous vegetables and greens in the Primal Fat Burner Plan. Also, however, early on in the EKA process you decrease your urinary excretion of uric acid. Potassium citrate (@99 mg/day) can also help the body get rid of uric acid. Not everyone needs it (males may need more than females). You can test for uric acid with a cheap urinary test strip. That said, it's also important to use a little extra unrefined Himalayan or Celtic sea salt, which contains a full spectrum of trace minerals, on your food so that you maintain a healthy sodium balance. In conjunction with drinking plenty of water, it should help remedy constipation. Don't worry, you won't get bloated by using real full-spectrum salt—that happens from refined sodium chloride and a high-carbohydrate diet. Please be sure *not* to use regular refined table salt: this is *highly* pro-inflammatory. Stick to the full-spectrum salt in its most natural, balanced state for best and healthiest results.

It's also important to consider magnesium. High-carbohydrate diets tend to cause a depletion of intracellular magnesium levels, and so most people are already magnesium-depleted when they shift to a fat-burning diet. If this gets coupled with loss of water, sodium, and potassium, you can experience muscle cramps. I recommend quality magnesium supplementation during the three-week plan (and thereafter only as needed). Please look for liquid ionic magnesium (I like Mineralife brand) or transdermal (topical) magnesium oil preparations that you apply to the skin, or simply enjoy soaking in Epsom salts (magnesium sulfate) dissolved in bathwater, which tends to allow for the transdermal absorption of some of the magnesium and is very relaxing. Magnesium citrate supplements (sold as pills or flavored powders) tend to have more of a laxative effect, for better or worse, but they don't improve your intracellular magnesium levels significantly. The best approach for rapidly correcting significant intracellular magnesium depletion is a series of what are called "Myers cocktails"—an inexpensive and highly replenishing IV solution that must be administered by a health care provider.

COCONUT OIL AND MCT OIL

Coconut oil and/or a supplemental derivative known as MCT (medium-chain triglyceride) oil can be taken off a spoon (working up to 1 to 2 tablespoons) or mixed into a smoothie and can be useful additives to your daily regimen early on to provide a very readily usable fat-based energy supply that cannot easily be stored as body fat. A favorite of mine is a particular brand of C8-type MCT oil called Brain Octane, made by Bulletproof (see "Nourishing Resources" on page 285). One to two tablespoons per day (start with less, maybe a teaspoon, and work your way up) can help combat fatigue experienced in the beginning by some not yet adapted to the use of ketones as a

primary source of fuel. MCT oil is commonly sold as a bodybuild-
ing supplement since it so readily facilitates fat burning. Bulletproof
Brain Octane generates 3 to 5 times more ketones than regular MCT
oil, at a savings. Please don't cook with it, as it isn't very heat-stable.

Be sure to get sufficient omega-3 supplementation from (preferably) Antarctic krill oil (I like the one sold through www.mercola.com).
The amounts people need can vary. If you have inflammation or suffer
from depression or autoimmune conditions, you should at least double or triple the standard recommendations on the label. These can be
energizing, anti-inflammatory, and mood-stabilizing, too. The standard Western diet is notoriously deficient in omega-3 fatty acids (EPA
and DHA), and most folks can benefit from some supplementation.
Start with following the directions on the label and increase if needed.

WATER

Drinking ample purified water is important and easily overlooked. There
are a few desktop or smart phone apps that will remind you periodically
(at whatever designated interval you select) to take a drink of water.
Something like this might be really useful for those who tend to forget
to hydrate regularly throughout the day. The rule of thumb is to calculate
your body weight in kilograms (divide your weight in pounds by 2.2) and
drink that number of ounces of water per day, ideally sipped at regular
intervals. (Note to those Down Under: 1 ounce is just about 30 ml.)

GREEN JUICE

Increasing your intake of unsweetened green veggie drinks during this
time can help support the detoxification process quite a bit. They will
also supply ample potassium to support your electrolyte balance as your
body sheds excess water weight. Don't load the juice with apples or other
fruit. (A few drops of liquid Stevita brand stevia can sweeten the drink
if you like, or use lemon or ginger. If you have to use apple, try to limit
that to no more than one-quarter of a more tart Granny Smith apple.)

EXERCISE

If you already follow a regular workout regimen, there is no reason to
change it during the plan. You might find that it is harder to exercise

for the first few days, so consider taking it easy. Most people find that exercise begins to feel much easier after about the two-week mark—but this is just an average estimate. Elite athletes are going to need three to six weeks to feel like they are fully back on top of their game, and possibly then some. It's always good if you can give yourself a couple of months to fully adapt before a competitive event. If you don't already have a regular routine, I recommend using this time of change to get out for a thirty minute or so brisk daily walk (minimum), which will support all aspects of well-being, including detoxification.

SLEEP

Give yourself the gift of a good eight hours of quality sleep during these weeks. Make sure your bedroom is as dark and quiet as possible. Purchase an inexpensive sleep mask and earplugs if your sleeping space gets too much light or noise. Avoid sleeping next to plugged-in appliances, Wi-Fi routers, or your cell phone, especially if you have issues with less than optimal sleep. If you snore, get an evaluation for possible sleep apnea as soon as possible (find a specialist to evaluate you via www.aadsm.org). Being sleep-deprived can disrupt your circadian rhythms and hormones and make it far more difficult to lose weight!

OPTIONAL AND SPECIALTY ITEMS

These optional items may be useful under certain circumstances.

KICK-START SUPPORT

L-carnitine (2 to 5 grams per day) can be helpful to prompt the body to start using fats for energy. If you're feeling stuck or slow to start, L-carnitine might help. It's an optional extra to enhance the Primal Fat Burner Plan. If you know or suspect you have low thyroid function, you'll want to limit L-carnitine use to no more than 2 grams (2,000 mg) per day.

HYPOGLYCEMIA SUPPORT

If you happen to have significant issues with clinical or garden-variety reactive hypoglycemia (i.e., low blood sugar symptoms), then you will absolutely need supplemental support to ease this transition. Three supplements to consider are L-glutamine powder (which your brain is able to use for energy in lieu of glucose, something like bicycle training wheels), used in small amounts (½ teaspoon or so) under the tongue throughout the day, a herb called *Gymnema sylvestre* (helpful for carb cravings when taken in doses of 4 to 8 grams of whole herb or 400 mg standardized extract per tablet/capsule three times a day while cravings last), and Bulletproof Brain Octane MCT oil (a source of fats that quickly convert to ketones and can be used preferentially for energy). Coconut oil can also be used as a source of at least some ketone-generating naturally occurring MCTs and has the added benefit of naturally occurring anti-microbial lauric acid, plus you can cook with it.

SUGAR OR STARCH CRAVINGS

If you suspect that cravings for sugar or starch will be an issue for you, try using *Gymnema sylvestre* at a dose of roughly 4 to 8 grams (4,000 mg) of whole herb or 400 mg of standardized extract per tablet/capsule three times a day while cravings last.

KETONE METERS

Though this is far from essential for achieving and sustaining a fat-burning metabolism, a quality ketone meter can be an indispensable tool for people who are really struggling with effective ketosis or who want to monitor their adaptation process with more precision. It isn't essential (unless you happen to be diabetic), but if you're a data geek or a bio-hacker looking to tangibly measure your progress, this is one way to do it. A "gold standard" blood ketone meter such as Precision Xtra (the most accurate, affordable, and convenient tool at the time of writing this book) measures beta-hydroxybutyrate, the most important ketone, along with blood sugar if you use different test strips. The meter is cheap, but the strips do add up; however, you may not need to use it for long, only until you get confident with your fat-burning program. Keeping your ketone levels between 1 and 3 mmol is the standard goal, though slightly higher is still okay. Up to 7 mmol is fine during fasting. Ketone levels don't become problematic before 15 to 25 mmol (a concern for type 1 diabetics). If you're testing your blood sugar, strive for a goal of 70 to 85 mg/dL for fasting blood glucose. If you are hypoglycemic, diabetic, or prediabetic, then this gizmo is the one for you. Use it daily to monitor your ketone and blood sugar levels.

One other useful method for determining whether you have officially arrived at a state of effective ketogenic adaptation (EKA) is the Glucose Ketone Index (GKI) calculator, developed by Dr. Thomas Seyfried of Boston College and his colleagues. It measures your ratio of blood glucose to ketones (specifically, beta hydroxybutyrate) and gives you a single number that tells you whether you're in that optimal "fat-burning zone" or not. It takes a little rudimentary math, so keep a calculator handy. First, you need to calculate your blood glucose results using your Precision Xtra glucose/ketone meter; then you convert that number (expressed in mg/dL) to mmol by dividing it by 18. Then take that glucose number and divide it by your ketone reading results (which are automatically expressed in mmol, or Mm) to get your GKI. Your goal is to get into the zone of between 0.7 and 2.0. Getting a 1 is spot-on. So, say you have a blood sugar reading of 75 mg/dL. Divide that number by 18 to get 4.16. Then say your blood ketone reading is 3.0 mmol. Take 4.16 and divide by 3.0. The result is 1.386. BAM. That's your GKI—and you're square in the zone!

Another option is a breath ketone meter. The Ketonix meter costs about $100 and requires no additional expenditure. Very portable, it recharges by USB and is about the size of a cigar tube. You can't get precise values with it, only approximate ones—it measures levels as low, medium, or high—and it measures just acetone, but experts I've consulted with find that it is generally reliable as a crude, correlary litmus test of whether or not you are "in the zone."

Please don't bother with measuring useless urinary ketone levels; this can be terribly misleading and in the long run not that useful as a measurement of actual progress. Save your money and avoid those.

FOOD JOURNAL

Keeping a log of your meals, snacks, and drinks during the plan is an extra step that can be incredibly helpful to show you any patterns that may emerge with certain foods. Make notes about any changes in mood or energy and any other notable physical symptoms (discomfort, digestion, aches, etc.). If you need to troubleshoot stubborn weight loss or any other problems, this journal will be an invaluable tool for any nutritional therapy practitioner, qualified natural health care provider, or functional medicine specialist.

Setting Your Expectations (and Preparing for Bumps)

As you get ready to start, let's address any bumpiness that may come up along the way. Some people breeze through the transition to a fat-burning metabolism almost as if nothing could be more natural to them. Others experience what has occasionally been called the "keto-genic flu," characterized by a feeling of general malaise, fatigue, head-aches, and brain fog for a few days. There can also be some temporary constipation. Making this adaptation fully can take time (even up to a couple of months), though most people start feeling much better within just a few short days. By the end of the first week, the majority of people start to feel significantly improved, though efforts at exercise may be a bit of a strain at first. But don't be discouraged if it takes you a while to feel comfortable; that's normal, too. Positive adaptation (that is, changing to a better way of doing things) is a *process*, not a single event. You may need to be patient with yourself and this approach in order to arrive at the best possible outcome. A lot depends upon what your former habits were and what your health challenges might be at the outset of this transition. If you are a bit older or suffer from a variety of health problems, then expect this to take a little longer than if you are younger and mostly healthy. You are making some rather significant alterations to your physiological makeup, and your body—not to mention your psychology—will need to adjust, especially when you've spent a lifetime doing things very differently.

Discomfort or flu-like symptoms are attributable to a couple of different factors. Number one, you are depriving yourself of the fuel your body and brain have grown used to—sugar—and you have not yet developed the ability to make efficient use of ketones, which you are undoubtedly producing in response to eliminating the sugar and starch. It's a bit of a temporary "metabolic purgatory"—you're no longer fully sugar burning and you're not yet fully fat burning, and though you may be producing ketones, you are not yet fully utilizing them. In some cases, the exorphins (morphine-like compounds) in grains reveal their true impact: coming off grains, you might experience withdrawal, with flu-like symptoms or agitation. If it sounds like coming off a narcotic, that's apt, because when it comes to dropping your reliance on gluten or sugar, you are doing just that! See "Sugar Blues" on page 173 for ideas about how to tackle this.

Second, you are also basically detoxifying, so any consequential bumpy feelings won't last long. Pay close attention to your body and your mental and emotional state as you go through your transition, and stay with it! Using a quality infrared sauna to help better facilitate this detox process, along with extra hydration, can help a lot (see Infrared Sauna in "Nourishing Resources" on page 285). Once you have adapted to the utilization of ketones and free fatty acids as your primary sources of fuel, however, you are much more likely to feel substantially improved across the board. You might notice a positive change in energy levels, moods, and cravings; excess weight is beginning to drop off; you may feel less stiffness in the morning and fewer aches and pains during the day or at night. These are all indicators that you are shifting to a much more efficient and anti-inflammatory fat-burning state.

The Detox Effect

When you begin to focus on eating food from unadulterated and untainted sources, especially if you are more accustomed to a standard American diet, you might initiate a significant measure of detoxification. It's as if the body finally gets the green light to do some housecleaning; now that the fatty tissue is beginning to be mobilized, the cumulative glut of toxins stored there will work their way out. If your avenues of elimination and detoxification are compromised in some way (i.e., through constipation or liver/biliary issues), then this can feel a little cruddy—active detoxification can certainly mimic a tired and run-down state. This is why extra hydration (adding an extra quart or two of water per day) and quality magnesium supplementation (preferably liquid ionic magnesium, Myers cocktails via IV, or transdermal forms) are so important in the early stages of this program. Magnesium is required for both phase I and phase II liver detoxification and can go a long way toward helping ease this part of the transition. Other signs you may not be getting enough magnesium can include muscle spasms, cramping, headaches, and insomnia. In addition, toning down your expectations, being kind to yourself, and giving yourself the rest you require will go a long way. You are clearing the decks and making way for a whole new standard of real health and metabolic freedom. You are effectively "re-booting" yourself!

If uncomfortable symptoms persist throughout the full three weeks, it might be time to assess whether something might be awry in your body. By "cleaning off the windshield," so to speak, certain long-standing imbalances can sometimes finally be revealed. There may be underlying metabolic, gastrointestinal, hormonal, or immune conditions that a simple change of diet is not going to automatically fix. Be open to finding a knowledgeable specialist in functional medicine to help diagnose certain conditions that may be present. Further testing may eventually be required to better clarify what's going on if certain sticking points come up. Don't *expect* this to happen to you—just be mindful that it *could*, and be open to what your body may be telling you.

Sugar Blues

If cravings or hypoglycemic symptoms are a problem during the plan, start taking or increase the dose of *Gymnema sylvestre* and/or L-glutamine. If this isn't sufficient to kill your sugar cravings, then double your dose of gymnema: 400 mg of standardized extract or 4 grams of whole herb taken three times a day. In cases of especially resistant or extreme carbohydrate addiction, doubling the standard 4 grams tends to take care of things. With respect to L-glutamine, I typically recommend ½ to 1 teaspoon of the powder under the tongue two or three times a day during the process of ketogenic adaptation, or during times when you are experiencing or anticipating cravings or low blood sugar symptoms. For instance, if you know you are likely to crave a glass or two of wine in the evenings, taking a dose of L-glutamine right when you get home from work can help offset those cravings. Drop-offs in energy levels and increased tiredness, headaches, mood issues, and cravings tend to be more pronounced in those prone to hypoglycemia or reactive hypoglycemia or those who have a very strong sugar habit. Once you've achieved EKA, you will likely need neither gymnema nor L-glutamine. Think of these supplements as temporary "training wheels" that can help you get over that initial hump. Until then, though, keep them on hand to help stave off symptoms until you better adapt to a more effective state of ketosis. You won't be needing them for long!

Supporting Your Body

During this transition you may experience one or more typical symptoms that can be less than pleasant. All can be fairly easily resolved.

> *Constipation.* Add more full-spectrum salt to your diet and
> use magnesium. Drink plenty of water.
> *Breath and body odor.* During this time your body is beginning
> to increase its production of ketones. You may not yet
> have the capacity to make efficient use of these ketones for
> fuel, so they are likely being handled as a waste product.
> As such, it is possible to notice changes in breath and
> body odor that may be mildly unpleasant. This is very
> temporary. If it becomes problematic for you, consider
> picking up some chlorophyll tablets and consume more
> green drinks during this time (with added parsley), which
> can help neutralize odors considerably.
> *Gas.* For those sensitive to some of the indigestible sugars
> found in cruciferous vegetables, you might try adding a
> digestive aid called Beano to meals containing these foods.
> (If gas persists, see the second tip in the "Troubleshooting
> Corner" section below.)

Troubleshooting Corner: Lessons from a Clinical Nutritionist

This section is a little advanced, but it may help if you come up against obstacles either during or after your three-week plan. These are three of the most common issues that come up for people who become primal fat burners.

UNEXPLAINED WEIGHT GAIN OR STUBBORN SLOWDOWN IN WEIGHT LOSS

A single slip-up (like a piece of birthday cake or a slice of pizza at the office party) can cause fat burning to come to a screeching halt for easily a good three days, or more if food sensitivities are involved. It can also result in quite a bit of water retention, adding significant weight seemingly overnight. Hidden carbohydrates are also a frequent problem. Dried fruits, such as raisins, dates, and figs, are especially problematic: they may seem healthful, but they are adding concentrated sugar to your diet. Although I am not categorically against the notion of having a glass of wine with dinner here and there, if you have weight to lose, then by drinking that wine you are effectively adding lighter fluid to the fire you are trying to put out, and it will likely constitute a backslide for you. I'm just saying. One company, dryfarmwines.com, carries wines that are carb-free and also free from undesirable additives.

Excess protein consumption is another frequently seen issue. If you have been a dyed-in-the-wool sugar burner for the better part of your life, then your body has become extremely efficient at making sugar any way it can. Protein in excess of what you need to meet your physiologic, rebuilding, and regeneration requirements can be converted to sugar in your body and used for ketone-thwarting fuel. I see this issue quite often, and people tell me that as soon as they cut back on the protein to where it should have been and added a little more fat, the weight finally came off. Overconsumption of bone broth can also lead to plateaus.

Many people don't realize that anything that causes an inflammatory response will typically result in temporary weight gain. I am not a fan of bathroom scales as a general rule, but they can be useful as a crude tool to help you ferret out problem foods. If you monitor your weight daily and discover you are two pounds heavier today than yesterday, you need to question whether something you ate yesterday incited an inflammatory response. This can be a very strong indicator of undiagnosed food sensitivities. Keeping a food journal can make any needed detective work much easier, helping you get to the bottom of problems such as this.

CHRONIC GAS AND BLOATING AFTER MEALS, EVEN WITHOUT THE SUGAR AND STARCH

This is a common situation, and it indicates that you may have one or more conditions that require some investigation:

- Small intestinal bacterial overgrowth (SIBO)
- Hydrochloric acid (HCl) insufficiency (often also paired with pancreatic enzyme insufficiency)
- Biliary stasis/gallbladder problems

SIBO is a condition that has been discovered and researched only in recent years. It is frequently found in those having immune reactivity to gluten or a history of alcoholism, but it is also commonly the result of some form of neurological compromise. Chronic neuroinflammation, deterioration, traumatic brain injury, stroke, or advancing dementia can lead to a loss of vagal tone that causes a dysregulation of ileocecal valve function (the otherwise selective gateway between your lower small intestine and your upper colon). When this happens, it can cause even the "good" bacteria in your colon to back up into your small intestine, where they most decidedly do not belong. This can cause plenty of symptoms like gas/bloating or IBS and lead to even bigger issues such as leaky gut. Ironically, many of the things people do to support their colon health (eating extra fiber or taking prebiotics like FOS, Arabinogalactan, or inulin) will actually make SIBO worse. The management of this condition typically requires you to completely avoid even low-sugar, low-starch fibrous vegetables for a period of time, along with anything else that could possibly feed your gut bacteria (save for Acacia gum/Acacia senegal, which is the acceptable exception), though treatment requirements may vary depending upon what the underlying cause of this condition happens to be in a given individual. For more information about this condition, see www.siboinfo.com.

In the case of something like hydrochloric acid insufficiency (also known as hypochlorhydria), you may require supplementation with HCl capsules for a period of time—or possibly even over the long term, depending on the circumstances. Taking extra supplemental pancreatic enzymes can also help. See "Hydrochloric Acid" in Chapter 6.

For information on gallbladder issues, see the "Gallbladder" section in Chapter 6.

UNEXPECTED THYROID LEVELS

Once you've fully made the transition to EKA, it is entirely normal for your T3 (active thyroid hormone) levels to drop slightly and to see small elevations in what is called "reverse T3." This will *not* typically be accompanied by elevations in TSH. This is merely an expression of improved thyroid efficiency that occurs in tandem with perfectly healthy ketogenic adaptation; in fact, it is even a common longevity marker! Think of it as having reached your most efficient orbit and not needing as much rocket fuel to boost you up anymore. It is not remotely pathological or any source of concern, no matter what you might read in the blogosphere. If you are experiencing actual symptoms of low thyroid, you may want to get the appropriate testing, which should of necessity include thyroid antibody markers to ascertain that you are not dealing with an autoimmune condition. Sometimes, too, improving your healthy foundations can result in what I call a "clean windshield effect," which can make previously unnoticed symptoms suddenly more obvious. Remember, however, that association is not necessarily causation. There is nothing in a healthfully adapted, nutrient-dense, quality ketogenic diet that is harmful to your thyroid or anything else, for that matter.

ADRENAL ISSUES

If you feel you might have adrenal fatigue, I urge you to read my ebook *Rethinking Fatigue: What Your Adrenals Are Really Telling You and What You Can Do About It*. It provides rich, detailed information about what it takes to identify and address possible adrenal issues. If your cortisol is chronically low for some reason, then you may experience more stubborn sugar cravings and low blood sugar symptoms.

CHAPTER 11

The Primal Fat-Burning Food Guide

WHAT TO BUY AND HOW TO USE IT
TO ENSURE OPTIMAL HEALTH

There are lots of foods to enjoy when you eat like a primal fat burner—rest assured your plate or bowl will be full on this plan. Here is a quick rundown of what to look for when shopping. Turn to the "Nourishing Resources" section on page 285 for my favorite sources.

Basic Guidelines: Pasture-Raised, Wild-Caught, Organically Grown, Minimally Processed

Meat

Make whatever effort you can to procure meat from 100% organic grass-fed and grass-finished sources. The organic part protects you against the use of GMO alfalfa and the herbicide glyphosate on pastures, which is on the rise. Meats from fully pastured animals are nutritionally superior because green grass and forage are the natural foods for ruminants and herbivores. Fully pastured (and organically raised) animals are not fed GMOs, cheap fillers, antibiotics, hormones, gum wrappers, stale candy, cement dust, or other questionable or harmful additives, therefore the meat, organs, and fat of pastured animals are the most healthful for you. It's also a far more humane, sustainable, and environmentally friendly option.

Beware of the new, more lax laws leading to confused language in this arena. Those not wanting to fuss and bother with quality care and ethics are now allowed to make misleading claims concerning the manner in which their meat was raised. Remember: All cattle spend most of their lives on pasture, but most then go to feedlots, where even a short time gorging on grains changes everything. It is what happens in the last few weeks of the animal's life that determines the fatty acid and fat-soluble nutrient content of the meat you eat! Most grocery markets sell grain-finished meat. Read the labels in the meat case very carefully, or better yet, ask the butcher, "Did the animal from where this meat came spend 100 percent of its life on untreated pasture, or was it grain/feedlot finished?" Be brave and speak up! Grocery stores and restaurants will not change what they try to sell you until consumers uncompromisingly and vocally demand it!

Chicken

Ideally, source fully pastured, or at least free-range and organic, poultry. Pastured chickens are allowed to naturally eat bugs and grasses, which give them the optimal nutritional profile. Organic chicken will at least be fed nonpesticided, non-GMO feed.

Fish

As noted in the section "Staying Strong in a Toxic World" in Chapter 3, because of extensive marine contamination issues I personally tend to avoid most seafood sources from the Northern Hemisphere (even Alaskan waters). Wherever possible I look for wild-caught seafood from pristine Southern Hemisphere waters (Tasmania/New Zealand), where contaminants are likelier to be minimal. Check with your local quality fishmonger. Never, ever eat any fish or shrimp that has come out of the Gulf of Mexico (and yes, it is being sold in markets and restaurants everywhere right now) because of the risk of exposure to petroleum contamination, other chemicals, and especially Corexit (the stuff that BP—in defiance of the EPA's concerns about extreme toxicity—sprayed all over the Gulf to basically hide the oil slick). Farmed fish are frequently exposed to antibiotics, GMO feed, and unsanitary conditions, and they often put wild fish populations at risk. See "Nourishing Resources" on page 285 for information on quality wild-caught or uniquely high-quality farmed fish.

Vegetables, Greens, Nuts, and Sprouts

It's important to strive to consume organic produce, as it minimizes your exposure to GMOs and pesticides and tends to have better nutrient content.

Pantry Goods

Go for minimally processed, preservative-free products with pronounceable ingredients! Make sure that condiments such as mustard are clearly marked "gluten-free." Look for products that are certified GMO-free. Seek out foods that are free of trans fats, hydrogenated/partially hydrogenated fats, and interesterified fats (avoid fractionated oils and palm oil), and always avoid products containing soybean or canola oil. Make sure the products you buy are nonirradiated, contain no MSG, and are free of sugar, starch, and high fructose corn syrup. See "Your Primal Shopping List" at the end of the book.

The Foods to Eat

PROTEINS

Meats

Alpaca
Beef
Bison
Chicken
Cornish hen
Duck
Elk

Emu

Goat

Goose

Guinea fowl

Kangaroo

Lamb

Mutton

Ostrich

Partridge

Pork

Quail

Rabbit

Squab

Turkey

Venison

Wild boar

Yak

Organ Meats and Offal

Blood pudding/blood sausage (make sure these don't include
some starchy filler!)

Brain

Braunschweiger

Gizzards (from poultry)

Headcheese (traditionally, a terrine made with flesh from the
head of a calf or pig, mixed with other organ meat trimmings)

Heart (beef, chicken)

Kidneys (beef, lamb)

Liver (beef, calf, pork, poultry)

Liverwurst

Spleen

Sweetbreads

Tongue (typically beef)

Tripe

Trotters (pigs' feet)

Seafood

As I've noted, most farmed seafood is of highly questionable quality and sustainability, but there are exceptions. One such exception is Ōra King salmon from New Zealand, uniquely farmed in the best possible way; ask your fishmonger if it can be ordered for you. There are some other fish-farming operations in Tasmania and New Zealand, and possibly elsewhere, that seem to do a good job of feeding their fish (i.e., salmon, trout, tilapia) naturally. Be extremely cautious about this, and always ask to see a listing of what the farmed fish are being fed. If a source is questionable at all, avoid it.

Anchovies
Sardines
Trout
Walleye

VEGETABLES

Artichokes
Asparagus
Beets (cultured)
Bok choy
Broccoli
Broccoli rabe
Broccolini
Brussels sprouts
Cabbage (red and green)
Carrots (raw)
Cauliflower
Celery
Cilantro
Collard greens
Cress
Cucumber

Eggplant*
Fennel
Garlic
Garlic spears (sort of like big chives with a bulb attached;
    prepare like asparagus)
Green onions (scallions)
Green or yellow beans
Kale
Kohlrabi
Jicama (raw)
Leeks
Mustard greens
Onions
Parsley
Peppers (bell and hot)*
Purslane
Radishes
Rhubarb
Shallots
Snap peas
Snow peas
Spinach
Swiss chard
Tomatillos*
Tomatoes*

*If you have inflammatory issues, you might attempt a trial of avoiding tomatoes and other nightshades (all tomatoes, bell peppers, hot peppers, eggplant, and goji berries) for a time.

Note: I tend to recommend avoiding most root vegetables, as they have a high starch content that can boot you out of ketosis fast and create a significant glycemic response/increased blood sugar. The exception would be small amounts of raw carrot and jicama.

SALAD GREENS

Lettuces
  Arugula
  Boston lettuce
  Butter lettuce
  Endive
  Escarole
  Frisée
  Green leaf lettuce
  Iceberg (poor in nutrients)
  Lovage
  Mâche
  Mizuna
  Oak leaf lettuce
  Radicchio
  Red leaf lettuce
  Romaine
  Watercress
Sprouts (broccoli, sunflower)
Watercress

Grow Your Own: Why You Should Develop a Sprout Habit

Sprouts are a vegetable-world superfood: cheap, easy to grow yourself, and extraordinarily rich in enzymes (up to a hundred times the amount in raw vegetables and fruits) that allow your body to extract more vitamins, minerals, amino acids, and essential fats from other foods. They are highly detoxifying and help protect the body against numerous environmental contaminants. Add a handful onto your salads, blend some into your smoothies, and accent pretty much any meal you like with them—they're a worthy compliment to fabulous fermented veggies. See "Nourishing Resources" on page 285 for more info.

FRUITS

Any sweet fruit (even those somewhat lower in sugar) should probably be avoided by those having metabolic issues, such as obesity,
diabetes or other blood sugar problems, gout or high uric acid levels,
and inflammation. While fruit isn't essential to the Primal Fat Burner
Plan, fresh berries are an optional inclusion for those without blood
sugar issues, metabolic challenges, or inflammation. Wild blueberries
in particular—the skins being especially rich in sirtuin-enhancing
pterostilbene (better than resveratrol)—are certainly an acceptable and
potentially health-enhancing treat for most.

Avocado
Berries
    Blackberries
    Blueberries (preferably wild)
    Cranberries (only unsweetened)
    Gooseberries
    Marionberries
    Raspberries
    Salmonberries
    Strawberries (only organic)
Lemons
Limes
Olives

HERBS AND SPICES

All herbs and spices (fresh or dried) are fine to use, as long as they are
organic and nonirradiated. Fresh herbs can be grown inexpensively in
your own garden.

NUTS AND SEEDS

Almonds
Brazil nuts
Cashews
Coconuts
Hazelnuts (filberts)
Macadamia nuts
Pecans
Pili nuts (sold by Wild Mountain Paleo; see "Nourishing
    Resources" on page 285)
Pine nuts
Pistachios
Walnuts
Seeds
        Chia seeds (in small amounts)
        Flax seeds (in small amounts)
        Hulled hemp seeds (only organic, nonirradiated)
        Pumpkin seeds (pepitas)
        Sesame seeds
        Sunflower seeds (sparingly, due to high omega-6 content)

Note: Most seeds (except flax and chia) are extremely high in inflammatory omega-6s and should be minimally consumed and/or
balanced with dietary omega-3s. Chia and flax, however, are fairly
estrogenic and should be kept to a minimum. Most hemp seeds are
routinely irradiated.

MUSHROOMS

My personal favorites to cook with are shiitake and maitake mushrooms for their excellent flavor and their uniquely beneficial health
properties. The least nutritious are the button, cremini, and portobello
varieties (which also happen to be the most commonly sold). For
excellent educational information on mushrooms and many of their

extraordinary healing properties, as well as to learn which can be easily grown at home, go to www.fungi.com.

Chanterelles
Chestnut
Enokitake (enoki)
Field
King brown
Lion's mane
Lobster
Maitake (hen of the woods)
Matsutake
Morels
Oyster
Pine
Porcini
Portobello
Reishi
Shiitake
Swiss browns (cremini)
Truffles (very expensive)
White or button
Wood ear

FATS FOR COOKING AND EATING

Avocado oil*
Black seed/black cumin oil* (I recommend the one from Pure Indian Foods)
Chicken fat (schmaltz)**
Duck fat**
Goose fat**
Organic virgin coconut oil
Cultured ghee (the one safe for dairy sensitivities is sold exclusively by Pure Indian Foods)

Pastured, non-hydrogenated lard
Macadamia nut oil* (rich in palmitoleic acid—a newly
    discovered omega-7 fatty acid—fabulous for weight loss
    and improving insulin sensitivity, great on salads and
    drizzled over cooked meats/fish/veggies)
Extra-virgin olive oil*
Sesame oil (in small amounts)
Grass-fed tallow

 *Best used on salads or with very low heat
**Best used with low to medium heat

SWEETENERS

Whole-leaf or unrefined stevia (I like Stevita brand)
Monk fruit extract (lo han guo)

The Foods to Avoid

SEAFOOD AND OTHER OCEAN PRODUCTS

The risk of contamination by mercury, PCBs, radionuclides, Corexit, and other harmful substances means that you should avoid the following types of seafood:

North Pacific seafood in general, and anything from the Gulf
    of Mexico
Atlantic salmon (always farmed)
Chilean sea bass
Grouper
Mackerel (especially king mackerel)
Monkfish
Orange roughy
Shark

Shellfish: clams, crab, lobster, oysters, mussels, scallops, and
  shrimp, unless from verifiably wild, pristine Southern
  Hemisphere sources
Swordfish
Tilefish
Tuna

Avoid kombu, due to its high natural MSG content. Also, at this
time I do not recommend other seaweed or sea vegetables from the
Northern Hemisphere due to potential contamination issues.

OTHER FOODS

Fast food
Grains: amaranth, barley, buckwheat, bulgur, corn, millet,
  oats, quinoa, rice and rice milk, rye, sorghum, spelt,
  tapioca, teff, and wheat
All GMOs
Processed food
Protein bars, powders, or energy bars
Sugar
Sodas
Juices
Sports drinks
Hot dogs
Bologna and other processed lunch meats
Nitrate- and sugar-laced bacon (nitrate-free, sugar-free bacon
  is okay)
Conventionally cured ham, salami, and pepperoni (fats may
  be rancid)
Peanuts and peanut butter (peanuts are a legume, a common
  allergen, and prone to aflatoxin)
Refined table salt, iodized or non-iodized (it will say "sodium
  chloride" on the label)
Figs

Nonorganic papaya

Dried fruit

Legumes

> Chickpeas (garbanzo beans)
>
> Black beans
>
> Broad beans
>
> Kidney beans
>
> Lentils
>
> Lima beans
>
> Navy beans
>
> Peas
>
> Pinto beans
>
> Soybeans and soy products such as soy milk and soy sauce
>
> Tofu
>
> White beans

Dairy

> Milk
>
> Cream
>
> Sour cream
>
> Dairy and/or store-bought yogurt
>
> Ice cream
>
> Cheese
>
> Butter (contains milk solids that can lead to inflammatory response for those immune reactive to them)
>
> Regular ghee (contains milk solids; only the Pure Indian Foods Cultured Ghee and Turmeric Super Ghee are certified as free of dairy proteins)

No More Milk

Butter, cream, and raw milk cheese from cows, sheep, or goats can be absolutely delicious and full of valuable fats. But immune reactivity and inflammatory responses to dairy fats are much more significant and common than most people realize; you may not recognize that you're having immunologic reactions to them until it's too late (as was unfortunately true for me). If you have a dairy sensitivity, it's not just about avoiding glasses of milk; cheese, butter, cream; even most forms of ghee can cause issues, even if the label says it's raw and not pasteurized. Goat, sheep, and cow sources are all potentially cross-reactive with one another, and for many people, simply avoiding casein is not enough, as other dairy proteins can generate a big inflammatory response, too! As a clinical nutritionist, I see a growing problem in which fully half of those with gluten sensitivity are also reactive to dairy foods. Considerable literature in immunology supports the concern that dairy contributes to the growing autoimmunity epidemic in general[1] and multiple sclerosis in particular.[2] Commercial dairy products carry the additional potential for contamination with pesticides, herbicides, GMOs, rBGH, other hormones, and antibiotics.

Finally, and crucially, full-fat milk of any kind or source is still an extremely high-carbohydrate food. The conglomeration of fats and sugars in the same liquid food source has the potential to stall or sabotage any weight loss efforts. (Cow's milk is designed by nature to make a baby cow grow very big very quickly!) This is why I tend to recommend taking it out of the diet entirely. But if I could have my wish for you, dear reader, I would have you test for dairy sensitivity through the only truly accurate laboratory available in the world, Cyrex Labs,[3] before you decide to let dairy products be part of your regular diet. If you test negative for a dairy food sensitivity with them (and only them; see the "Helpful Resources" section), then look for fully pastured, minimally processed sources. If you are interested in the health benefits of raw milk and/or colostrum but want to avoid most of the potential for immune reactivity, you may want to consider camel's milk (mostly indistinguishable in taste to regular cow's milk). It is uniquely nonantigenic (or at least only rarely) in humans due to the molecular similarity to human milk. It has more health benefits than bovine, sheep, or goat sources, with few of the risks, but it is also more costly. It is best used in small amounts as a healing supplement (the brand I recommend is Desert Farms).

Sugars

    Agave (please avoid all of it)

    All artificial sweeteners (see www.doctoroz.com/article/
        list-names-artificial-sweeteners for a complete list)

    Amazake (made from rice)

    Barley malt

    Beet sugar

Birch syrup

Brown sugar

Cane sugar

Coconut nectar or sugar

Corn syrup

Date sugar

Fruit juice concentrate

Honey (yes, honey—unless using the high-MGO manuka
variety for a sore throat)

Maple syrup

Molasses

Palm sugar

Raw sugar

Rice syrup

Sorghum syrup

Sucanat

Turbinado sugar

White table sugar

Xylitol (may be GMO and has a delayed glycemic response)

Sweet Cheats

Research suggests that artificial noncaloric sweeteners such as aspartame and saccha-
rine contribute to obesity even more than refined sugar![4] They increase your cravings
for carbohydrates and your appetite and increase the amount of fat your body stores.
Two key amino acids in aspartame—phenylalanine and aspartic acid (which make up
about 90 percent of aspartame, sold under the names NutraSweet and Equal)—have
been shown to rapidly stimulate the two key hormones that regulate your fat stores
in an adverse way: insulin and leptin. Interestingly, pure, unrefined stevia (a non-
carbohydrate sweetener derived from the leaves of the South American stevia plant)
did not have the same negative effect on insulin levels.[5] Still, stevia is extremely sweet
and can keep you looking for more of that sweet taste if you overuse it. Avoid the overly
processed commercial versions of stevia commonly sold (they are bleached and contain
chemical additives—read all labels). I personally use Stevita brand liquid stevia.

Processed oils

    Canola oil (never—not even the supposedly organic variety)

    Corn oil

    Cottonseed oil

    Grapeseed oil (extracted using hexane)

    Hemp oil

    Margarine

    Palm oil/red palm/palm kernel oil (may cause gut inflammation,[6] is frequently interesterified, and is environmentally unsustainable)

    Peanut oil

    Rice bran oil

    Safflower oil

    Soybean oil

    Sunflower oil

    Wheat germ oil (also contains gluten)

    All processed commercial vegetable oil blends

When Good Fats Go Bad: Using Fats Safely

Though primal fat burners do love fat dearly, our love is not unconditional. It's very important to avoid fats that have become rancid and/or oxidized, which happens when fats and oils are overprocessed, improperly stored, stored for too long, or overheated. Any of these things can generate especially aggressive, damaging free radical activity in the body. Remember, fat and fat-soluble nutrients have a profound effect upon your mitochondria and mitochondrial DNA and may even affect your nuclear DNA, initiating or modifying gene expression and gene transcription. This power can work for you or against you, depending upon the quality and relative balance of those fats and fat-soluble nutrients. A rancid fat is more likely to generate a genetic mutation than to support optimal health. Follow these five rules for using fats safely.

Rule #1: Store Them Well, Use Them Quickly

Fats naturally present within meats, nuts, and seeds are far safer within the matrix of their natural home than they are when separated from it. Once a fat has been removed from its natural source, it should either be used immediately or stored properly in a cool, dry place away from sunlight (ideally in a dark-colored glass container) or kept refrigerated or frozen. Once the container is opened, fat varies quite a bit in stability. Coconut oil and tallow are pretty stable and can last a few months unrefrigerated. Vegetable oils such as olive and avocado oils are less stable and once opened should be used up within a couple of months. Other more fragile oils need some means of proper preservation: vitamin E, rosemary oil, and vitamin D. Check the label.

If that open bottle of olive oil has been sitting in your cupboard for more than a couple of months, it may very well not be worth keeping around. Better to buy smaller bottles and use them relatively rapidly than that big "bargain bottle" of olive oil that sits in your cupboard oxidizing for a year.

Rule #2: Never, Ever Overheat Fats

Practicing safe cooking methods is incredibly important when it comes to retaining the quality and integrity of the fats you consume and ensuring they help your health, not harm it. It's always safest to cook at low or medium heat (unless you are boiling water). If you do fry or sauté using higher heat, pick the right fat or oil and pay careful attention to the smoking point. This is the temperature threshold where fatty acids and other volatile compounds undergo rapid degradation and also produce toxic, volatile, noxious, peroxidized, potentially damaging, and even carcinogenic compounds (such as free radicals and various toxic aldehydes). Signs that you have passed the threshold include actual smoke rising from the pan, an associated acrid odor, or a darkened color. Abort mission! Immediately discard the heated fat (pour it into a glass jar until it's cool enough to go into the trash), and if possible, avoid food cooked in such damaged oil.

This may sound extreme, but the potential consequences of consuming spoiled fats are serious.

Most saturated fats and oils will hold up fine up to 350°F (medium heat). Butter tends to burn at lower temperatures, often between 250° and 300°F, because of its relatively high protein (milk solids) content. Cultured ghee, free of proteins, is more forgiving. Refined olive oil may burn at temperatures as low as 325°F. The smoke point varies depending on how refined the oil is, so use your eyes and nose. If you fry or sauté, it's safest to use lard or cultured ghee. I personally never heat any fat above medium heat. Most of the cooking I do is right at about 250° to 275°F.

Boiling or poaching fatty meats and fish—fully immersing the protein in boiling water—greatly minimizes the potential for unhealthy oxidation. As long as you don't overdo it and you melt a great oil on top (or my fabulous Primal Gaucho Chimichurri), the results are terrific. (The new trend of sous-vide cooking takes this to melt-in-your-mouth, gourmet extremes.)

To truly safeguard your health when cooking, invest in an induction-based cooking technology. It eliminates a lot of risk and guesswork by giving you exact temperature control when frying, simmering, sautéing, searing, barbecuing, melting, and grilling. There are even affordable, freestanding induction hot plates. Ever since I got mine, I don't use the regular stove anymore.

Rule #3: Not All Oils of the Same Kind Are Equal

It is wise to have both quality refined and unrefined coconut and olive oils on hand. Use the cold-processed, organic, unrefined, or virgin oil for raw use (salads, flavorings, etc.), and you'll get their antioxidant and nutritional goodness. But the presence of naturally occurring organic particulate matter makes the unrefined versions vulnerable to damage when heated, so use the refined versions (or just lower the heat) for frying or sautéing.

Rule #4: Minimize Aged Fats

Aged fats refers to deli meats and fatty meats preserved with nitrates or nitrites. Bacon needs to be carefully sourced. Seek fully pastured and non-GMO-fed pork that has been processed without sodium and sugar. I always cook my low-sodium, sugar-free, nitrate-free bacon in the oven at 350°F for about twenty minutes, give or take. I season it myself, and it is to die for. I promise that once you have tried this using an oven you will never look back. The bacon turns out perfect every time and the fats are not overheated. You can even save the bacon fat for a couple of days and use it to sauté on low heat if you want, but don't keep it any longer than that or heat it any higher. Conventional brands of bacon are to be avoided because they use nitrates or nitrites (either industrial sources or the seemingly innocent "celery powder" sources of these same sketchy compounds), lots of commercially refined salt (which is *highly* inflammatory), and a ton of sugar. The animals are also frequently fed GMO feed. It pays to be fussy with bacon.

Rule #5: Watch Out for Trans Fats and Interesterified Fats

The science is clear that industrialized oils like canola and soy are "trash oils"—they're often extracted with toxic solvents, GMO sourced, lose omega-3s in the hydrogenation/interesterification process, and go rancid when exposed to heat. Yet many if not most restaurants cook with them, because they are dirt cheap! They are pervasive in grocery store delis (including at supposedly "natural" food stores) and in most processed foods (check the label of your mayonnaise). Ask restaurants and delis what they use for cooking and dressings. If it's "vegetable oil," canola, or soy, go elsewhere and tell them why that concerns you. Better restaurants will often specially cook your food in olive oil (hopefully at a lower heat) and will bring olive oil and balsamic vinegar for salads if you request them.

CHAPTER 12

The Primal Fat Burner
Meal Plan and Recipes

This meal plan is designed to help you achieve a fat-burning state fairly easily. There are no calorie counts or absolutely precise portion sizes to eat, because this isn't a one-size-fits-all approach to eating. Your portion size, mainly when it comes to protein, depends upon how much you weigh and other factors such as activity level, age, and other unique demands that may accompany illness. This plan is about *eating*, and eating well! You'll find sixty truly delicious fat-burning recipes; use them daily for twenty-one days, or as you get in the swing of things, go freestyle by making meals of simply cooked protein, served according to the guidelines below, with lots of vegetables filling your plate or bowl and ample fats eaten till satiety.

What You Can Eat

At each meal, eat no more than 2 to 3 ounces (60 to 90 grams) of protein, such as a small chicken thigh, several slices of beef or pork, a lamb chop, or a small fish fillet. To calculate your approximate total daily protein needs, see "Protein Math" on page 199. Try to get close to that total each day. If after a month or two you start feeling as though you are not getting enough protein in your diet (you feel fatigued, have brittle nails, are losing hair, have stopped menstruating, or feel continually hungry), the problem is more likely to be poor digestion than not enough protein. Follow the guidelines for HCl supplementation (see "Hydrochloric Acid" in Chapter 6) to improve the digestion and utilization of the protein you are consuming. You might also want to incorporate proteolytic pancreatic enzymes with this, in addition to adding some highly absorbable and utilizable Vital Proteins Collagen Peptides to your diet. They can be added to any liquid, sauce, or soup. (But be sure to count that protein!)

It is generally better to err on the side of a little *less* protein than a little too much (except for those categories of people listed at the bottom of "Protein Math"). In fact, the latest research on cancer initiation suggests significantly less protein than what I outline below, using 0.5 gram per kilogram of body weight instead of 0.8 gram. Read about why this is important in the section "Cancer: A New Approach to a Uniquely Modern Problem" in Chapter 8.

Fill your plate or bowl with abundant vegetables, greens, and sprouts at each meal. You may use a handful of nuts and a few seeds here and there. If you stick to the approved foods listed in Chapter 10, it will be almost impossible to exceed the 50 to 60 grams of carbs per day that is the threshold for fat burning. That will free you of the need to track carb intake—it's liberating!

Cook and finish your foods with as much fat as you need to feel satiated. This will vary from person to person and from day to day. Sauté foods in plenty of coconut oil, Pure Indian Foods Cultured Ghee (your best choices in the beginning if you're trying to lose weight as well as using macadamia nut oil), rendered tallow from pastured beef or mutton, lard from pastured pigs, or duck, chicken, or goose fat. (Be mindful of the temperature you cook with, and try not to ever exceed medium heat, except with quick searing, as you don't want to risk having the oil go rancid during cooking. See "When Good Fats Go Bad" in Chapter 11.) Add avocados, olives, and chopped nuts like macadamias to your plate. Be generous with drizzling fats (extra-virgin olive, avocado, and macadamia nut oils) on your salads and cooked vegetables. A drizzle of sesame oil in stir-fries is fine.

Protein Math

The one piece of homework you have to do diligently at first is learning what a "moderate" serving of protein is for your needs. Worry not; this brief calculation is as easy as 1, 2, 3. It requires about sixty seconds and a basic calculator. And if you are following the recipes, the math has mostly been done for you. If you are cooking something on your own from scratch, here's the basic formula:

1. Estimate what you think of as your ideal body weight (it might be different from your current weight).

2. Convert that number from pounds to kilograms by dividing by 2.2. For example, if you weigh 300 pounds but know your ideal weight is 140, then use the number 140. Divide this by 2.2, which is 63.63 kilograms. Round up to the closest whole number, 64, for the sake of simplicity.

3. Take this number, 64, and multiply that by 0.8,* which in this case gives you 51.2. Round off to 51. This is how many grams of protein you need to shoot for *in a whole day*. Don't eat all of this at once, but instead spread that amount over two or three meals.

4. To calculate portion sizes of meat, fish, and eggs—which are high in protein but also have a lot of other things in them, like fat (hopefully), water, vitamins, minerals, and other nutrients—you have to count the hidden grams of protein. I strongly recommend using an inexpensive digital scale that measures in ounces and grams at first (soon you will be familiar enough with your portion sizes that you won't need it). Weigh your meat or fish raw, before cooking, for the most accurate measurement. Then, use the following guide:

    i. One ounce (or 30 grams) of raw meat or fish contains about 7 grams of protein. This means that 2 to 3 ounces of meat or fish is appropriate for each meal for most people. This is a piece of meat or fish about the size of a deck of playing cards or the palm of your hand.

    ii. A chicken egg contains roughly 6 to 7 grams of protein (depending on the size). Thus you should have a maximum of 3 eggs per meal.

    iii. A cup of homemade bone broth contains close to 7 grams of protein.

    iv. Two ounces of most nuts contain close to 7 grams of protein.

5. Armed with this information, you can cook a meal from scratch and keep your portion sizes in check. (The recipes in this book have all been designed so that each portion is around 2 to 3 ounces.) Come back to this exercise every so often, as it's easy to get a little loose and increase protein sizes unconsciously.

*Elite athletes, women who are pregnant or trying to become pregnant, and nursing mothers should multiply by 1.5 instead of 0.8 to better meet their increased protein demands. Children and teens who may be using the Primal Fat Burner Plan either for therapeutic needs or for weight loss (under the guidance of a knowledgeable health care provider and/or knowledgeable parent) should also multiply by 1.5, as growing young people should *not* overly restrict their protein intake.

The Meal Plan

The 21-day meal plan included here offers general guidelines to help you get your total daily nutritional requirements without going over your carb threshold. It is not carved in stone, of course. If you aren't hungry enough to eat Hearty Breakfast Hash in the morning, as recommended on a certain day, don't! Feel free to swap out any breakfast menu items with another recipe. Or make breakfast out of last night's dinner leftovers, if you'd prefer. As time goes on you might find that you are less hungry in the mornings and satisfied with a cup of warm broth to kick off your day. This is absolutely fine. You may also make your own simple meals based on the Primal Fat Burner Plan, as already mentioned. In this case, ensure that your ingredients are nutrient-dense, based on the food lists in Chapter 11. Take a moment to check your protein serving size, heap your plate or bowl with approved vegetables, and have a liberal hand with fats (for cooking and raw serving). You will stay in your primal fat-burning zone this way.

You will find that you eventually become less hungry on this dietary plan than you have been used to. Skipping one meal a day is fine, *but be sure to meet your daily protein requirements, and eat enough fat!* Without enough fat you will find yourself becoming hungrier and may become more vulnerable to cravings. Also, I encourage you to be adventurous and eat organ meats at least two or three times per week, which will help tremendously in getting you the quality protein and key fat-soluble and other nutrients your body requires.

Special note for vegetarians: If you are presently following a vegetarian or vegan way of eating and are trying to reincorporate more animal foods into your diet, I urge you to stick to bone broths and broth-based recipes for at least the first two weeks—up to a month—to ease your body into making use of complete, animal-source protein again. By avoiding animal proteins you may have lost your ability to produce enough hydrochloric acid and may experience digestive discomfort until your body gets used to making it again. Consider adding a scoop of Vital Protein Collagen Peptides to those broth-based meals in order to enhance the digestibility and absorbability of the available protein and provide extra assistance with gut healing. Each scoop contains 9 grams of protein, so adjust the amount of protein you eat accordingly.

Other tips:

- If you are trying to lose weight, then be careful how much protein you eat. Be generous with the coconut oil or Pure Indian Foods Cultured Ghee, as some of their short- and medium-chain fats convert to ketones more readily and may be easier on your gallbladder than longer-chained saturated fats if you aren't used to them. Use macadamia nut oil on your salad

- If you are trying to lose *a lot* of weight, eat your larger meals at lunch and lighter meals (salads, Breakfast Broth, etc.) for an early dinner most nights. Try to eat most of your meals within a six- to eight-hour window, and don't eat anything in the three or four hours before going to bed. This can give you many of the added benefits of intermittent fasting while helping maximize your weight loss.

- If you are underweight or don't want to lose weight, then liquid calories may be a better choice. Be sure to use the Power Breakfast Smoothie, puree soups with added coconut milk, and use nut butters (like my Almond-Cardamom Ambrosia) as a snack or add them to smoothies. Consuming a bit more bone broth and adding some Vital Protein Collagen Peptides, which contains a number of nutrients useful for healing leaky guts (something not uncommon in those who are underweight and may have malabsorption issues) can be helpful.

- If you have an autoimmune disease, such as Hashimoto's, rheumatoid arthritis, multiple sclerosis, asthma, psoriasis, celiac disease, or type 1 diabetes, you *may* need to further restrict certain foods to avoid immune reactivity. The most common culprits are eggs, nuts and seeds (including sometimes coconut), and nightshade vegetables (tomatoes, bell and other peppers, and eggplants). You might try systematically eliminating these to see if your symptoms improve. If after a couple of weeks you continue to have inflammatory symptoms or aren't losing any weight, start keeping a food journal to track your daily food intake, paying special attention to any symptoms that arise, such as fatigue, stomach upset, brain fog, headaches, joint pain, or other signs of inflammation. Once you have identified a suspect food, try eliminating it from your diet for at least two weeks to see if that is the food causing the problem. If you're not sure after two weeks, try eating a lot of that food all at once (if, say, you're testing eggs, then eat a big omelet made with two or three eggs; if it's nuts, try eating a big handful or a couple of tablespoons of nut butter). Wait two or three days. If you feel an increase in any of your symptoms during that time (or see a jump up in weight on the bathroom scale), then you'll have your answer. You should simply eliminate that food from your daily menu.

To get to the bottom of troublesome or more elusive food sensitivities much more quickly and in the most detail, ask your qualified health care provider to order food sensitivity testing for you through Cyrex Labs (www.cyrexlabs.com).

DAY 1

BREAKFAST: Spinach Egg Bake or Power Breakfast Smoothie (if you don't want to lose weight)

LUNCH: Mixed green salad (see A Road Map for a Composed Salad and Easy Primal Dressing) with ½ sliced avocado and 2 to 3 olives (whole, chopped, or sliced)

DINNER: Thai Chicken Curry Stir-Fry

DAY 2

BREAKFAST: Roasted Marrow Bones (2 half marrow bones), 2 to 3 tablespoons Primal Cultured Vegetable Kraut

LUNCH: Best Ever Chicken Salad on a bed of mixed greens

DINNER: Primal Zoodles

DAY 3

BREAKFAST: Breakfast Broth, with added greens and yellow curry (meat optional)

LUNCH: Primal Ground Beef Salad

DINNER: Chicken Thigh Skillet Supper with steamed broccolini or asparagus and a drizzle of olive or avocado oil

DAY 4

BREAKFAST: Primal Power Breakfast

LUNCH: 1 cup leftover Best Ever Chicken Salad or 1 cup Hearty Primal Chili

DINNER: Primal Chicken Marsala with Sautéed Wild Mushrooms and Vegetables, Primal Cauliflower Fried Rice, 2 to 3 tablespoons Primal Cultured Vegetable Kraut

DAY 5

BREAKFAST: Primal Omelet

LUNCH: Breakfast Broth for lunch: add 1 to 2 ounces raw ground beef while simmering, plus a bit of salsa, ½ to 1 clove minced garlic (or ⅛ teaspoon garlic powder), and Himalayan/Celtic sea salt to taste

DINNER: Primal Roast Chicken (about 2 ounces of cooked chicken), Cauliflower Mashers, 2 to 3 tablespoons Primal Cultured Vegetable Kraut

DAY 6

BREAKFAST: Slow Cooker Vegetable Stew *or* Power Breakfast Smoothie (if you don't want to lose weight)

LUNCH: Mixed vegetable salad (see A Road Map for a Composed Salad and Easy Primal Dressing) topped with ½ sliced avocado and 2 ounces leftover Primal Roast Chicken

DINNER: Primalritos

DAY 7

BREAKFAST: Breakfast Broth with seasonings and vegetables or greens of choice *or* Power Breakfast Smoothie (if you don't want to lose weight)

LUNCH: Primal Cauliflower Fried Rice with vegetables of choice and 2 ounces leftover Primal Roast Chicken, or Breakfast Broth for lunch (see Day 5)

DINNER: Hearty Burgers with Mushrooms, Cauliflower Mashers, 2 to 3 tablespoons Primal Cultured Vegetable Kraut

DAY 8

BREAKFAST: Primal Huevos Rancheros with Primal Greek Spinach

LUNCH: Bone Broth with 2 ounces leftover cooked meat, ⅛ teaspoon garlic powder, ⅛ teaspoon ginger, 1 teaspoon curry powder, and a splash of coconut milk *or* leftover Best Ever Chicken Salad, mixed vegetable salad (see A Road Map for a Composed Salad and Easy Primal Dressing) topped with ½ sliced avocado and a chopped hard-boiled egg

DINNER: Primal Kālua Pork, Lithuanian Red Cabbage

DAY 9

BREAKFAST: 1 cup Breakfast Broth with 2 to 3 tablespoons of salsa *or* Power Breakfast Smoothie (if you don't want to lose weight)

LUNCH: Thai Salad with Spicy Dressing

DINNER: Cumin Pork Stir-Fry, Primal Cauliflower Fried Rice

DAY 10

BREAKFAST: Primal Breakfast "Fondue" with coconut oil or
Primal Gaucho Chimichurri

LUNCH: Amazing Coconut Thai Soup

DINNER: Carnitas Salad

DAY 11

BREAKFAST: Breakfast Sausage Patty with Sautéed Greens, 2 to 3
tablespoons Primal Cultured Vegetable Kraut

LUNCH: Coconut-Lemon Yogurt Soup or leftover Amazing
Coconut Thai Soup

DINNER: Larb Wraps

DAY 12

BREAKFAST: 1 or 2 hard-boiled eggs with salty seasoning of
choice *or* leftover Amazing Coconut Thai Soup or Power
Breakfast Smoothie (if you don't want to lose weight)

LUNCH: Mixed vegetable salad (see A Road Map for a Composed
Salad and Easy Primal Dressing) topped with ¼ sliced
avocado and meat if desired

DINNER: Lamb Chop Skillet Supper, Primally Raw Cauliflower
Tabouli

DAY 13

BREAKFAST: Breakfast Broth with or without added meat or salsa
or Power Breakfast Smoothie (if you don't want to lose weight)

LUNCH: Grilled Caesar Salad

DINNER: Liver and Bacon, Cauliflower Mashers, Lithuanian Red
Cabbage, steamed broccoli drizzled with olive or avocado oil

DAY 14

BREAKFAST: Hearty Breakfast Hash

LUNCH: Breakfast Broth with meat, greens, and seasonings of choice

DINNER: Wild-Caught Trout or Walleye Almondine, Primal
Greek Spinach

DAY 15

BREAKFAST: Primal Power Breakfast

LUNCH: Mixed vegetable salad (see A Road Map for a Composed
Salad and Easy Primal Dressing) topped with ½ sliced
avocado, meat if desired, and 1 to 2 tablespoons pine nuts if
desired

DINNER: Chicken Heart Anticuchos, The Best Kale Salad with
½ sliced avocado on the side and seasoned to taste with
Himalayan/Celtic sea salt

DAY 16

BREAKFAST: Roasted bone marrow, sautéed greens, Primal Greek
Spinach, 2 to 3 tablespoons Primal Cultured Vegetable Kraut

LUNCH: Curried Lamb and Chicken Gizzard Stew

DINNER: Primal Zoodles with a mixed vegetable salad (see A
Road Map for a Composed Salad and Easy Primal Dressing)
topped with ½ sliced avocado

DAY 17

BREAKFAST: Breakfast Sausage Patty with Sautéed Greens, 2 to 3
tablespoons of Primal Cultured Vegetable Kraut on the side

LUNCH: Hearty Primal Chili

DINNER: Best Ever Grilled Steak, Cauliflower Mashers, steamed
asparagus drizzled with melted duck fat, olive oil, or avocado oil

DAY 18

BREAKFAST: Primal Breakfast "Fondue"

LUNCH: Lithuanian Šaltibarščiai Soup, large salad of mixed
greens and chopped veggies with hard-boiled egg or leftover
chicken or steak and Easy Primal Dressing

DINNER: 3 ounces Crispy Pork Belly, Primal Greek Spinach or
Lithuanian Red Cabbage, 2 to 3 tablespoons Primal Cultured
Vegetable Kraut

DAY 19

BREAKFAST: Primal Huevos Rancheros

LUNCH: Coconut-Lemon Yogurt Soup

DINNER: Fish Tacos, 2 to 3 tablespoons of Primal Cultured
Vegetable Kraut

DAY 20

BREAKFAST: Coconut Yogurt with a handful of blueberries or
Power Breakfast Smoothie (if you don't want to lose weight)

LUNCH: Large chopped vegetable salad with sliced avocado,
artichoke hearts, a sprinkle of walnuts or pine nuts, and
sliced meat if desired

DINNER: Braised Chicken Thighs with Mushrooms

DAY 21

BREAKFAST: Pan-seared chicken livers with sautéed spinach and
pine nuts

LUNCH: Coconut-Lemon Yogurt Soup

DINNER: 2 to 3 ounces sliced Best Ever Grilled Steak topped
with Primal Gaucho Chimichurri and sautéed onions and
mushrooms, The Best Kale Salad, 2 to 3 tablespoons Primal
Cultured Vegetable Kraut

The Recipes

The Basics: The "Fatisfying" Dishes to Always Have On Hand

Please be sure to use all-organic ingredients wherever possible and
fully pastured (i.e., grass-fed and grass-finished, non-factory-farmed)
meats and poultry for every recipe. See "Nourishing Resources" on
page 285 for information on finding fully pastured meats and wild-
caught fish.

Primal Gaucho Chimichurri
Makes about 3 cups

Here's the ultimate dipping sauce—or even a salad dressing! Slather this version of the South American favorite over steamed or roasted vegetables for an easy meal. Use it as an elegant sauce with roasted or grilled beef, pork, chicken, or fish. It's also terrific spooned over eggs or even spread into a coconut wrap for an on-the-go pick-me-up. Make your first batch a little thicker until you get the hang of your preferred consistency. You can always thin it out with more olive oil when you drizzle it over salads and vegetables. The sauce won't freeze well, but it will keep in the fridge for up to a week.

1 cup packed fresh cilantro leaves

1 cup packed fresh flat-leaf parsley leaves

8 medium garlic cloves

¼ cup raw unfiltered cider vinegar (such as Bragg)

3 tablespoons fresh oregano leaves

3 tablespoons fresh lemon juice

2 tablespoons minced red onion

Up to 2 teaspoons red pepper flakes

1 teaspoon ground black pepper

½ teaspoon Himalayan or Celtic sea salt

Up to 2 cups extra-virgin cold-pressed olive oil

1. Place the cilantro, parsley, garlic, vinegar, and oregano in a food processor fitted with the chopping blade. Cover and pulse until finely chopped but not liquefied. Scrape the contents into a medium bowl.
2. Stir in the lemon juice, onion, red pepper flakes, black pepper, and salt. Then stir in 1 cup oil until combined. Drizzle in more oil, up to 1 additional cup, stirring all the while, until the mixture reaches the texture of pesto, a wetter dipping sauce, or even a salad dressing. Store, covered, in the refrigerator for up to 1 week but bring back to room temperature before serving.

Primal Bone Broth

Makes 2½ to 3 quarts

I love making bone broth. But I like to make a giant batch and freeze it. This recipe's for a more manageable amount, but you can always double or even triple it. What's the difference between a broth and a stock? A broth is typically eaten as is or lightly garnished, while a stock is used in the preparation of other dishes, like sauce and soups. If you can find chicken feet, use them to add more gelatin to the broth (which is extremely nourishing and adds more body to the soup). You can also use 1 to 2 scoops of Vital Proteins Gelatin, lightly sprinkled onto the broth and stirred in as it's cooking (note that this adds 9 grams of extra protein to your recipe per scoop). I use new canning jars and lids to store the broth in the freezer in 1- or 2-cup servings. Do not use recycled jars: they can break in the freezer. Fill the jars just three-quarters full, as the broth will expand in the freezer.

> 1 leftover roasted organic free-range chicken carcass,
>   cut into several pieces
> 1 pound organic free-range chicken feet, cleaned
>   (see Note), organic free-range chicken necks
>   and/or wings, or 1 to 2 scoops Vital Proteins
>   Gelatin
> 2 large yellow or white onions, peeled and quartered
> 1 large head garlic, separated into cloves and peeled
> 1 medium lemon, halved and seeded
> ¼ cup raw unfiltered cider vinegar (such as Bragg)
> 1 tablespoon black peppercorns
> 2 bay leaves
> 2 teaspoons Himalayan or Celtic sea salt

1. Place the chicken carcass and chicken feet in a large stockpot. Add the onions, garlic, lemon, vinegar, peppercorns, and bay leaves. Pour in enough water to submerge the ingredients, then cover

them by at least 2 more inches of water, perhaps 4 to 6 quarts. Refrigerate for 1 hour.

2. Set the uncovered stockpot over high heat and bring it to a full boil. Skim and discard any scum that rises to the surface. Cover, reduce the heat to very low, and simmer for 6 hours. If you are using the gelatin instead of the feet or chicken parts, sprinkle it over the liquid and stir in.

3. Strain the broth through a colander set over another large pot or a very large bowl. (For the clearest broth, line the colander with cheesecloth.) Stir in the salt. The broth can be refrigerated, covered, for up to 4 days (it will gel), or frozen.

Note: To clean chicken feet, fill a large bowl with 2 quarts water and 2 cups raw unfiltered apple cider vinegar. Add the feet, stir well, and set aside for 10 minutes. Drain in a colander and rinse thoroughly with cool tap water to remove any grit.

MORE

This broth can be used in a multitude of ways: on its own, as a stock base for soups or chili, as an enhancer for sauces, for deglazing skillet-prepared recipes, or on its own as a warm and nourishing meal. You can also modify this recipe to include beef, pork, or lamb bones (or a combination of these).

To doctor this broth for lunch or dinner, place a small amount of chopped and stemmed leafy greens, perhaps a few small broccoli florets, maybe chopped green beans or asparagus, some leftover roast chicken or pork, sliced mushrooms, or even just a couple of stems of fresh herbs like rosemary or tarragon in a bowl. Heat 1 to 2 cups broth to a low simmer, then ladle over these ingredients. Wait a minute or two for them to wilt or heat through.

Easy Primal Dressing

Makes about 1½ cups

Finish every salad with this easy dressing! Then take it way beyond chopped lettuces. Drizzle it over avocado halves or thinly sliced fennel. Or use it as a condiment with roasted, steamed, or even raw cauliflower or broccoli. Better yet, spoon a little over just about any protein off the grill: fish, chicken, pork, or beef. It's as versatile as it is delicious!

    1 cup avocado oil, macadamia nut oil, or extra-virgin cold-pressed
        olive oil (or a blend of these)
    ¼ cup organic balsamic vinegar
    1½ tablespoons raw unfiltered cider vinegar
    1 tablespoon organic whole grain mustard
    ½ teaspoon ground black pepper
    ¼ teaspoon Himalayan or Celtic sea salt

Put all the ingredients in a small bowl; whisk until well combined and emulsified. Use immediately or cover and store in the refrigerator for up to 2 weeks (return to room temperature before whisking again).

Primal Cultured Vegetable Kraut

Makes about 1½ quarts

We don't have to turn on the stove to make the best cultured vegetable sauerkraut! First, remove the hard center core from the cabbage, then cut the vegetable into thin slices, which you can separate and chop into shreds. Or use a food processor with the slicing blade to create shreds from cored cabbage quarters. To ward off possible contamination, wear latex, nitrile, or vinyl gloves when working with sauerkraut. Once the sauerkraut is ready, serve it alongside any roasted meat. Or mix it into a chopped vegetable salad—you won't need any additional dressing. Or fork up a bit during the day for a burst of energy.

> 1 medium cabbage (about 3 pounds), such as red, green, Savoy or
>   Napa, cored and shredded
> 1½ tablespoons Himalayan or Celtic sea salt
> 1 tablespoon minced fresh ginger, caraway seeds, dried dill, fennel
>   seeds, or thinly sliced green chiles such as jalapeño or serrano
>   (optional)

1. Put the cabbage in a large bowl; sprinkle with the salt. Put on a pair of latex, nitrile, or vinyl gloves and rub and squeeze the salt through the cabbage, tossing and mixing constantly, until the vegetable starts to release its juices and becomes quite soft, about 10 minutes. Mix in the ginger or other seasoning, if using.

2. Divide the mixture between 2 sterilized 1-quart mason jars, tamping the cabbage down after each addition. Make sure each jar has 1 inch of space at the top.

3. Cover the mouth of each jar with a double layer of cheesecloth; secure with a rubber band. Set the jars on a rimmed baking sheet or in a baking pan in case the mixture bubbles up and the liquid comes over the top of the jars. Store in a cool room, around 65°F.

4. For the first 24 hours, occasionally remove the cheesecloth and press down on the cabbage mixture with gloved fingers to encourage the vegetable to release more moisture. After 24 hours, the cabbage should be submerged in liquid. If not, whisk 1 teaspoon of sea salt into 1 cup of water in a small bowl, then add as much of this brine to the jars as needed to submerge all the cabbage.

5. Cover the jars again with cheesecloth and return them to the cool room for 3 to 10 days, until the cabbage has a pleasantly sour flavor. The longer the cabbage sits, the softer and more sour it will become. Once the sauerkraut is to your liking, stop the fermentation process by covering the jars tightly with canning lids or plastic wrap and a rubber band and then storing in the refrigerator for up to 1 month.

Note: To sterilize mason jars, either submerge the empty jars in a big pot of boiling water for 10 minutes or run them through an *empty* dishwasher *with no detergent* on an extra-hot cycle followed by the heated drying cycle. Set the jars upside down on paper towels on a heat-safe surface to dry for at least 15 minutes before using.

MORE

See my website primalfatburner.com for a more advanced bulk cultured vegetable recipe!

Beet Kvass
Makes 2 pints (1 serving = 4 ounces)

If you don't want to make beet kvass, a fermented beverage, you can buy it at health food stores. Zukay.com makes an excellent beet kvass as well as other fermented and cultured beverages. But once in a while it's great (and more affordable) to try it on your own! The beverage is strained from the beets and imbibed in small amounts as a daily tonic. Use kvass as you would vinegar in salad dressings and marinades. Or use it as the base of a cold soup, like my delicious and medicinal Lithuanian Šaltibarščiai Soup (page 239).

>   1½ pounds red beets
>   4 teaspoons Himalayan or Celtic sea salt

1. Without peeling them, scrub the beets, and chop them into ½-inch chunks. Be careful to include the part where the bulb connects to the stems (it contains a concentration of healthy bile-thinning properties). Place the beets in a 2-quart sterilized mason jar.
2. Add the salt. Pour enough water into the jar to cover the beets and leave a 2-inch headspace at the top of the jar.
3. Cover the jar with a double layer of cheesecloth and secure it with a rubber band. Agitate a little and place in a cool room, about 68°F,

to ferment, agitating the jar every day, for 1 to 2 weeks, depending on your taste preference. Sample a little after 1 week and see how it tastes to you. The longer the beets ferment, the more sour (sort of like yogurt or kefir) they'll become.

4. Skim off any surface mold or debris, then strain the kvass through a colander lined with more cheesecloth into one or more sealable containers or jars. Refrigerate for up to 1 week.

Note: Although beets themselves are typically high in sugar (most table sugar is made with GMO sugar beets, by the way, not sugar cane), the fermentation process actually removes most of the sugar from the finished product. The sugars are instead used to feed probiotic bacteria. The result is a healthful, low- or no-sugar probiotic beverage with all the inherent benefits associated with beets themselves. Beet kvass can be made in a couple of different ways: with a starter culture or in a wild fermentation that relies on naturally occurring bacteria from the soil and surrounding environment. Purchasing a culture isn't necessary, but there can be significant benefits if you use a really good one. Dr. Joseph Mercola sells one in particular that has some rather exciting benefits. Called Kinetic Culture, this probiotic culture is specifically formulated to boost vitamin K_2 production from the bacterial fermentation. Using a culture can also promote a bit more piece of mind, ensuring that only beneficial bacteria end up in the kvass.

Coconut Yogurt
Makes about 2 quarts

Learn to make coconut yogurt! Don't rely on a store brand. I've rarely seen one that doesn't include sugar, preservatives, or other additives. Besides, it's easy and inexpensive to make your own—you need only two ingredients. While I have several jury-rigged methods of holding this yogurt at the proper temperature until thickened, you can also make it in a standard home yogurt maker; pour it into sterilized jars and follow the manufacturer's instructions. Since I don't add any thickeners, there may be some separation of liquid at the bottom of the jars. Simply spoon the thickened yogurt off the top.

> 1 liter organic coconut cream with at least 22% fat, preferably Wilderness Family Naturals
> 3 (50 billion count) probiotic capsules or 3 tablespoons Inner-Eco probiotic dairy-free kefir

1. Pour the coconut cream into a large saucepan and set over low heat. Cook just until warm, about 100°F. Remove from the heat.
2. Open the probiotic capsules and stir the powder into the coconut cream, or stir in the kefir. Divide the mixture between 2 sterilized 1-quart mason jars. Cover and seal.
3. The best incubation temperature is 110°F. You have a few options beyond a yogurt marker. If you have a food dehydrator with a predictable temperature setting, remove the trays and set the temperature for 110°F. Set the filled jars in the dehydrator and heat for 12 to 24 hours, until the yogurt has thickened. Or if your oven has a bread proof setting, warm it to this mark, set the covered jars on a rimmed baking sheet, and warm for 12 to 24 hours. Or fill a large saucepan with very hot tap water, then set it aside to cool to 110°F. Place the sealed jars in a small, well-insulated cooler and pour in enough water so that it comes up above the level of the coconut mixture in the jars. Cover tightly and set aside for 12 to 24 hours.

MORE

I love this yogurt as a midday treat. Top a cup of this with a sprinkle of bee pollen or maybe a few blueberries. The yogurt can also be added to smoothies or even savory sauces for a creamy finish. And it can be used for recipes like my probiotic-rich Lithuanian Šaltibarščiai Soup (page 239) or Coconut-Lemon Yogurt Soup (page 238).

Nut Mylk
Makes about 1 quart

You'll need a large and powerful blender to create the creamiest nut mylk imaginable. Macadamia nuts will make a mild, gentle mylk, while almonds will offer more body and a somewhat more savory flavor.

> 1 cup unsweetened shredded coconut
> ⅓ cup raw macadamia nuts or almonds
> 1½ teaspoons non-GMO lecithin
> ⅛ teaspoon Himalayan or Celtic sea salt

Put the coconut, nuts, soy lecithin, and salt in a large blender and add 4 cups of water. Cover and blend for 2 minutes, or until smooth. Strain through a colander lined with a double thickness of cheesecloth or a nut mylk bag and into a large bottle or other sealable container with a spout for pouring. Cover and store in the refrigerator for up to 4 days.

Nondairy Creamer
Makes about 3¾ cups (use 2 to 3 tablespoons per serving)

My preferred morning beverage is a cup of hot tea with this home-made nondairy creamer. You will never miss half-and-half or heavy cream again. Plus, this takes just two minutes to make.

> 2 cups Nut Mylk (above)
> 1 (13½-ounce) can full-fat coconut milk
> 1 teaspoon alcohol-free vanilla extract

Pour nut mylk, coconut milk, and vanilla into a 1-quart glass jar. Cover and shake well. Store in the refrigerator for up to 1 week.

Note: If you like the cream frothy, you're in luck! I use a small electric Nespresso cream frother. I pour a little of this mixture in and hit the button. Voilà: in about 30 seconds you have a thick, rich, creamy, frothy ambrosia to add to your favorite black, green, or herbal tea. Or to your organic coffee, if you prefer.

Breakfast

Breakfast Broth
Makes 1 serving

This recipe is quick, nourishing, and comforting. The broth could even be taken with you in the morning in a small widemouthed thermos for a meal on the go. Save any leftover proteins from other meals in a sealed container in the fridge, have some greens on hand in the hydrator, and consider this your standard primal breakfast.

1½ cups Primal Bone Broth (page 209)
¼ cup baby kale leaves, baby spinach leaves, chopped bok choy,
   chopped watercress (any large stems removed), or frozen
   organic spinach, thawed
¼ cup chopped boned cooked chicken, ground beef, leftover
   steak, chopped boned turkey breast, or wild-caught trout or
   walleye
½ teaspoon curry powder, Italian seasoning blend, herbes de
   Provence, five-spice powder, ground turmeric, celery seeds, or
   dried thyme

Bring the broth to a simmer in a small saucepan set over medium-high heat. Stir in the kale, the protein, and the seasoning. Cover and set aside off the heat for 2 minutes, until heated through. Serve at once.

MORE

Enrich the Breakfast Broth with 2 tablespoons full-fat coconut milk or fresh salsa (mild or spicy) once it has been heated. For a mental boost, add 1 tablespoon virgin coconut oil after heating. Or add 1 scoop Vital Proteins Gelatin or Vital Proteins Collagen Peptides (but don't forget that these add 9 grams of protein per scoop).

Primal Power Breakfast

Makes 4 servings

This breakfast will set you up for the morning! You get a hearty bump of protein and lots of leafy greens, the perfect match to keep your energy high. For the best flavor, don't cook the chicken livers too long. They should still be slightly pink inside.

4 cups baby kale leaves

3 tablespoons organic cultured ghee

4 medium scallions, thinly sliced

1 tablespoon minced fresh ginger

1 teaspoon minced garlic

½ teaspoon yellow curry powder

12 ounces organic free-range chicken livers, chopped

1½ tablespoons coconut vinegar

¼ teaspoon Himalayan or Celtic sea salt

1. Place the kale in a large bowl. Set aside.
2. Melt the ghee in a medium skillet set over medium heat. Add the scallions, ginger, and garlic and cook, stirring constantly, for 30 seconds. Add the curry powder and cook, stirring, for about 20 seconds, or until fragrant.
3. Add the livers and cook, turning occasionally, for 3 minutes, until the livers are browned but pink at the center. Add the vinegar and salt; toss well over the heat for 30 seconds.

4. Scrape the contents of the skillet over the kale. Toss until the leaves begin to wilt.

Primal Huevos Rancheros
Makes 1 serving

This one's a simplified version of the classic, more in keeping with the primal way to eat. You can double the recipe in a large skillet—but you might want to have two medium skillets on the stove if you want to make four servings for the family meal.

1 tablespoon organic cultured ghee
¼ cup diced yellow or white onion (about ½ small)
¼ cup sliced oyster or maitake mushrooms (about 1 ounce)
¼ cup packed baby spinach leaves
2 to 3 large eggs, well beaten
2 tablespoons fresh salsa, mild or hot
½ Hass avocado, pitted, peeled, and thinly sliced
Himalayan or Celtic sea salt
Ground black pepper

1. Melt the ghee in a medium skillet set over medium heat. Add the onion and mushrooms and cook, stirring occasionally, for 4 minutes, or until softened. Add the spinach; stir for 10 seconds, until just wilted.
2. Pour in the eggs. Cook, stirring often, for 1 to 2 minutes, until scrambled and set. Transfer to a plate; top with the salsa. Place the avocado slices on the side and season with salt and pepper.

MORE

For fried eggs, do not beat the eggs in a small bowl. Instead, melt the ghee in the skillet over medium heat, then crack the eggs into the skillet and cook until the whites are set, flipping the eggs if desired.

Transfer to a plate. Cook the vegetables as stated in the recipe and spoon them on top of the eggs with the salsa. Place the avocado slices on the side and season with salt and pepper.

Spinach Egg Bake
Makes 2 to 4 servings

Here's a great hot breakfast when you've got to get out of the house! You can even take the egg muffins with you. Make sure you grease every bit of the inside of the muffin pan cups so the patties don't stick as they bake.

2 tablespoons organic lard or beef tallow, plus more for the
    muffin pans, preferably Fatworks

6 ounces shiitake caps or maitake mushrooms, chopped

3 cups packed baby spinach leaves

1 tablespoon minced fresh dill

2 teaspoons minced garlic

½ teaspoon ground allspice (optional)

½ teaspoon Himalayan or Celtic sea salt

½ teaspoon ground black pepper

4 large eggs

1. Position a rack in the center of the oven. Preheat the oven to 400°F. Lightly grease the inside of four ¾- to 1-cup muffin pans with a little lard on a paper towel.
2. Melt the lard in a large skillet set over medium heat. Add the mushrooms and cook, stirring often, for 2 minutes, or until they just begin to wilt at the edges. Add the spinach, dill, garlic, allspice (if using), salt, and pepper. Cook, stirring occasionally, for 1 minute, or until the spinach has wilted. The mixture should be moist from the liquid in the mushrooms. Divide among the four muffin pans, packing the mixture into place. Use the back of a spoon to

create a well in the middle of the mushroom mixture; crack one egg into each well.

3. Bake for 12 minutes, or until the eggs are set to your liking. Cool in the muffin pan for 2 or 3 minutes before serving.

MORE

Cook the mushroom mixture in an 8-inch oven-safe skillet. (You may need to add the spinach leaves in batches to wilt it properly.) Instead of using a muffin pan, pack this mixture down in the pan, then create the four wells with the back of a spoon. Add the eggs and bake as directed.

Primal Omelet

Makes 1 serving

Sure, an omelet is a great breakfast. But it's also terrific for lunch or even in the evenings for a quick dinner. An omelet is mostly about technique: scraping the eggs back from the edge of the pan, then folding the omelet over. If you don't get it perfect the first time, remember that there's nothing wrong with scrambled eggs!

2 tablespoons organic duck fat, preferably Fatworks

2 tablespoons minced red onion

½ teaspoon fennel seeds

2 ounces Swiss chard leaves, stemmed and chopped (about ½ cup)

1 teaspoon minced fresh oregano leaves

¼ teaspoon Himalayan or Celtic sea salt

¼ teaspoon ground black pepper

2 large eggs, well beaten

1. Melt the duck fat in a small skillet set over medium-low heat. Add the onion and fennel seeds and cook, stirring occasionally, for 20 seconds, or until the seeds begin to pop.
2. Add the chard, oregano, salt, and pepper. Stir well over the heat for 1 minute, or until the chard has just wilted.
3. Pour in the eggs. Cook undisturbed for 1 minute. Use a rubber spatula to pull the cooked bits from the perimeter toward the center, letting more of the uncooked egg flow into place. Cook about 1 minute, then repeat this operation. Cook about 1 more minute, or until the eggs are just about set. Fold the omelet closed and slip it from the pan to a plate.

MORE

Omit the duck fat. Instead, scoop out 2 tablespoons marrow from a cooked bone, melt it in the skillet, and use it to cook the omelet.

Primal Breakfast "Fondue"
Makes 2 servings

I've used this recipe as a satisfying breakfast when I feel too busy to make something fancier. It's sort of like a traditional Swiss fondue— except there you'd fry the bits of meat in fat, rather than simmering them in tasty bone broth. I save any leftover fat for a rich coconut-oil condiment, a real perk-up in the morning.

3 cups Primal Bone Broth (page 209)
6 ounces 100% grass-fed/finished boneless strip steak, organic
    pastured boneless leg of lamb, or organic free-range boneless,
    skinless chicken thighs, cut into ½-inch cubes
2 tablespoons virgin coconut oil, melted and cooled
¼ teaspoon ground turmeric
¼ teaspoon Himalayan or Celtic sea salt

1. Bring the broth to a boil in a small saucepan set over high heat. Drop in the protein of your choice, reduce the heat to medium, and cook for 2 minutes, or until cooked through.
2. Meanwhile, mix the oil, turmeric, and salt in a small bowl.
3. Use a slotted spoon to transfer the chicken pieces to 2 bowls. Drizzle each serving with half the seasoned oil. Pour the broth into 2 mugs and enjoy with the seasoned meat. You can even spear the meat and dip it in the broth as you enjoy your breakfast!

MORE

Add ¼ cup baby spinach or kale leaves to each cup before pouring in the hot broth. Or skip the seasoned coconut oil entirely and drizzle the meat with some Primal Gaucho Chimichurri (page 208).

Breakfast Sausage Patty with Sautéed Greens
Makes 2 servings

Finding a source for quality pastured, organic sausage can be tough. Even the best stuff often contains sugar or gluten of some sort. One high-quality brand, Mulay's Sausage—available in a number of flavors in both links and patties—is available for purchase online (also available for purchase in many natural markets—try asking your grocer to carry it). But it's also easy to make your own! In fact, you might want to triple or even quadruple this pork mixture, form it into small, 1½-ounce patties, and store them between sheets of wax paper in a sealed container in the freezer for up to 6 months. Set 2 frozen patties per serving on a plate in the fridge before you go to bed and you'll be ready for breakfast the next morning.

6 ounces ground organic, pastured pork, preferably fatty

¼ teaspoon fennel seeds

¼ teaspoon dried oregano

¼ teaspoon dried sage

¼ teaspoon Himalayan or Celtic sea salt

¼ teaspoon ground black pepper

2 tablespoons organic lard

1 tablespoon pine nuts

2 ounces spinach leaves, stemmed and chopped (about ½ cup)

2 ounces Swiss chard leaves, stemmed and chopped (about ½ cup)

2 ounces kale leaves, stemmed and chopped (about ½ cup)

1. Mix the pork, fennel seeds, oregano, sage, salt, and pepper in a medium bowl until the spices are uniform throughout. Divide this mixture into 4 patties.
2. Melt half the lard in a large skillet set over medium heat. Add the patties and cook, turning once, for 6 minutes, or until cooked through. Transfer to a plate.
3. Melt the remainder of the lard in the skillet. Add the pine nuts and cook, stirring often, for 1 minute, until lightly browned and aromatic. Add all the greens and cook, tossing often, for 1 to 2 minutes, or until wilted.
4. Divide the greens between 2 plates. Top each with 2 patties.

Note: I love all these greens! But you might not want to buy so many at once. All you really need is 1½ cups of stemmed and chopped leafy greens. But variety sure makes for a tastier breakfast!

MORE

Add 1 teaspoon minced garlic with the pine nuts. If desired, serve 2 tablespoons Primal Cultured Vegetable Kraut (page 211) on the side.

Roasted Marrow Bones

Makes 2 servings

Bone marrow from grass-fed cows is rich in quality fats and fat-soluble nutrients. Ask your butcher to cut long marrow bones in half lengthwise and to trim away any connective tissue on the bones. Serve a double portion for a hearty lunch.

2 (6- to 8-inch) organic grass-fed marrow bones, trimmed
   and split lengthwise
1 small shallot, minced
¼ teaspoon Himalayan or Celtic sea salt
¼ teaspoon ground black pepper
2 tablespoons olive oil
1 tablespoon fresh lemon juice

1. Position the rack in the center of the oven. Preheat the oven to 400°F.
2. Arrange the bones cut side up in a roasting pan or on a rimmed baking sheet. Sprinkle the shallots, salt, and pepper evenly over the bones.
3. Roast for 15 minutes, or until the marrow is browned and bubbling. Drizzle with the oil and lemon juice before serving. Serve with small spoons to dig all the marrow out.

MORE

Omit the shallot and sprinkle the marrow bones with minced garlic and chopped pumpkin seeds (as well as the salt and pepper) before roasting. Serve stir-fried, sautéed, or steamed vegetables on the side—or 2 tablespoons of Primal Cultured Vegetable Kraut (page 211).

Slow Cooker Vegetable Stew
Makes 4 servings

There's nothing quite like an aromatic stew, ready in the morning when you get up. This one's stocked with plenty of healthy vegetables and bold flavors. For an easier prep, look for bagged shredded organic red cabbage. You can also enjoy this paired with 2 ounces of any left-over meats you might have.

14 ounces cored and finely shredded red cabbage (about 4 cups)

12 ounces cauliflower florets, coarsely chopped (about 2 cups)

8 ounces oyster mushrooms, coarsely chopped

1 small red onion, thinly sliced and separated into rings

2 tablespoons organic whole grain mustard

1 teaspoon caraway seeds

1 teaspoon finely grated lemon zest

½ teaspoon Himalayan or Celtic sea salt

½ teaspoon ground black pepper

¼ teaspoon red pepper flakes (optional)

Mix all the ingredients in a 4- to 6-quart slow cooker. Cover and cook on low for 8 hours. Serve in bowls.

MORE

For a little more zip, sprinkle coconut vinegar over each serving. If you want a hearty breakfast, fry a large egg in duck fat and place it on top of each serving. And for even heartier fare, add the egg plus 1 tablespoon pine nuts and 1 tablespoon unsweetened shredded coconut.

Hearty Breakfast Hash
Makes 4 servings

This is a nice alternative to eggs and a way to get a few more vegetables into your morning meal. Also, the dish makes for a nice brunch on the weekends when you have a bit more time to prepare a larger meal.

12 ounces organic free-range ground chicken or organic
    pastured ground pork

2 teaspoons minced fresh sage leaves

1 teaspoon fresh thyme leaves

½ teaspoon Himalayan or Celtic sea salt

½ teaspoon ground black pepper

¼ teaspoon grated nutmeg

¼ teaspoon cayenne pepper (optional)

2 tablespoons organic duck fat or schmaltz (chicken fat),
    preferably Fatworks

1 small yellow or white onion, chopped

8 ounces sliced shiitake mushroom caps

8 ounces small Brussels sprouts, thinly sliced

4 ounces thin asparagus spears, chopped

1. Mix the ground meat with the sage, thyme, salt, black, pepper, nutmeg, and cayenne (if using) until uniform.
2. Melt 1 tablespoon of the duck fat in a large skillet set over medium heat. Add the meat mixture; cook, stirring occasionally and breaking up the mixture with the back of a wooden spoon, for 5 minutes, or until browned and cooked through. Scrape into a large bowl.
3. Melt the remaining 1 tablespoon duck fat in the skillet. Add the onion and mushrooms; cook, stirring often, 4 minutes, or until softened. Add the Brussels sprouts and asparagus; cook, stirring occasionally, 2 minutes, or until the Brussels sprouts begin to wilt.

4. Return the meat mixture to the skillet. Toss well for 1 minute, until hot. Divide among 4 plates.

Note: If you had to take the stems off the shiitakes, save those stems in a small, sealed bag in the freezer and add them with the bones to your next batch of Primal Bone Broth.

MORE

Substitute stemmed and chopped kale or cored and chopped escarole for the Brussels sprouts. Or substitute chopped green beans or broccoli florets for the asparagus.

Power Breakfast Smoothie
Makes 1 smoothie

Smoothies are a great way to pack a lot of nutrition into one serving. If you're trying to maintain your weight, smoothies can be really helpful. However, they're a bit less ideal for those seeking to lose weight, given all the tasty, heavier ingredients packed into a glass. Juiced green vegetables with some lemon juice or minced ginger and a drop or two of stevia for sweetness (but no added fruit) are a better choice for those trying to lose a few pounds. The green vegetables are a powerful source of detoxifying and nourishing phytonutrients and antioxidants.

In general, I am not a fan of protein powders, as (1) they are highly processed, (2) they tend to contain a number of questionable ingredients, (3) it's way too easy to overdo the protein, and (4) most protein powders use protein sources that tend to be antigenic for a lot of people. In this recipe I do recommend Vital Proteins Collagen Peptides, as they add quality gut-healing, connective tissue–building peptides from exclusively 100% pastured bovine sources, with no other additives. One scoop provides about 9 grams of highly digestible, assimilable, quality protein from a quality source.

½ small cucumber, thinly sliced

½ small Hass avocado, pitted and peeled

4 medium broccoli florets

¼ cup packed baby kale or spinach leaves

¼ cup broccoli sprouts

¼ cup frozen wild blueberries (do not thaw)

¼ cup shelled Brazil or macadamia nuts

1 large egg yolk

1 tablespoon macadamia nut oil or virgin coconut oil

1 scoop Vital Protein Collagen Peptides (adds 9 grams of
   protein)

2 teaspoons minced fresh turmeric root, or ½ teaspoon
   ground turmeric

2 drops liquid stevia, or to taste

Up to ½ cup full-fat coconut milk

3 medium ice cubes

1. Put the cucumber, avocado, broccoli, kale, broccoli sprouts, blueberries, nuts, egg yolk, oil, Vital Protein Collagen Peptides, turmeric, and stevia in a large blender.

2. Turn the blender on high and add enough coconut milk to get the ingredients blending. Add the ice cubes, cover, and blend until thick and slushy.

MORE

You can also add 1 to 2 tablespoons of nut butter for extra creaminess and calories.

Lunch

A Road Map for a Composed Salad
Makes 1 serving

This one's not a standard recipe. Rather, it's a way to think about building a satisfying salad for lunch (or maybe even dinner). Keep these ingredients in the refrigerator and the pantry so you can have an easy meal any day of the week. If you've got several people at the table, consider laying out the separate ingredients in bowls and letting everyone build their own salad at the table.

1. Make a layer of 1½ cups greens on a large plate, using one or a combination of the following:

    Baby kale leaves

    Baby spinach leaves

    Cored romaine lettuce

    Cored frisée

    Cored Boston lettuce

    Cored red leaf lettuce

    Cored butter lettuce

    Mesclun mix

2. Top the greens with ¾ cup of one or a combination of the following:

    Chopped broccoli florets

    Shredded carrots

    Sliced radishes

    Thinly sliced snow peas

    Thinly sliced sugar snap peas

    Peeled and diced cucumbers

    . . . And no matter what you choose, always add a handful
    of sprouts of your choice!

3. Add a layer of thinly sliced mushrooms, ¼ cup of one or a combination of the following:

    Shiitake mushroom caps

    Maitake mushrooms

Portobello mushroom caps

Oyster mushrooms

Chanterelle mushrooms

4. If desired, add 2 to 3 ounces chopped protein to the top of the salad, using one of the following:

Boned cooked chicken

Sautéed liver

Shredded pork

Boned cooked turkey

Grilled steak

Cooked ground beef

5. Whisk together a dressing in a small bowl, using 2 tablespoons of one of these oils, 1 tablespoon of one of these vinegars, and the remaining ingredients, then drizzle the dressing over the salad:

OILS

Extra-virgin cold-pressed olive oil

Avocado oil

Macadamia nut oil

VINEGARS

Coconut vinegar

Aged balsamic vinegar

REMAINING DRESSING INGREDIENTS

1 teaspoon organic coarse grain mustard

¼ teaspoon ground black pepper

⅛ teaspoon Himalayan or Celtic sea salt

Thai Salad with Spicy Dressing
Makes 2 servings

I've adapted this recipe from Pauli Halstead's wonderful cookbook *Primal Cuisine: Cooking for the Paleo Diet.* The red pepper flakes and jalapeño add lots of spicy heat to the salad, but since they're derived from nightshades, use them only if they fit your specific diet.

3 tablespoons toasted sesame oil

2 tablespoons coconut vinegar

1 tablespoon coconut aminos (gluten- and soy-free substitute for
    soy sauce or tamari)

2 teaspoons minced fresh ginger

2 teaspoons fresh lime juice

1 teaspoon minced garlic

¼ teaspoon red pepper flakes

¼ teaspoon Himalayan or Celtic sea salt

3 cups cored and shredded Napa cabbage

6 ounces organic free-range boned chicken, cooked and
    chopped

1 medium red bell pepper, seeded and cut into thin strips

1 cup mung bean sprouts

2 medium scallions, thinly sliced

Up to 1 small jalapeño, seeded and thinly sliced

¼ cup roasted macadamia nuts, finely chopped

2 tablespoons chopped cilantro leaves

1. Whisk the sesame oil, vinegar, coconut aminos, ginger, lime juice, garlic, red pepper flakes, and salt in a large bowl until well blended.
2. Add the cabbage, chicken, bell pepper, bean sprouts, scallions, and jalapeño. Toss well to coat in the dressing; divide between 2 plates. Garnish with the nuts and cilantro.

Grilled Caesar Salad

Makes 2 servings

Grilling lettuces gives them a savory, smoky flavor that can't be beat with this primal riff on a traditional Caesar dressing. The trick here is not to let the lettuces burn. Watch them closely. Once they begin to blacken at the leaves' edges, they're within a few seconds of being done.

2 tablespoons aged balsamic vinegar

1 small jarred anchovy fillet, minced

1 teaspoon minced garlic

1 teaspoon organic coarse grain mustard

¼ teaspoon ground black pepper

2 small heads romaine lettuce

¼ cup coconut oil, melted

1. Whisk the vinegar, anchovy, garlic, mustard, and pepper in a large bowl until uniform. Set aside.
2. Prepare a grill for high-heat direct cooking, or set a large grill pan over high heat for 1 or 2 minutes. Slice the romaine heads in half lengthwise through the core. Brush the cut sides with all the oil. Set the lettuce cut side down on the grate or in the grill pan. Grill for 4 minutes without turning, until well marked and a little charred.
3. Transfer the romaine halves to a large cutting board; slice into ½-inch-thick sections widthwise. Separate into shreds and drop these into the prepared dressing. Toss well to coat and divide between 2 plates.

MORE

For a bigger salad, sprinkle sliced radishes, sliced celery, shredded carrots, or diced, pitted, and peeled avocado over the salad on the plates. For a heartier meal, cook 6 ounces organic free-range boneless, skinless chicken breast on the grill or in the pan before you grill the lettuce; slice the meat into strips and toss with the lettuces to serve.

Primal Ground Beef Salad
Makes 4 servings

This meal is easy and quick! You won't believe how delicious the vegetables are when they've been cooked in a little animal fat. If you want to go all out, substitute beef tallow for the duck fat or schmaltz (chicken fat). I buy all my animal cooking fat from Fatworks (see "Nourishing Resources" on page 285).

2 tablespoons organic duck fat or schmaltz (chicken fat)

¾ cup chopped red onion (about ½ large)

8 ounces shiitake mushroom caps, chopped

2 teaspoons minced garlic

12 ounces organic grass-fed ground beef

6 cups cored and chopped butter or romaine lettuce

1 Hass avocado, pitted, peeled, and diced

1 cup canned or jarred organic artichoke hearts packed in water, drained

⅓ cup avocado oil or extra-virgin cold-pressed olive oil

2 tablespoons organic balsamic vinegar

1 tablespoon organic stone-ground mustard

¼ teaspoon Himalayan or Celtic sea salt

¼ teaspoon ground black pepper

1. Melt the duck fat in a large skillet set over medium heat. Add ½ cup of the onion; cook, stirring often, for 2 minutes, until barely softened.
2. Add the mushrooms and garlic; continue cooking, stirring occasionally, until the mushrooms release their liquid and the skillet dries out a bit again, about 4 minutes. Add the ground beef and cook, stirring often, for 4 minutes, until cooked through. Remove the skillet from the heat.
3. Divide the romaine among 4 plates. Spoon a quarter of the beef mixture over the lettuce on each plate. Divide the avocado, artichoke hearts, and the remaining ¼ cup onion among the plates.
4. Whisk the oil, vinegar, mustard, salt, and pepper in a small bowl until emulsified. Drizzle evenly over each salad.

MORE

Steam or sauté some diced asparagus, cored and chopped red cabbage, or chopped broccolini and add to the salad.

Best Ever Chicken Salad
Makes 4 servings

This recipe has been my closely guarded secret, but it's just too good not to share. I'm spreading the love. You may have leftovers. They'll store in a sealed container in the fridge for a couple of days. Try a serving for breakfast!

4 cups cored and finely shredded green cabbage (about 1 pound)

12 ounces organic free-range boneless, skinless chicken thighs, cut into ½-inch pieces

1 tablespoon organic duck fat or schmaltz (chicken fat), preferably Fatworks

1 small yellow or white onion, chopped

4 ounces shiitake mushroom caps, thinly sliced

2 teaspoons yellow curry powder

1 teaspoon minced garlic

½ teaspoon Himalayan or Celtic sea salt

¼ cup pine nuts

½ cup unsweetened shredded coconut

⅓ cup avocado oil, macadamia nut oil, and/or extra-virgin cold-pressed olive oil

1 tablespoon toasted sesame oil

2 drops liquid stevia (optional)

1. Place the cabbage in a large bowl and set aside. Bring a small pot of water to a boil, plunge the chicken into it, and cook for 5 minutes, or until cooked through. Drain in a colander and pour the hot chicken over the cabbage. Toss well so the chicken helps wilt the cabbage.

2. Melt the duck fat in a small skillet set over medium heat. Add the onion and mushrooms. Cook, stirring occasionally, for 2 minutes, until they just begin to soften. Stir in the curry powder, garlic, and salt, and cook about 15 seconds, until fragrant. Scrape the contents of the skillet into the bowl with the cabbage and chicken.
3. Set the skillet back over medium heat (there's no need to wash it). Add the pine nuts and cook, stirring occasionally, for 2 minutes, until lightly browned. Pour them onto the cabbage mixture, add the coconut, and toss well.
4. Add the avocado oil, the sesame oil, and the stevia, if using. Toss well one more time before dividing among 4 plates.

MORE

This amazing yet simple dish is fabulous spooned over a bed of greens and chopped fresh vegetables, served with chopped avocado, or even topped with sprouts.

Amazing Coconut Thai Soup
Makes 4 servings

This soup is heaven on wheels. Not only is it wonderfully comforting on a cold winter day, it's also chock-full of ingredients that can help support your immune function. If you have any left over, it keeps well in a sealed container in the refrigerator and may even taste better the next day. If you're feeling under the weather and are looking for the ultimate in comforting support, a cup of this ambrosia will lift your spirits while it supercharges your immune system!

1 tablespoon virgin coconut oil
1 medium yellow or white onion, diced
2 teaspoons minced garlic

6 cups Primal Bone Broth (page 209), preferably homemade
 chicken bone broth, or packaged organic free-range gluten-
 and MSG-free chicken broth (see Note)

8 ounces organic free-range boneless, skinless chicken thighs,
 chopped

2 cups full-fat coconut milk

1 cup cored and thinly sliced red cabbage (about ¼ small head)

4 ounces maitake mushrooms or shiitake mushroom caps,
 chopped

2 tablespoons sugar- and MSG-free fish sauce, preferably Red
 Boat brand

1 tablespoon organic, sugar- and gluten-free red curry paste

1 tablespoon minced fresh ginger

½ teaspoon ground turmeric

2 cups packed baby spinach leaves

2 tablespoons fresh lime juice

Chopped cilantro leaves

1. Melt the oil in a large pot or Dutch oven set over medium heat.
 Add the onion and garlic; cook, stirring often, for 3 minutes, until
 softened.

2. Add the broth, chicken, coconut milk, cabbage, mushrooms, fish
 sauce, curry paste, ginger, and turmeric. Stir well to dissolve the
 paste and bring to a full simmer. Reduce the heat to very low and
 simmer for 20 minutes.

3. Turn off the heat. Stir in the spinach and lime juice. Cover and
 set aside for 2 minutes to wilt the spinach. Ladle into bowls and
 sprinkle cilantro over each serving.

Note: Pacific brand makes a good one, to which you could add a couple of
tablespoons of Fatworks brand schmaltz to get more of the antimicrobial effect. Keep in mind that the long-fabled "Jewish penicillin" magic of chicken
soup lies mostly in the fat (which has natural anti-microbial effects)!

Coconut-Lemon Yogurt Soup
Makes 4 servings

This soup is uniquely healthy and delicious. Your taste buds, your family, and your internal microbiome will thank you. Making a habit of regularly including naturally cultured or fermented foods such as this and others on the Primal Fat Burner Plan adds surprising extra benefits to your digestive and brain function (see David Perlmutter's excellent book *Brain Maker* for more information).

This soup doesn't freeze well, but that just means you can have a bowl the next morning for breakfast!

1 tablespoon organic cultured ghee

1 medium yellow or white onion, chopped

1 teaspoon minced garlic

4 cups Primal Bone Broth (page 209), preferably chicken bone broth, or 1 quart packaged organic free-range gluten- and MSG-free chicken broth

4 ounces organic free-range boneless, skinless chicken thighs, diced

4 ounces shiitake mushroom caps, thinly sliced

½ teaspoon Himalayan or Celtic sea salt

2 cups Coconut Yogurt (page 214) or store-bought plain unsweetened organic coconut yogurt

¼ to ⅓ cup fresh lemon juice

1. Melt the ghee in a large saucepan over medium heat. Add the onion and garlic; cook, stirring often, for 3 minutes, or until softened.
2. Add the broth, chicken, mushrooms, and salt. Bring to a full simmer. Reduce the heat to low and cook uncovered for 5 minutes.
3. Remove from the heat and cool for 5 minutes. Stir in the coconut yogurt until well blended. Stir in the lemon juice to taste, starting with ¼ cup and adding more as desired.

Note: Chicken thighs are easiest to cut into small bits when they're still slightly frozen.

Lithuanian Šaltibarščiai Soup

Makes 1½ quarts (about 6 servings)

My Lithuanian mother made a version of šaltibarščiai (*shahl-barsh-tay* or cold beet soup) during the summer. It's more traditionally made with fresh cooked beets and lots of sour cream or buttermilk, not a combination I recommend for anyone wanting to lose weight. But there is a way of making it the Primal Fat Burner way that avoids the pitfalls in the old way of preparing it and even makes it a bit of a tonic (for the gut, liver, and gallbladder)!

> 2 cups Beet Kvass (page 213)
> 2 cups Coconut Yogurt (page 214)
> 1 large cucumber, peeled, seeded, and diced
> ¼ cup minced fresh dill
> 2 teaspoons Vital Choice Beef Gelatin (optional)
> 2 drops liquid stevia (optional)
> 6 hard-boiled eggs
> Minced fresh chives

1. Whisk the kvass and coconut yogurt in a large bowl until smooth. Stir in the cucumber and dill, as well as the gelatin and stevia, if using. Cover and refrigerate for at least 2 hours, or up to 2 days before serving.
2. To serve, peel and quarter a hard-boiled egg. Place the pieces in a small bowl; top with 1 cup kvass mixture. Sprinkle with chives. Prepare more bowls as needed.

Note: This dish packs quite a probiotic punch, being made from not one but two probiotic-rich cultured foods. It also helps support biliary health.

If you're looking for the perfect meal to advance the healthy population of your microbiome and support your fat digestion, this is it! Traditionally, Šaltibarščiai is made using the actual beets and not kvass, so it typically contains far more natural sugar. I asked my culinarily astute, intrepid Lithuanian friend Carolyn Rush (author of the amazing food budget–saving book *Primal Tightwad*) to test this recipe out for me to see if it passed a die-hard Lithuanian cuisine fan's muster—and it did, with flying colors! Note, however, that this recipe may be a bit too potent for some people having digestive challenges, particularly those unaccustomed to cultured foods. Start with a small serving, see how you feel, and resist the temptation to eat a big serving in one sitting. If you can tolerate a little, indulge in a larger serving on another day, but try to keep it to a cup at a time.

Hearty Primal Chili
Makes 4 servings

With chili, the longer you simmer it the better and more flavorful it becomes. Serve this dish with a generous pinch of raw onions on top, some pico de gallo, or even just a drizzle of aged balsamic vinegar. It makes for a filling and satisfying meal, especially on a cold day! I add more broth than a standard chili, so this is a bit soupier. But the flavors are even better with all that bone broth!

1 tablespoon organic duck fat, schmaltz (chicken fat), or beef tallow, preferably Fatworks

1 large yellow or white onion, diced

1 fresh jalapeño, seeded and diced

1 pound maitake mushrooms and/or shiitake mushroom caps, chopped

¾ pound organic grass-fed ground beef, buffalo, chicken, or turkey

2 tablespoons chili powder

2 teaspoons minced garlic

4 cups Primal Bone Broth (page 209), preferably chicken bone
   broth, or 1 quart packaged organic free-range gluten- and
   MSG-free chicken broth
1 (14-ounce) can diced fire-roasted tomatoes
1 (6-ounce) can organic tomato paste
½ teaspoon Himalayan or Celtic sea salt

1. Melt the duck fat in a large pot or Dutch oven set over medium heat. Add the onion and jalapeño; cook, stirring often, for 3 minutes, or until softened.
2. Add the mushrooms. Cook, stirring occasionally, for 5 minutes, or until they give off their moisture and it mostly evaporates.
3. Crumble in the ground meat. Cook, stirring once in a while, for 3 minutes, or until it loses its raw, pink color. Stir in the chili powder and garlic; cook for 15 seconds, or until fragrant. Stir in the broth, diced tomatoes, tomato paste, and salt until the paste dissolves.
4. Bring to a full simmer, then reduce the heat to low and cook uncovered for 30 to 60 minutes, or until thickened to your taste.

MORE

To make this chili in a slow cooker, reduce the broth to 2 cups. Complete the recipe through step 3, then pour the contents of the pot into a 5- to 6-quart slow cooker. Cover and cook on low for 7 hours.

Curried Lamb and Chicken Gizzard Stew
Makes 4 servings

Here's the heartiest lunch, a bold mix of flavors! Chicken gizzards are most often sold cleaned; however, if you've bought them from a local farmer or even at a farmers' market, they may need to be cleaned at home. To be certain, ask the provider. To clean them, cut each gizzard open and remove any fibrous material inside. Wash thoroughly to remove grit, then peel off the inner linings.

10 ounces organic pastured boneless lamb stew meat, cut into
   1-inch pieces

2 ounces organic free-range chicken gizzards, cleaned and diced

2 teaspoons minced garlic

1 teaspoon ground cumin

1 teaspoon ground coriander

1 teaspoon ground ginger

¼ teaspoon cayenne pepper

¼ teaspoon Himalayan or Celtic sea salt

1 pound Brussels sprouts, halved

1 (14-ounce) can diced fire-roasted tomatoes

1 large red onion, halved and thinly sliced

Minced fresh chives

1. Put the lamb stew meat, gizzards, garlic, cumin, coriander, ginger, cayenne, and salt into a 4- to 6-quart slow cooker. Stir until the meat is thoroughly coated in the spices.
2. Add the Brussels sprouts, tomatoes, and onion. Toss well. Cover and cook on high heat for 3 hours or on low for 5 hours, or until the lamb is tender. Serve in bowls with the chives as a garnish.

MORE

Top the servings with a little Coconut Yogurt (page 214).

Dinner

Hearty Burgers with Mushrooms
Makes 4 burgers

Beef heart offers a wonderfully savory spark to these burgers. And a small amount of liver sneaks some nourishing organ meat into the mix. You don't want the burgers to be too lean. The fat not only improves the flavor but also helps hold the patties together. You don't need a meat grinder; a food processor will do the job. Buy a whole heart from the butcher and cut it up into 2-inch chunks. Put the pieces in a storage container and freeze until you need them. I like to serve these burgers on top of a simple bed of chopped lettuces, dressed with a bit of olive oil and fresh lemon juice or balsamic vinegar and a grinding of salt and pepper. The juices from the burger add their own dressing to the salad.

    2 tablespoons organic beef tallow, preferably Fatworks
    2 tablespoons minced red or yellow onion
    2 ounces maitake or oyster mushrooms, minced
    1 teaspoon minced garlic
    ¼ teaspoon Himalayan or Celtic sea salt
    ¼ teaspoon ground black pepper
    4 ounces organic grass-fed beef heart, cut into chunks and
        partially frozen
    2 ounces organic grass-fed beef liver, cut into chunks and partially
        frozen
    6 ounces organic grass-fed ground beef, preferably 80% lean or
        fattier

1. Melt 1 tablespoon of the tallow in a small skillet set over medium heat. Add the onion and cook, stirring constantly, for 1 minute. Add the mushrooms, garlic, salt, and pepper. Continue cooking, stirring often, for 1 minute more, or until softened. Scrape into a medium bowl and cool for 10 minutes.

2. Gently pulse the heart and liver pieces in a food processor until finely ground but not pureed. Add this mixture to the bowl along with the ground beef. Stir until well combined. Or use your clean, dry hands to mix the ingredients together. Form the mixture into 4 patties.

3. Melt the remaining 1 tablespoon tallow in a large grill pan or cast-iron skillet over medium heat, or prepare a grill for high, direct-heat cooking. Set the burgers in the pan or on the grate. Cook for 8 minutes, turning once, until cooked to medium doneness. The longer you cook the burgers, the more pronounced the liver flavor will be.

MORE

Drizzle a small amount of aged balsamic vinegar over the top of each patty as a sweet, tangy condiment, or use a sugar-free, whole grain mustard. If you want an even heartier meal, use 2 extra-large portobello mushroom caps as buns. Lightly brush the gill side of the caps with olive oil; add some minced garlic and sea salt. Set them in the grill pan or on the grill gill side down and cook for 3 minutes without turning. Set them gill side up on plates and set a patty on each.

Best Ever Grilled Steak
Makes 4 servings

Who says you can't be primal and have a dinner party? These steaks are a great way to set an elegant table. Serve these with Cauliflower Mashers (page 268) and have a big, crunchy salad on the side.

4 (2½-ounce) filets mignons or rib eye

½ teaspoon Himalayan or Celtic sea salt

½ teaspoon ground black pepper

2 tablespoons organic beef tallow, preferably Fatworks

1 large shallot, minced

3 ounces shiitake mushrooms caps, chopped

2 ounces organic free-range chicken livers, chopped

1 tablespoon organic coarse grain mustard

1 teaspoon fresh thyme leaves, minced

⅓ cup Primal Bone Broth (page 209), preferably chicken bone broth, or 1 quart packaged organic free-range gluten- and MSG-free chicken broth

1. Season the steaks with salt and pepper. Melt the fat in a large skillet, preferably cast iron, set over medium heat. Add the steaks; cook, turning once, for 5 minutes, or until an instant-read meat thermometer inserted into the center of one steak registers 130°F for medium-rare or 140°F for medium. Transfer to 4 plates or a platter.

2. Add the shallot and mushrooms to the skillet. Cook, stirring often, for 1 minute, or until the shallot just turns translucent. Add the liver; cook, stirring often, for 1 minute. Add the mustard and thyme; stir about 10 seconds, until fragrant.

3. Pour in the broth; bring to a full simmer, scraping up any browned bits in the skillet. Cook, stirring often, for 1 minute, or until somewhat reduced, about like a sauce. Spoon over the steaks to serve.

MORE

Omit the beef tallow and scoop the marrow from a 2-inch uncooked beef marrow bone. Use this as the fat in the recipe.

Primal Kālua Pork
Makes 16 servings

Call it pulled pork Hawaiian style! *Kālua* means "to cook underground." But you don't have to go out in your backyard and dig a pit. All you need is a slow cooker. The important thing here is the salt. It makes the dish! Many recipes for Kālua Pork also call for liquid smoke. I actually prefer this version with plenty of herbs and seasonings. Don't forget: you must start this recipe in the morning since it takes a long time. It also makes a lot. Consider freezing individual servings in small, sealed containers for meals in minutes.

> 1 (4-pound) organic pastured boneless pork shoulder roast, skin removed (do not trim the fat)
> 2 tablespoons Hawaiian black or red sea salt
> 1 tablespoon minced garlic
> 2 teaspoons cumin seeds or black cumin seeds
> 1 teaspoon coriander seeds
> ½ teaspoon ground black pepper

1. Place the pork in a 5- to 6-quart slow cooker. Use the point of a paring knife to poke holes all over the meat.
2. Combine the salt, garlic, cumin seeds, coriander seeds, and pepper in a small bowl. With clean, dry hands, rub this mixture all over the pork, pushing it down into the holes you've made but leaving some on the surface of the cut.
3. Cover and cook on low for 6 hours. Turn the meat, cover, and continue cooking on low for 6 more hours, or until the pork is fork-tender.

MORE

Strain the liquid into a large saucepan and use it to braise chopped, stemmed kale or collard greens over low heat until tender, about 20 minutes. No other seasoning will be required!

Cumin Pork Stir-Fry
Makes 4 servings

Cumin stir-fries are a Chinese favorite—and turned primal with this rather simple preparation. Make sure the wok is hot so that it cooks the ingredients without too much caramelization. Keep everything moving as it cooks. A wooden spoon in each hand is best!

2 tablespoons virgin coconut oil

2 teaspoons cumin seeds, preferably black cumin seeds

½ teaspoon red pepper flakes

12 ounces organic pastured boneless center-cut pork loin, thinly sliced

1 pound baby bok choy, coarsely chopped

2 tablespoons minced fresh ginger

2 teaspoons minced garlic

2 tablespoons coconut vinegar

2 tablespoons coconut aminos

2 teaspoons toasted sesame oil

1. Melt the oil in a large wok or skillet set over high heat. Add the cumin seeds and red pepper flakes; stir-fry for 10 seconds, or until aromatic. Add the pork; stir-fry for 3 minutes, or until it loses any raw, pink color.
2. Add the bok choy, ginger, and garlic; stir-fry for 2 minutes, or until the bok choy wilts and the pork is cooked through. Stir in the vinegar and coconut aminos; stir-fry for 1 minute, or until everything's well coated in the sauce. Remove from the heat and drizzle with the sesame oil before serving.

Note: Baby bok choy can be sandy. To wash it, fill a cleaned sink about halfway with cool tap water, then drop in the bok choy. Agitate well, then leave the bok choy to soak for 10 minutes to let the grit fall to the bottom of the sink. Use a slotted spoon to scoop the vegetables into a colander, then drain the sink and rinse the vegetables one more time.

Crispy Pork Belly
Makes 4 servings

Look no further for the ultimate primal meal! The juicy pork belly with its crisp skin attached will surely be one of your new favorite foods. You'll want to slice the skin into tiny bits to enjoy with each forkful of the meat. Serve with wilted greens or set the meat and vegetables over slices of roasted or grilled fennel. The onions and garlic will get quite charred, a sophisticatedly bitter contrast to the sweet pork.

1 pound skin-on pastured organic pork belly

3 tablespoons olive oil

½ teaspoon Himalayan or Celtic sea salt

½ teaspoon ground black pepper

1 large yellow onion, sliced into thin half-moons

5 garlic cloves, peeled and left whole

1. Use a sharp knife to score the skin of the pork in a crisscross pattern without cutting through into the meat below. Rub the meat with 1½ tablespoons of the oil, then the salt and pepper.
2. Preheat the oven to 450°F. Toss the onion, garlic, and the remaining 1½ tablespoons oil in a small roasting pan or a 9 x 13-inch baking dish. Place the prepared pork on top of the vegetables.
3. Roast for 20 minutes. Turn the heat to 275°F; continue roasting for an additional 2 hours, or until the skin is crispy and browned, occasionally stirring the vegetables and basting the meat with the pan juices. Transfer the meat to a cutting board; rest for 10 minutes. Slice into chunks to serve with the charred onions and garlic from the pan.

Larb Wraps
Makes 4 servings

Larb is practically the national dish of Laos! It's a spicy pork mixture that's folded into lettuce wraps, a super dinner when you want a more casual vibe. For the best texture, rock a chef's knife through the beef or pork heart on a cutting board, gathering the pieces together several times and changing the knife's direction to make tiny bits that resemble the texture of the ground pork.

2 tablespoons toasted sesame oil

10 ounces organic pastured ground pork

2 ounces organic pastured beef or pork heart, minced

6 medium scallions, thinly sliced

2 tablespoons minced fresh ginger

2 tablespoons minced lemongrass

2 tablespoons sugar- and MSG-free fish sauce

1 tablespoon fresh lime juice

3 drops liquid stevia

2 Boston lettuce heads, separated into leaves

Fresh jalapeños, seeded and thinly sliced

Pine nuts

1. Melt the oil in a large skillet set over medium-high heat. Add the ground pork and minced heart. Cook, stirring often, for 5 minutes, until cooked through and brown.
2. Add the scallions, ginger, and lemongrass; cook, stirring constantly, for 1 minute, or until fragrant. Stir in the fish sauce, lime juice, and stevia. Cook for 30 seconds, or until bubbling. Remove the skillet from the heat and cool for a couple of minutes.
3. To serve, spoon 1 to 2 tablespoons of the pork mixture into each lettuce leaf. Sprinkle with 1 or 2 jalapeño strips and just a few pine nuts as a garnish before folding closed.

Liver and Bacon
Makes 6 servings

Here's a hearty lunch that'll keep you working all afternoon, or a rejuvenating dinner at the end of a long, hard day at the office. The bacon and liver are a sweet, savory, and salty blend of primal flavors. This recipe is wonderful served on top of Cauliflower Mashers (page 268)! Or enjoy it with a side salad or seasoned, steamed greens with avocado oil drizzled on top.

4 slices organic nitrate-free thick-cut bacon, cut into ½-inch
    pieces
Organic pastured lard, as necessary
8 sage leaves
1 medium shallot, thinly sliced and separated into rings
1 pound organic pastured calf or beef liver, cut into 6 equal
    pieces
4 cups Primal Bone Broth (page 209), preferably chicken
    bone broth, or 1 quart packaged organic free-range
    gluten- and MSG-free chicken broth
Ground black pepper

1. Put the bacon in a large skillet and set over medium heat. Cook, stirring occasionally, for 4 minutes, or until crisp. Use a slotted spoon to transfer the bacon to a plate lined with paper towels. At this point, you'll need 3 tablespoons rendered fat in the skillet. Either discard any more bacon fat from the skillet or add a little lard to make sure you have enough.
2. Add the sage leaves and fry, stirring often, for 2 minutes, or until crispy. Remove them with a slotted spoon and drain on the plate with the bacon.
3. Add the shallot and cook, stirring often, for 2 minutes, or until softened. Transfer the shallot to the plate.
4. If the pan is dry, add up to 1 tablespoon reserved bacon fat or additional lard. Add the liver; reduce the heat to medium-low. Cook,

turning once, for 5 minutes, or until well browned but still slightly pink in the center.

5. Return the bacon and sage to the skillet. Pour in the broth; cook for 1 minute, or until reduced to a thick sauce. Spoon onto serving plates. Crumble the sage leaves over the meat; season with pepper.

Note: For better texture and a milder flavor, soak the liver strips in a bowl of cool tap water with the juice of a medium lemon or 2 tablespoons raw unfiltered cider vinegar for 20 minutes. Drain, then pat dry.

Primal Roast Chicken
Makes 8 servings

Skip the supermarket's rotisserie birds. Here's the best roast chicken, a Sunday dinner ready any night of the week. The ghee adds a mellow butteriness that would befit a Parisian bistro. Serve with steamed cauliflower florets and some soaked/sprouted (i.e., activated) cashews or toasted pine nuts, if you can have them. And save those giblets for Best Ever Grilled Steak (page 244), Chicken Heart Anticuchos (page 258), or other recipes that add a touch of organ meat.

⅓ cup Pure Indian Foods Cultured Ghee

2 tablespoons minced chives

2 teaspoons minced garlic

1 teaspoon Himalayan or Celtic sea salt

1 teaspoon ground black pepper

1 (3-pound) organic free-range whole chicken, giblets and neck removed from the inner cavities

1 small yellow or white onion, halved

1 small lemon, halved

1. Position the rack in the center of the oven. Preheat the oven to 375°F.

2. Mix the ghee, chives, garlic, salt, and pepper in a small bowl until a wet paste. With clean, dry fingers, separate the skin from the meat over the breast and thighs without tearing or removing the skin. It should stay attached around the edges and toward the back of each section. Smear a little more than half the ghee paste over the meat and under the skin in these places. Then spread the remaining ghee mixture over the outside of the bird, patting the skin into place. Push the onion and lemon into the cavity.

3. Set the chicken breast side up in a small roasting pan or a large oven-safe skillet. Roast for 45 minutes. Baste well with any pan juices.

4. Continue roasting, basting more frequently, for another 45 minutes, or until an instant-read meat thermometer inserted into a thigh and the thickest part of the breast without touching bone registers 165°F. Set aside on a carving or cutting board for 10 minutes. Remove the onion and lemon before carving and serving.

Note: The easiest way to "carve" a roast chicken is with poultry shears. You can cut the bird in half, remove the legs, and even remove the thighs. Don't forget to save the meatless carcass for bone broth!

Chicken Thigh Skillet Supper
Makes 4 servings

Here's a family meal that can keep you eating primal any night of the week. It's an old-fashioned skillet supper that you can set on a trivet right at the table. Save those fennel stems and fronds in a sealed bag in the freezer to use in your next batch of bone broth.

2 tablespoons toasted sesame oil

4 (5-ounce) organic free-range bone-in chicken thighs

1 small yellow or white onion, chopped

1 small fennel bulb, trimmed of its fronds and stems, then chopped

1 medium lemon, thinly sliced and seeded

⅓ cup pitted black olives

1 teaspoon fennel seeds

2 (4-inch) fresh rosemary sprigs

½ cup Primal Bone Broth (page 209), preferably chicken bone broth, or packaged/organic free-range gluten- and MSG-free chicken broth

½ teaspoon Himalayan or Celtic sea salt

½ teaspoon ground black pepper

1. Position the rack in the center of the oven; heat the oven to 375°F.
2. Melt the oil in a large, oven-safe skillet set over medium-high heat. Add the chicken and brown well, turning once, about 4 minutes. Transfer the chicken to a plate.
3. Add the onion and fennel; cook, stirring often, for 4 minutes, or until softened. Add the lemon, olives, and fennel seeds. Cook about 20 seconds, or until fragrant.
4. Return the chicken to the skillet. Tuck the rosemary sprig into the sauce. Pour the broth over the dish; sprinkle with the salt and pepper. Set in the oven and bake for 20 minutes, or until the chicken is tender and cooked through. Cool for 5 minutes before serving.

Primal Chicken Marsala with Sautéed Wild Mushrooms and Vegetables

Makes 4 servings

To pound chicken thighs flat, place each one between sheets of wax paper, then use the bottom of a heavy saucepan or the smooth side of a meat mallet to create ¼-inch thick cutlets. Strike the chicken with firm but not hard comma-like arcs.

4 (3-ounce) organic free-range boneless, skinless chicken thighs,
  pounded flat

½ teaspoon Himalayan or Celtic sea salt

½ teaspoon ground black pepper

¼ cup organic duck fat or schmaltz (chicken fat), preferably Fatworks

1 small yellow onion, chopped

8 ounces thin asparagus spears, chopped

4 ounces maitake mushrooms, thinly sliced

2 ounces shiitake mushroom caps, thinly sliced

½ cup baby spinach leaves

2 teaspoons chopped fresh oregano leaves

2 teaspoons chopped fresh rosemary leaves

1 teaspoon minced garlic

¼ cup Marsala wine or Primal Bone Broth (page 209)

¼ cup organic coconut cream with at least 22% fat, preferably
  Wilderness Family Naturals

1. Season the chicken with the salt and pepper. Heat 2 tablespoons of the duck fat in a large skillet set over medium-low heat. Add the chicken and cook, turning once, for 5 minutes, until well browned. Transfer the chicken to plates or a platter.

2. Melt the remaining 2 tablespoons duck fat in the skillet. Add the onion and cook, stirring often, for 2 minutes, or until it just begins to soften. Add the asparagus; cook, stirring often, for 2 minutes, or until the asparagus is bright green.

3. Add both mushrooms and cook, stirring once in a while, for 3 minutes, or until they give off their liquid. Add the spinach, oregano, rosemary, and garlic. Cook, tossing constantly, for 1 minute, until the spinach wilts.

4. Pour in the Marsala and the coconut cream. Stir well to combine. Cook for 1 minute, or until hot and bubbling. Spoon this sauce and vegetables over the chicken to serve.

Note: Any alcohol content in the Marsala wine will evaporate with 20 to 30 seconds of simmering. Also, there is only an estimated 2.3 g of sugar in

¼ cup of Marsala wine, as used in this recipe, amounting to 0.57 g of sugar per serving—roughly the same natural sugar content as in just over ¼ pound of steamed broccoli (0.48 g) or ¼ cup of almonds (0.43 g). I offer the broth option for those extra concerned about unnecessary sugar intake, but the amount present in the Marsala option is really quite minimal and the unique flavor it imparts is marvelous.

MORE

For a "more surf than turf" twist on this recipe, you can substitute four 3-ounce pieces of salmon fillet for the chicken (using Ōra King brand king salmon from New Zealand—see "Nourishing Resources" on page 285 for sourcing info).

Braised Chicken Thighs with Mushrooms
Makes 4 servings

Here's old-fashioned comfort fare turned primal! The lard will deepen the flavors of the dish considerably. If you want a brighter flavor, squeeze a wedge of lemon over each serving.

4 (3-ounce) organic free-range boneless, skinless chicken thighs

½ teaspoon Himalayan or Celtic sea salt

½ teaspoon ground black pepper

2 tablespoons organic pastured lard

2 medium shallots, thinly sliced and separated into rings

8 ounces shiitake mushroom caps, thinly sliced

2 teaspoons minced garlic

1 teaspoon herbes de Provence

1 teaspoon mild paprika

½ cup Primal Bone Broth (page 209), preferably chicken bone broth, or packaged organic free-range gluten- and MSG-free chicken broth

1. Season the chicken with the salt and pepper. Melt half the lard in a medium skillet set over medium heat. Add the thighs and cook, turning once, for 4 minutes, or until browned but not cooked through. Transfer the chicken to a plate.
2. Melt the remainder of the lard in the skillet. Add the shallots; cook, stirring constantly, for 1 minute, or until just barely softened. Add the mushrooms, garlic, herbes de Provence, and paprika. Cook, stirring often, for 1 minute, until the mushrooms just begin to soften.
3. Pour in the broth. Return the chicken to the skillet, cover, reduce the heat to very low, and simmer for 20 minutes, or until the chicken is tender.

MORE

Substitute yellow curry and turmeric, or thyme and coriander, or marjoram and rosemary for the herbes de Provence and paprika.

Thai Chicken Curry Stir-Fry
Makes 4 servings

This meal has a little of everything to please your palate, satisfy your appetite, and make your budget happy. If you close your eyes and inhale the intoxicating aroma, you can almost imagine yourself on a vacation in Phuket.

    2 tablespoons virgin coconut oil
    1 small red onion, halved and sliced into thin half-moons
    1½ cups chopped broccoli (about 12 ounces)
    1 cup fresh snap or snow peas (about 4 ounces)
    1 cup thinly sliced asparagus spears (about 4 ounces)
    12 ounces organic free-range boneless, skinless chicken thighs,
        sliced into thin strips

1 tablespoon minced fresh ginger

2 teaspoons yellow curry powder

1 teaspoon minced garlic

½ teaspoon Himalayan or Celtic sea salt

4 ounces shiitake caps or maitake mushrooms, thinly sliced

¼ cup packed baby spinach leaves

2 tablespoons shredded unsweetened coconut

½ cup full-fat coconut milk

1 tablespoon sugar- and MSG-free fish sauce

1 tablespoon fresh lime juice

Sesame oil or hot chile sesame oil

1. Melt the coconut oil in a very large skillet or a wok set over medium-high heat. Add the onion, stir-fry for 1 minute. Add the broccoli, peas, and asparagus; stir-fry for 2 minutes, or until the vegetables turn bright green.

2. Add the chicken; stir-fry for 4 minutes, or until the chicken is cooked through. Add the ginger, curry powder, garlic, and salt. Cook, tossing constantly, for 15 seconds, or until aromatic.

3. Add the mushrooms, spinach, and shredded coconut; stir-fry for 2 minutes, or until the spinach wilts. Pour in the coconut milk, fish sauce, and lime juice. Stir-fry for 1 minute, or until bubbling and hot. Divide among 4 bowls; drizzle each with a little sesame oil.

Note: For those concerned about BPA, guar gum, or xanthan gum, the brand Wilderness Family Naturals coconut milk and cream come in a carton. If you suffer from GI symptoms in general (especially IBS), you can go to www.importfood.com and order the Aroy-D all-natural coconut milk or cream in a carton (no BPA, guar gum, or xanthan gum added).

Chicken Heart Anticuchos

Makes 4 servings (2 skewers each)

Inspired by my recent travels through Peru, this South American specialty is real primal fare! I've added Brussels sprouts for their slightly bitter flavor, a great contrast to the full-flavored marinade. Make sure the coconut oil has cooled to room temperature before you use it. Otherwise, the marinade will begin to cook the chicken hearts too soon.

12 ounces organic free-range chicken hearts

2 tablespoons virgin coconut oil, melted and cooled

2 tablespoons raw unfiltered cider vinegar (such as Bragg)

2 teaspoons dried oregano

1 teaspoon mild paprika

1 teaspoon minced garlic

½ teaspoon Himalayan or Celtic sea salt

¼ teaspoon cayenne pepper

24 small Brussels sprouts (about 10 ounces), trimmed

8 bamboo skewers (no need to soak)

1 cup Primal Gaucho Chimichurri (page 208)

1. Toss the chicken hearts, oil, vinegar, oregano, paprika, garlic, salt, and cayenne in a medium bowl until the chicken hearts are well coated in the spices. Refrigerate for 2 hours to blend the flavors.
2. Prepare a grill for high-heat direct cooking, or set a large grill pan over medium-high heat for a couple of minutes. Alternately thread the chicken hearts and Brussels sprouts onto the bamboo skewers, dividing the ingredients evenly among the skewers.
3. Grill, turning several times, for 10 minutes, or until lightly charred and cooked through. Spoon 2 tablespoons Primal Gaucho Chimichurri over each skewer to serve.

Lamb Chop Skillet Supper
Makes 4 servings

Lamb chops made a great dinner! They're meaty and satisfying, with a bold flavor that can stand up to this aromatic sauce. Reduce the artichoke mixture until the tomatoes break down and the sauce has a thick, rich consistency.

> 8 (3-ounce) organic pastured bone-in lamb rib or loin chops
>   (2 chops yield about 3 ounces of meat)
> ½ teaspoon Himalayan or Celtic sea salt
> ½ teaspoon ground black pepper
> 2 tablespoons organic lard or beef tallow, preferably Fatworks
> 9 ounces frozen artichoke heart quarters, thawed
> 6 ounces small cauliflower florets
> 1 teaspoon dried thyme
> ½ teaspoon dried dill
> 1 (14-ounce) can diced fire-roasted tomatoes
> ¼ cup Primal Bone Broth (page 209), preferably chicken bone
>   broth, or packaged organic free-range gluten- and MSG-free
>   chicken broth

1. Season the lamb chops with the salt and pepper. Melt the lard in a large, oven-safe skillet set over medium heat. Add the lamb chops; brown well, turning once, about 4 minutes. Transfer to a plate.
2. Add the artichokes, cauliflower, thyme, and dill. Cook, stirring constantly, for 1 minute. Pour in the tomatoes and broth; bring the sauce to a full simmer. Cook, stirring occasionally, for 10 minutes, or until somewhat thickened.
3. Return the lamb chops and any juices to the skillet. Cook for 1 to 2 minutes, or until warmed through, spooning the sauce over the lamb chops as they warm up.

Primal Zoodles
Makes 4 servings

Zoodles are really spaghetti made from zucchini. There are different vegetable noodle–making gizmos that you can purchase, such as the Spiralizer, the Benriner tool from Japan, or even a handheld vegetable julienne tool from OXO. You can also make zoodles with a mandoline or even a standard vegetable peeler for wider, longer noodles when you run either all the way down the length of the vegetable. For a simpler meal without this ragù, stir-fry the zoodles in a little pure cultured ghee with minced garlic and chopped fresh parsley.

3 large zucchini

3 tablespoons pure cultured ghee

1 small yellow or white onion, chopped

1 large portobello mushroom cap, chopped

2 teaspoons minced garlic

12 ounces organic grass-fed ground beef, preferably 80% lean

1 (14-ounce) can diced tomatoes

1 teaspoon dried oregano

1 teaspoon dried thyme

¼ teaspoon grated nutmeg

¼ teaspoon Himalayan or Celtic sea salt

1. Use a vegetable peeler or another specialty kitchen tool to make long, flat strips down the length of the zucchini.
2. Melt 1½ tablespoons of the ghee in a very large skillet set over medium heat. Add the zucchini and cook, tossing often, about 1 minute, or until tender but still with a little toothy texture. Divide the zucchini among 4 servings bowls or place it all on a platter.
3. Melt the remaining 1½ tablespoons ghee in the skillet over medium heat. Add the onion; cook, stirring often, for 3 minutes, or until softened. Add the mushrooms and garlic; cook, stirring

often, for 2 minutes, until the mushrooms just begin to give off their liquid.

4. Crumble in the ground beef. Cook, stirring occasionally and breaking up any chunks with the back of a wooden spoon, for 4 minutes, or until the ground beef loses its raw, pink color.

5. Stir in the tomatoes, oregano, thyme, nutmeg, and salt. Bring to a simmer, then reduce the heat to low and cook, uncovered but stirring often, for 5 minutes, or until somewhat thickened. Ladle the sauce over the noodles.

MORE

If you want a Parmesan-like garnish, sprinkle a little nutritional yeast on top. Or drizzle a little aged balsamic vinegar on top for a little sweet-tangy zip.

Carnitas Salad
Makes 1 serving

This recipe gives leftover Primal Kālua Pork a south-of-the-border twist. You'll create a single-serving chopped salad, a fast meal any night of the week. Double, triple, or even quadruple the recipe as needed, building enough plates of salad for everyone.

2 cups cored and shredded romaine lettuce

½ cup cored and finely shredded red cabbage

½ Hass avocado, pitted, peeled, and sliced

1 very thin red onion slice, separated into rings

3 ounces leftover Primal Kālua Pork (page 245)

2 tablespoons pico de gallo

1 tablespoon avocado oil

1 tablespoon fresh lime juice

Minced seeded fresh jalapeño, garlic pepper, and Himalayan or
    Celtic sea salt

1. Place the romaine, cabbage, avocado, and onion on a dinner plate. Gently toss, if desired, or simply leave in layers.
2. Scatter the pork over the vegetables. Spoon the pico de gallo over the pork. Drizzle the oil and lime juice over the salad. Garnish with jalapeño, garlic pepper, and salt, if desired.

Note: You can find bags of organic, pre-shredded lettuces and cabbages at most large supermarkets these days.

MORE

The pork can be warmed before adding it to the salad. Place 2 to 3 ounces per serving in a small skillet and cook over medium heat, stirring often, until warmed through, about 2 minutes.

Primalritos
Makes 4 servings

You've never had burritos like these! Primalritos make an unbelievably satisfying meal. This one's an absolute favorite around my house!

2 cups cored and shredded lettuce (such as romaine, butter, or Boston)

1 cup broccoli sprouts (about ¾ ounce)

2 medium Hass avocados, pitted, peeled, and diced

2 tablespoons fresh lemon juice

2 tablespoons avocado oil

½ teaspoon Himalayan or Celtic sea salt

½ teaspoon ground black pepper

2 tablespoons virgin coconut oil

1 medium yellow or white onion, chopped

8 ounces organic grass-fed ground beef, preferably 80% lean or
    fattier

4 ounces organic grass-fed beef liver, minced

2 teaspoons chili powder

2 teaspoons minced garlic

7 ounces enoki mushrooms, coarsely chopped

3 ounces Swiss chard leaves, stemmed and chopped

1 (14-ounce) can diced fire-roasted tomatoes

4 coconut wraps

1. Toss the lettuce, broccoli sprouts, avocado, lemon juice, avocado oil, salt, and pepper in a large bowl until well combined.
2. Melt the coconut oil in a large skillet set over medium heat. Add the onion; cook, stirring often, for 3 minutes, or until softened. Crumble in the ground beef and add the liver. Cook, stirring occasionally and breaking up the ground beef with the back of a wooden spoon, for 4 minutes, until the meat loses its raw, pink color.
3. Stir in the chili powder and garlic; stir over the heat for 15 seconds, until fragrant. Add the mushrooms and chard; cook, stirring often, about 1 minute, or until the chard begins to wilt.
4. Pour in the tomatoes and bring the mixture to a simmer. Reduce the heat to low and cook, stirring often, for 5 minutes, or until somewhat thickened.
5. Divide the meat mixture among the 4 wraps on plates. Fold or roll the wraps closed. Top with the lettuce mixture to serve. Optional: garnish with a high-quality fresh salsa.

Wild-Caught Trout or Walleye Almondine
Makes 4 servings

Here's a recipe almost anyone who loves seafood will find delicious. It calls for quite a bit of almond flour, but you won't use it all. You want enough to get an even coating across the fillets without the remainder getting too gummy in the process.

  2 tablespoons virgin coconut oil

  2 large yellow or white onions, sliced into thin rings

  2 teaspoons minced garlic

  4 (3-ounce) trout or walleye fillets

  ½ teaspoon Himalayan or Celtic sea salt

  ½ teaspoon ground black pepper

  1 cup finely milled almond flour (such as Bob's Red Mill)

  6 tablespoons organic duck fat, preferably Fatworks

  ½ cup slivered almonds or pine nuts

  2 tablespoons minced fresh basil, cilantro, or parsley leaves

  1 tablespoon minced fresh chives

  4 lemon wedges

1. Melt the oil in a large skillet set over very low heat. Add the onions and cook, stirring often, for 40 minutes, or until golden brown, very soft, and very sweet. Should the onions brown too deeply, reduce the heat even further.
2. Add the garlic. Cook, stirring often, for 2 minutes, or until fragrant. Set aside off the heat.
3. Season the fillets with the salt and pepper. Spread the almond flour on a large plate and dredge the fillets in it, patting them down to get an even coating but shaking off any excess.
4. Melt the duck fat in a second large skillet set over medium heat. Add the fish and cook for 6 minutes, turning once, until crisp and cooked through. Transfer to 4 serving plates.
5. Add the nuts to the skillet and toast, stirring often, for 1 minute, or until fragrant. Set aside off the heat.
6. Spoon the onions over the fish; sprinkle the nuts and herbs over the onions. Offer a lemon wedge to squeeze over each serving as a garnish.

Fish Tacos
Makes 4 servings

There may be no better meal for the deck or patio when the weather turns warmer. If you've got lots of friends over, double or even triple the recipe and bring the vegetables and garnishes to the table so everyone can assemble their own tacos.

4 (3-ounce) trout or walleye fillets

1 tablespoon chili powder

½ teaspoon Himalayan or Celtic sea salt

2 tablespoons toasted sesame oil

8 coconut wraps

4 cups cored and chopped butter lettuce, cored and finely shredded green cabbage, and/or broccoli sprouts (a combo of two is preferred)

2 medium Hass avocados, peeled, pitted, and sliced

½ cup chopped red onion (about 1 small)

½ cup fresh cilantro leaves

1 cup Primal Cultured Vegetable Kraut (page 211), optional

Up to 2 medium jalapeños, seeded and minced (optional)

½ cup avocado oil

8 lemon wedges

1. Season the fillets with the chili powder and salt. Heat the oil in a large skillet set over medium heat. Add the fillets and cook, turning once, for 4 minutes, or until cooked through. Transfer the fillets to a cutting board and slice into 1-inch-thick sections.
2. Lay the coconut wraps on a clean, dry work surface. Divide the fish pieces among them. Top evenly with the lettuce, avocado, onion, and cilantro, as well as the sauerkraut and jalapeños, if desired. Drizzle each with 2 tablespoons of the avocado oil and squeeze a lemon wedge over each before folding closed.

Side Dishes

The side dishes in the 21-day meal plan are merely suggested pairings for main course entrees but you can mix or match these to your own liking, as you wish!

The Best Kale Salad
Makes 4 servings

By massaging a little lemon or lime juice into kale leaves, you can soften them a bit and make them even tastier! It doesn't take much more to turn them into a great side salad that can go with just about any cut of protein off the grill or out of the oven. If you ever make this for a potluck, you'll always be asked to bring it!

¼ cup chopped pecans or pine nuts

8 ounces baby kale leaves or chopped large kale leaves

2 tablespoons fresh lemon or lime juice

½ teaspoon Himalayan or Celtic sea salt

½ teaspoon ground black pepper

1 large Globe tomato, diced

3 tablespoons extra-virgin cold-pressed olive oil

1. Set a dry medium skillet over medium-low heat. Add the pecans, toast, stirring occasionally, for 5 minutes, or until lightly browned and aromatic. Pour into a large bowl to cool while you prepare the salad.
2. Place the kale in a large bowl. Add the lemon juice, salt, and pepper. With clean, dry hands, gently massage the juice and seasonings into the kale leaves to help break them down a bit, about 30 seconds for the baby leaves or up to 2 minutes for the larger leaves. Add the toasted nuts, tomato, and oil. Toss well to serve.

MORE

Reduce the olive oil to 1 tablespoon. Mash a small, pitted, peeled Hass avocado into the oil to create a creamy dressing.

Primally Raw Cauliflower Tabouli
Makes 4 to 6 servings

I first learned about this recipe from an Australian friend, Dr. Ron Ehrlich, a biological dentist and a nutritional expert with his own podcast, *The Good Doctors*. A devotee of all things primal, Ron is also a great home cook. I've adapted his original a bit to keep the flavors intact but simplify the preparation.

1 small cauliflower head (about 1¼ pounds), leaves removed, the
    remainder coarsely chopped
8 ounces small broccoli florets, either raw or very lightly steamed
    (still crunchy), as you prefer
1 small red onion, finely chopped
1 small cucumber, peeled, seeded, and chopped
1 cup lightly packed fresh parsley leaves, finely chopped
½ cup extra-virgin cold-pressed olive oil
3 tablespoons fresh lemon juice
1 teaspoon Himalayan or Celtic sea salt
½ teaspoon ground black pepper

1. Place the cauliflower and broccoli in a large food processor fitted with the chopping blade. Pulse repeatedly until finely ground. Work in batches as necessary.
2. Transfer the ground vegetables to a large bowl. Add the onion, cucumber, parsley, oil, lemon juice, salt, and pepper. Toss well before serving.

Note: To seed a cucumber after peeling it, halve it lengthwise, then use a serrated grapefruit spoon or even just a teaspoon to scrape out the tiny seeds and their pulp.

Cauliflower Mashers
Makes 4 to 6 servings

This is the quintessential alternative to mashed potatoes, and (in my humble opinion) far more flavorful! It is also largely carb-free yet contains fiber and a nourishing blend of highly beneficial nutrients. Use it as you would mashed potatoes and never miss potatoes again!

1 large cauliflower head (about 2½ pounds), leaves removed, the
    remainder cut into large chunks
¼ cup organic coconut cream with at least 22% fat, preferably
    Wilderness Family Naturals, or 3 tablespoons Kite Hill almond
    cream cheese
2 tablespoons fresh lemon juice
2 tablespoons pure cultured ghee or organic duck fat, preferably
    Fatworks
1 medium garlic clove
1 teaspoon Himalayan or Celtic sea salt
½ teaspoon ground black pepper
Up to ¼ cup Primal Bone Broth (page 209), preferably chicken
    broth, or packaged organic free-range gluten- and MSG-free
    chicken broth
Minced fresh chives

1. Set a large vegetable steamer over 1 inch of simmering water in a large saucepan. Add the cauliflower chunks, cover, and steam for 10 minutes, or until tender.
2. Transfer the cauliflower to a large food processor fitted with the chopping blade. Add the coconut cream, lemon juice, ghee, garlic, salt, and pepper. Cover and process, drizzling in the broth through

the feed tube, until the mixture resembles mashed potatoes, not soup. Garnish the servings with chives.

MORE

Turn this side dish into a main course by topping it with sliced yellow onions and chopped shiitake or maitake mushrooms that have been cooked until soft in a little pure cultured ghee or organic duck fat.

Primal Cauliflower Fried Rice
Makes 4 servings

You can use this as a side dish for almost any protein or serve it alongside stir-fries as you would rice. It's great with the Primal Kālua Pork (page 245). Or use it as a base in the bowls for the Thai Chicken Curry Stir-Fry (page 256).

3 tablespoons virgin coconut oil

4 medium scallions, thinly sliced

1 tablespoon minced fresh ginger

2 teaspoons minced garlic

1 small cauliflower head (about 1¼ pounds), leaves removed, the remainder grated through the large holes of a box grater or run through the shredding blade of a food processor

2 tablespoons coconut aminos

1. Melt the oil in a large wok or skillet set over medium-high heat. Add the scallions, ginger, and garlic; stir-fry for 30 seconds, or until fragrant.
2. Add the cauliflower. Stir-fry for 3 minutes, or until tender but still a little crunchy. Add the coconut aminos and toss to blend well before serving.

MORE

For a heartier meal, chop 3 to 6 ounces leftover Crispy Pork Belly and add these with the scallion mixture.

Lithuanian Red Cabbage

Makes 4 servings

My parents came from Lithuania. Among the many Lithuanian culinary delights I grew up with was something similar to this dish. I hope my mother will forgive me for the liberties I've taken to make it primal, but I think you'll agree that this dish is as delicious as it is healthy!

   2 tablespoons organic duck fat, preferably Fatworks
   ½ large red cabbage (about 2½ pounds total weight), cored and
      finely chopped
   6 ounces shiitake mushroom caps, thinly sliced
   2 tablespoons aged balsamic vinegar
   ½ teaspoon Himalayan or Celtic sea salt

1. Melt the duck fat in a large skillet set over medium heat. Add the cabbage and cook, stirring often, for 6 minutes, or until wilted but with some crunch.
2. Add the mushrooms and vinegar. Cook, stirring often, for 2 minutes, or until the mushrooms have softened. Stir in the salt before serving.

Primal Greek Spinach

Makes 4 servings

Opa! Okay, I'm not Greek. But I love Greek food. Here's my heartier take on horta, a Greek classic.

2 tablespoons organic duck fat or schmaltz (chicken fat),
 preferably Fatworks

1 medium yellow or white onion, finely chopped

⅓ cup pine nuts

4 cups stemmed, chopped large spinach leaves

2 teaspoons minced fresh oregano leaves

1 teaspoon fresh thyme leaves

2 tablespoons extra-virgin cold-pressed olive oil

2 tablespoons fresh lemon juice

½ teaspoon Himalayan or Celtic sea salt

1. Melt the duck fat in a large skillet set over medium heat. Add the onion and pine nuts. Cook, stirring often, for 4 minutes, or until the onion softens. Add the spinach and cook, tossing constantly, for 2 minutes, or until it begins to wilt.
2. Pour in ¼ cup of water. Cover the skillet, reduce the heat to low, and simmer for 5 minutes, or until the spinach is tender. Stir in the oregano and thyme. Continue cooking, stirring all the while, for about 1 minute, or until any additional liquid evaporates.
3. Remove from the heat. Drizzle the top of the dish with the oil and lemon juice. Sprinkle with salt before serving.

On-the-Go Snacks or Meals

Use these "to-go" recipes for occasions when you may not have the time or ability to make bigger meals at home, have a busy day, or are traveling. They're your backup plan—insurance for unpredictable moments! Pack small containers of these goodies and slip them into the hotel refrigerator or a cooler while on the go. Since they are nutrient-dense and many are high in protein, I refer to them as "meals," as they would tend to replace regular entrées with their protein content. It's easy enough to find a salad on the road (ask for olive oil and balsamic vinegar, or a lemon wedge or two), so many of the following foods can be used to supply critical fats, complete protein (save for the nuts), and fat-soluble nutrients if you cannot find healthy, grass-fed sources of meat or poultry. The Primal Keto-Coconut Pemmican makes for an amazingly mouthwatering and satisfying snack (a spoonful or two will do you) if you find yourself hungry between meals—and kids love the stuff.

Ground Beef Jerky

Makes 32 mini-patties

This is the most incredible-tasting jerky I've ever eaten! Making the patties with sea salt will yield a cleaner, brighter flavor, while using the coconut aminos will add a teriyaki flavor to the mix.

1½ tablespoons raw unfiltered cider vinegar (such as Bragg)

4 teaspoons Himalayan or Celtic sea salt, or coconut aminos

2 teaspoons chili powder

1½ teaspoons garlic powder

1½ teaspoons onion powder

1½ teaspoons ground ginger

1½ teaspoons ground black pepper

3 drops liquid stevia

2 pounds organic grass-fed ground beef, preferably 80% lean

1. Stir the vinegar, salt, chili powder, garlic powder, onion powder, ginger, pepper, and stevia in a medium bowl until well blended. Add the ground beef and stir until uniform.
2. Form this mixture into 1-ounce patties, about 2 tablespoons per patty (but use kitchen scales for the best accuracy). Flatten the patties to ¼-inch thickness.
3. Set a 5-tray dehydrator on the highest setting (145° to 155°F). Fill the drying racks with the patties. Dry for around 5 to 10 hours, rotating the trays about halfway through, until the patties are cooked through and a little leathery. Cool and store in a sealed container in the refrigerator for up to 1 week.

Note: Eat no more than three of these patties as a serving. They aren't potato chips! If you've had these as a snack, stick to a big chopped salad for your next meal and skip the protein altogether.

Primal Keto-Coconut Pemmican

Makes about 3 pounds. Most folks will find 2 to 3 tablespoons of this amazingly rich collection of healthy fats and flavors quite filling.

This is a tasty snack for athletes, students, or those on the go look-ing for an ultra-quick mental and physical energy source they can take with them almost anywhere and enjoy as a snack without add-ing too much to their protein load. Be forewarned, though, that the ingredients for this can be a bit pricy. On the plus side, this recipe will make enough to last you a *long* while. Unfortunately, this rec-ipe is not for you if you have an immune reactivity to tree nuts or coconut.

1 (25-ounce) jar virgin coconut oil

8 ounces coconut butter

4 ounces cacao butter

½ cup almond flour (such as Bob's Red Mill)

½ cup hazelnut flour

¼ cup coconut flour

1 to 2 tablespoons ground cinnamon

1 tablespoon alcohol-free vanilla extract

3 drops liquid stevia

1½ cups unsweetened shredded coconut or coconut flakes

1½ cups chopped activated macadamia nuts, almonds,
   Brazil nuts, skinned hazelnuts, pumpkin seeds, and/or
   chia seeds

1. Melt the oil, coconut butter, and cacao butter in a medium sauce-pan set over low heat. Set aside to cool for 5 minutes.

2. Pour the melted fats into a large blender. Add the almond flour, hazelnut flour, coconut flour, cinnamon, and stevia, if using. Cover and blend until smooth. Pour into a large bowl.

3. Stir in the shredded coconut and the nuts and/or seeds. Pour the blended mixture either into silicone-based ice cube tray molds (to portion it out into bite-size servings) or into small canning jars that can be sealed. Refrigerate or freeze until set. Enjoy as individual portions or right out of a jar, at home or on the go! This keeps well at room temperature but can be refrigerated as well. If you choose to refrigerate it, you may want to leave it out for an hour to soften a bit before digging in.

MORE

Add up to ¼ cup maca powder with the other flours. Add up to ½ cup cacao nibs with the coconut and nuts or seeds.

Stuffed Grape Leaves

Makes about 24 stuffed leaves (having 1½ ounce of meat each)

Durga Fuller, a devotee of low-carb and paleo-friendly cuisine, shared this recipe with me, and I adapted it for a great go-to primal snack. For a full meal, serve these grape leaves with Primal Greek Spinach (page 270) or Cauliflower Mashers (page 268) and a salad of sliced tomatoes and pitted black olives. You can also pack a cooler with these to take on the go, as it is delicious cold and makes a great take-along finger food, as well as a delicious and tantalizing appetizer at parties!

4 tablespoons pure cultured ghee, plus more for the casserole

2 small yellow or white onions, minced

½ cup very finely chopped celery leaves or stemmed mustard greens

4 teaspoons minced garlic

1 pound organic grass-fed ground lamb or beef

¼ cup packed fresh flat-leaf parsley leaves, finely chopped

¼ cup pine nuts

3 tablespoons packed fresh oregano leaves, finely chopped

1 teaspoon Himalayan or Celtic sea salt

½ teaspoon ground black pepper

40 jarred grape leaves, drained and rinsed

At least 2 cups Primal Bone Broth (page 209), preferably beef
   broth, or packaged organic free-range gluten- and MSG-free
   beef broth

½ cup fresh lemon juice

1. Position the rack in the center of the oven. Preheat the oven to 350°F. Lightly grease the inside of a covered 2- to 4-quart round or oval casserole with a little ghee spread on a paper towel.

2. Melt 2 tablespoons of the ghee in a medium skillet set over medium-low heat. Add the onions; cook, stirring often, for 3 minutes, or until just softened. Add the celery leaves and garlic; cook, stirring often, for 2 minutes, or until just wilted. Set aside off the heat to cool for 15 minutes.

3. Stir the contents of the skillet into the ground meat in a large bowl. Mix in the parsley, pine nuts, oregano, salt, and pepper until uniform.

4. Use the smallest grape leaves to make a thin cover across the bottom of the casserole. Place a large grape leaf shiny side down on a clean, dry work surface. Snip off the stem, if visible. Place a rounded tablespoon of the meat mixture in the center of the leaf. Fold in the sides and roll the leaf closed. Place the seam side down in the casserole. Continue stuffing more grape leaves, making two layers if necessary.

5. Pour 2 cups broth and the lemon juice over the top. Add more broth to the casserole as necessary so the liquid just covers the stuffed grape leaves below. Dot with the remaining 2 tablespoons ghee. Lay a thin layer of grape leaves across the top of the casserole, covering the stuffed ones below.

6. Cover and bake for 1 hour. Cool in the cooking liquid until room

temperature. Remove the top layer of grape leaves. Store the covered casserole in the fridge for up to 5 days. Serve the stuffed grape leaves without the cooking liquid in the pot.

Primal Pâté

Makes 6 servings

Pâté is a mixture of cooked meats and fats. It makes a convenient snack or meal. Serve alongside fresh vegetables and Primal Gaucho Chimichurri (page 208). It is easy to make and great for parties. This version is adapted from one in *Nourishing Traditions* by Sally Fallon.

6 tablespoons duck fat or schmaltz (chicken fat), preferably Fatworks

1 medium yellow or white onion, chopped

12 ounces shiitake mushroom caps, maitake mushrooms, and/or portobello mushrooms, chopped

2 teaspoons minced garlic

1 pound organic free-range chicken (and/or other poultry) livers, trimmed and rinsed

1 teaspoon minced fresh rosemary leaves

1 teaspoon ground black pepper

½ teaspoon dry mustard powder

½ teaspoon dried dill

½ teaspoon Himalayan or Celtic sea salt

⅔ cup bone broth

5 to 10 drops liquid stevia

2 tablespoons fresh lemon juice

1. Melt 3 tablespoons of the duck fat in a large skillet set over medium heat. Add the onion; cook, stirring often, for 2 minutes, until the edges just soften. Add the mushrooms and garlic; cook, stirring often, for 6 minutes, or until the mushrooms give off their liquid and it mostly evaporates.

2. Add the livers and cook, stirring often, for 4 minutes, or until lightly browned. Stir in the rosemary, pepper, mustard powder, dill, and salt. Cook for 20 seconds, until just aromatic.

3. Pour in the broth, stevia, and the lemon juice. Simmer, stirring occasionally, for 10 minutes, or until the liquid has almost evaporated. Cool for 10 minutes.

4. Pour and scrape the contents of the skillet into a large food processor fitted with the chopping blade. Add the remaining 2 tablespoons duck fat. Cover and process until smooth. Transfer to a bowl. Cover and refrigerate for at least 6 hours before serving or up to 4 days.

Golden Mylk Elixir
Makes 2 servings

This über-healthy, comforting, and anti-inflammatory beverage is adapted from one that my friends serve at the Roadhouse in Byron Bay, Australia.

1 (1½-inch) piece turmeric root (about ½ ounce), grated through the large holes of a box grater

1 (1½-inch) piece fresh ginger (just under 1 ounce), grated through the large holes of a box grater

¼ teaspoon ground cinnamon

¼ teaspoon ground black pepper

2 cups filtered water

1 cup Nut Mylk (page 216)

1 tablespoon MCT oil or coconut oil

2 drops liquid stevia (optional)

1. Warm the turmeric, ginger, cinnamon, and pepper in a medium saucepan over low heat for 1 minute, or until very fragrant.

2. Pour in the water, raise the heat to medium, and bring to a full

simmer. Cook for about 8 minutes, or until the mixture has reduced to half its original volume.

3. Stir in the Nut Mylk, reduce the heat to low, and stir for 1 minute
to bind the fat-soluble compounds in the turmeric to the Nut
Mylk.

4. Strain into two mugs. Stir ½ tablespoon MCT oil and 1 drop stevia, if desired, into each mug before serving.

MORE

If you want to add a luscious frothy finish to this recipe, put an ounce
or two of the nondairy creamer in your milk frother to create a vel-
vety topping for the beverage. You can add a sprinkle of nutmeg or
cinnamon on top before serving for that special finishing touch.

Almond-Cardamom Ambrosia

Makes 28 (1-tablespoon) servings

This stuff is delicious! If you're struggling with sugar cravings, have a
tablespoonful to ward off hunger pangs (unless you have a sensitivity
to tree nuts or a total lack of self-restraint). Or smear it on organic
strawberries. Or add it to your morning smoothie. Each tablespoon
contains 3 grams of protein.

   1 (16-ounce) jar organic unsalted creamy lightly toasted almond
       butter
   1 tablespoon MCT oil or macadamia nut oil
   2 teaspoons ground cardamom
   2 teaspoons Himalayan or Celtic sea salt
   1 teaspoon alcohol-free vanilla extract
   2 drops liquid stevia (optional)

1. Pour off the almond oil at the top of the jar. Add the MCT oil.
Plunge a dinner knife into the center of the almond butter and stir

it inside the jar, working to get even the bits at the bottom of the jar into the mix, until fairly creamy.

2. Add the cardamom, salt, vanilla, and stevia, if desired. Continue stirring with the knife until smooth and uniform. Put the lid back on the jar and store in the refrigerator for up to 2 weeks.

HELPFUL RESOURCES

Ongoing Primal Fat Burner Support and Education: www.Primal FatBurner.com and www.PrimalBody-PrimalMind.com. My own websites, filled with articles, resources, recipes, and more, designed to support, delight, and educate primal fat burners everywhere!

Nutritional Therapy Association (NTA): A quality introductory source of certified education in nutritional therapy, with an emphasis on physiology, human evolutionary history, and the work of numerous acclaimed nutritional pioneers. Highly recommended. www .NutritionalTherapy.com

Hunt Gather Grow Foundation: www.huntgathergrowfoundation .com. A newly established foundation dedicated to bringing the "Real Food" communities together. Committed to democratic, bottom-up governance and the wisdom of Weston Price and other nutritional pioneers past and present. Offering numerous resources and regional chapters for community support.

Price-Pottenger Nutritional Foundation: www.ppnf.org. A non-profit education foundation committed to reversing the trend of declining health in our modern world. The organization teaches public and health professionals the proven principles from nutrition pioneers including Weston A. Price, Francis M. Pottenger Jr., and others.

Nourishing Australia: www.nourishingaustralia.org.au. Nourishing Australia is a not-for-profit organization dedicated to educating and inspiring people about the critical importance of nourishing soil, water, plants, animals, people, communities, and ultimately our planet.

The Ancestral Health Society: www.ancestryfoundation.org/AHS .html. The Ancestral Health Society fosters interdisciplinary collaboration among scientists, health professionals, and laypeople who study and communicate about the human ecological niche in modern health from an ancestral perspective.

MINDD Foundation: www.mindd.org. Centered in Sydney, Australia, the MINDD Foundation helps practitioners and patients discover and implement effective treatments for metabolic, immunologic, neurologic, digestive, and developmental conditions that often affect the mind. Their focus is on pediatric disorders such as ADHD, asthma, allergies, autism, chronic illness, depression, learning and language delay, and digestive and behavioral disorders. They also offer a list of MINDD-affiliated practitioners and other resources.

The Institute for Responsible Technology: www.responsibletech nology.org/GMFree/Home/index.cfm. Your number one source for comprehensive, clear, science-based, and hugely important information about GMOs. Please spend time on this website and support this organization!

The Center for Food Safety: www.truefoodnow.org. Works to protect human health and the environment by curbing the proliferation of harmful food production technologies and by promoting organic and other forms of sustainable agriculture. Say no to industrial agriculture and yes to real food!

THINCS: The International Network of Cholesterol Skeptics: www.thincs.org. A noncommercial organization of doctors and scientists providing information opposing the prevalent dogma about cholesterol and heart disease.

Nutrition and Metabolism Society: www.nmsociety.org. The Nutrition and Metabolism Society is a 501(c)3 nonprofit health organization that provides research, information, and education in the application of fundamental science to nutrition. The society is particularly dedicated to the application of low-carbohydrate nutrition toward resolving issues surrounding obesity, diabetes, cardiovascular disease, and other metabolic diseases.

Weston A. Price Foundation: www.westonaprice.org. Originally founded by Sally Fallon and the late Mary Enig, PhD, the organization promotes certain aspects of Weston Price's work and food activism. There are numerous regional chapters, which may be a good source for finding local organic/pastured foods in your area.

The Savory Institute: www.savory.global. An organization teaching Holistic Management to ranchers and landowners. It seeks to restore natural systems, healthy soils, healthy watersheds, and environmental diversity (plus a certain measure of global climate stability) through the healthy systematic restoration of ruminants to the land and the most natural approach to managing them.

Cyrex Labs: www.cyrexlabs.com. The only truly accurate and comprehensive lab offering for food sensitivity and immunologic testing anywhere. Available as of 2015 only in the United States, Canada, the United Kingdom, and Ireland. More locations in other countries soon to come.

Primal Tightwad: www.primaltightwad.com. Your guide to making primal eating more affordable. With tips and ideas to amaze even the most thrift-savvy consumer, Primal Tightwad proves that eating optimally well in no way means having to be wealthy and shows how you will literally save money compared to the standard American diet!

Eat Wild: www.eatwild.com. This is the definitive source for all things grass-fed, including links to many local sources, farmers, and ranchers near you!

Find a Spring: www.findaspring.com. This is a resource you can use to find clean, natural spring water near you. Many of these available sources of deep-aquifer, artesian natural spring water are either free or a low-cost means of obtaining the cleanest, purest water nature has to offer.

Information about SIBO (small intestinal bacterial overgrowth): www.siboinfo.com. SIBO expert Dr. Allison Siebecker's detailed, informative, and definitive website on the subject.

In addition, conferences such as Paleo(f)X and the Ancestral Health Society Symposium are incredible for educating, inspiring, and opening your eyes to the range of resources (including foods) available.

NOURISHING RESOURCES

Fatworks: https://fatworks.wazala.com. The world's finest source of truly organic pastured animal fats for cooking, including tallow, lard, and duck fat. Imitated by some, but unmatched in its uncompromising quality and meticulous sourcing.

Pure Indian Foods: Cultured Ghee (batch-tested to contain less than 0.25% lactose and 2.5 ppm casein/whey) at www.pureindianfoods .com/Grassfed-Organic-Cultured-Ghee-p/cg.htm. (Cultured) Turmeric Superghee (batch-tested to contain less than 0.5% lactose and less than 5 ppm casein/whey) at www.pureindianfoods.com/turmeric -superghee-p/tsg7.htm.

Antarctic krill oil: I recommend the one from Mercola.com, at http://shop.mercola.com/catalog/omega-3s,418,0,0.htm.

In case of accidental gluten/dairy exposure: A product called E3 Advanced Plus offered by gluten expert Dr. Tom O'Bryan is a gluten- and other antigenic-trace protein-digesting formula uniquely designed with powerful enzymes, prebiotics, and probiotics to break down gluten proteins by targeting both internal and external peptide bonds. This product is shown to produce 99 percent digestion of all eight major antigens (wheat, dairy, soy, egg, nuts, fish, hemp, pea) within 90 minutes. Note: This is *not* a "morning-after pill" for pizza night, but is instead helpful for taking before or immediately after eating in restaurants and other situations where trace gluten or dairy contamination is suspected, or some extremely minute amount is accidentally eaten. http://thedr.com/products-page-2/nutrition-formulas.

Vital Proteins brand Gelatin and Collagen Peptides: www.vital proteins.com.

Walkabout emu oil: www.walkabouthealthproducts.com (in the United States) and www.Baramul100.com (in Australia). The rare genetic strain of this particular emu oil and its superior natural feeding and meticulous quality control make all the difference!

US Wellness Meats: www.grasslandbeef.com. An online resource for top-quality pastured meats and other related products. Delivers 100% grass-fed/grass-finished meats right to your door (in the United States).

Mulay's Sausage Company: https://mulayssausage.com. This company's sausages are made with antibiotic-free pork that is humanely raised. They are all certified gluten-free, with no nitrates, no nitrites, no MSG, no sugar, no soy, no dairy. They are also delicious! Mulay's offers the best ground breakfast sausage (for making patties or adding to Breakfast Broth) I have ever tasted. They also offer mild and spicy Italian sausage as well as chorizo, both ground and in links.

Kinetic cultured veggie started culture (30 servings per container): http://shop.mercola.com/product/kinetic-culture-30g-1-bottle, 1275,417,0.htm. Enhances the vitamin K_2 content of your home-cultured and fermented foods!

Cultures for Health: www.culturesforhealth.com. High-quality yogurt, kefir, kombucha, and cultured veggie starters, equipment, and how-to videos.

Walleye Direct: www.walleyedirect.com. An online source of quality, wild-caught Canadian freshwater fish.

Ōra King healthfully farmed salmon: http://orakingsalmon.co.nz. Although I am typically the first to dissuade consumers from ever purchasing farmed fish, there is a new breed of fish farming emerging that is far more healthful and sustainable and does not threaten wild populations. One such company offering a high-quality alternative to questionable or potentially tainted wild Pacific salmon fisheries comes from New Zealand and is called Ōra King. These king salmon (the richest in omega-3 fats of any salmon species) are fed a natural diet rich in omega-3s and astaxanthin. They are never exposed to chemicals, antibiotics, or GMO feed, and they are raised under utterly pristine conditions that can no longer be guaranteed through wild Pacific Ocean sources. Monterey Bay Aquarium's globally respected consumer guide Seafood Watch has rated New Zealand's marine-farmed salmon, including Ōra King salmon, as "green," meaning it is a "Best Choice" for consumers. The Ōra King website offers sourcing information, and you can contact your local fish market to request that they order Ōra King salmon.

Wild Mountain Paleo Market: www.wildmountainpaleo.com. A great source for wild volcanic pili nuts—the ultimate primal fat burner nut—plus quality 100% organic "Galactic Hog Skins," pastured pork rinds for snacking in a variety of flavors. Wild Mountain Paleo Market offers a huge selection of foods, supplements, books, and lifestyle products that meet the most stringent guidelines. Their mission is to be a highly trusted source of the best products, providing a "health over profits" alternative to the entrenched natural foods industry.

Wilderness Family Naturals: www.wildernessfamilynaturals.com. A superb resource for top-quality coconut milk, coconut cream, coconut oil, and coconut butter/"spread," plus a variety of organic, preactivated nuts and much more. There is no better-quality coconut milk or cream anywhere.

Dr. Ron's Ultra-Pure Supplements: www.drrons.com. Home of Dr. Ron's brand Organ Delight and other additive-free supplements. Also a source of Unique E, as recommended elsewhere in this book.

Zukay: www.zukay.com. A source for high-quality raw, cultured kvass and salad dressings (also available from Wild Mountain Paleo Market).

Bulletproof "Brain Octane" C-8 MCT Oil: www.bulletproof.com /nutrition/quality-fats.

Sprouting supplies: http://sprouthouse.com/organic-sprouting-seeds.

Infrared Sauna (for excellent and effective daily detoxing). I have one of these and swear by it. The lowest EMF and most researched infrared sauna on the market. Fantastic for daily detoxing! Go to www.sunlighten.com. (Full disclosure: I receive a small fee if you tell them I referred you.)

For additional recommended and helpful products and other, more specific supplement recommendations, please see my store web page: www.primalbody-primalmind.com/store.

YOUR PRIMAL SHOPPING LIST

A few regular items you will want to stock your refrigerator and/or pantry with that are mostly included in the 21-day meal plan recipes include:

Coconut aminos (Coconut Secret brand is widely available and quite good). This is a marvelous substitute for gluten- or soy-containing soy or tamari sauce.

Stevita brand liquid stevia: In my opinion, the best and purest source of liquid stevia on the market. It's just the juice squeezed out of the leaves with a touch of grapefruit seed extract as a natural anti-microbial preservative. Available on my website through an Amazon link: www.primalbody-primalmind.com/store. This is quite possibly the only truly (and even beneficial) healthful, natural, non-glycemic sweetener available. Use it to sweeten dishes and/or your morning tea instead of table sugar or honey.

Organic, virgin centrifuge-extracted coconut oil: There are a number of fine brands available, including Wilderness Family Naturals brand (see "Nourishing Resources" on page 285 for ordering info), Nutiva brand, Dr. Bronner's, and others. Please avoid "liquid" fractionated forms! Omega Nutrition makes a slightly refined organic coconut oil that has no coconut smell or taste, either for those who don't like the flavor or for when you don't want everything you cook with it to taste like coconut.

Coconut milk and cream: The best I have found is Wilderness Family Naturals brand (see "Nourishing Resources" on page 285 for ordering info).

Himalayan or Celtic sea salt: Never, ever purchase refined pure sodium chloride table salt.

Coconut wraps: my favorite Pure Wraps brand (you can get this from Wild Mountain Paleo Market—www.wildmountainpaleo.com). Also comes in a delicious curry flavor!

Fully pastured animal fats for cooking: Tallow, pastured lard, and duck fat are all available through Fatworks or US Wellness Meats (see "Nourishing Resources" on page 285).

Organic cooking herbs and spices: The best sources include Pure Indian Foods (www.pureindianfoods.com/popular-indian-spices -s/31.htm)—they also have rare black cumin seed, in addition to the highest-quality curcumin-rich turmeric, along with other organic, nonirradiated exotic herbs and spices. I also like the Simply Organic brand (which has a good chili powder, too) and the Morton & Basset brand (found in most natural grocery markets—I especially like M&B's yellow curry powder). Red Ape cinnamon is also great.

Nut flours: Nutiva makes great organic nut flour (including coconut flour). Also, Bob's Red Mill brand.

Raw apple cider vinegar: I like the Bragg brand. They have a wonderful herb seasoning mix and nutritional yeast, too.

Balsamic vinegar: I like Napa Valley Naturals, but any organic, gluten-free balsamic vinegar will do.

Coconut vinegar: Made from coconut sap. Coconut Secret brand is a really good one.

Organic salsa: Salsa de Casa is a good-tasting, organic, and widely sold brand; it comes in mild, medium, and hot.

Fish sauce: Red Boat brand fish sauce is an all-natural, first press, "extra-virgin" Vietnamese fish sauce. It does not contain added water, preservatives, or MSG. Made from a two-hundred-year-old, chemical-free, artisanal process. See more at http://redboatfishsauce .com/#sthash.Hg8D8FER.dpuf.

Vanilla: Simply Organic brand and Singing Dog make a very good-quality organic alcohol-free liquid vanilla extract. Bulletproof (www.bulletproof.com) has the finest pure, finely ground vanilla bean (VanillaMax).

Raw, organic cacao butter: The best brand I've come across is the Stirs the Soul brand.

Sesame oil: Napa Organics is a great brand.

Avocado oil: Hands-down the best is Ava Jane's.

Olive oil: I like Bariani brand organic, unfiltered olive oil.

Macadamia nut oil: I use Taylor's Pure and Natural brand; you can get it on Amazon.com. (Note: I personally tend to avoid Spectrum Naturals brand oils. Let's just say I am fussy about my fats and oils.)

Prepared organic mustard: OrganicVille is widely available in up-scale national food markets and makes an organic stone-ground variety (my personal favorite), a Dijon, and also a plain yellow mustard. No gluten or other "nasties" in them. I avoid their other products, however, as they tend to be sweetened with agave syrup. Always be sure to read labels!

BBQ sauce: Most commercial BBQ sauces are loaded with sugar, gluten, canola or soybean oil, and a plethora of other unspeakable "nasties." Trinity Hill Farms brand is the only one I have found that is "nasties-free," and it really tastes wonderful. It is sweetened only with stevia! Although there are no BBQ recipes in the 21-day meal plan, I wanted to supply a quality source of BBQ sauce, as sooner or later you will want to fire up the grill to make your own baby back ribs or BBQ chicken. You can purchase this BBQ sauce on Amazon if you can't find it in a store near you.

Tomato paste: Bionaturae makes an excellent organic one.

Packaged organic, free-range chicken broth: Pacific brand makes a decent enough one that is gluten-free for use as a quick soup stock in a pinch (get the low-sodium version, then use your own Himalayan/Celtic sea salt instead)—though you are always better off making your own!

AFTERWORD:
WELCOME TO THE TRIBE!

You've made it to the end of the 21-day fat-burning plan. Congratulations! If you have followed it diligently, you are well on your way to adopting a fat-burning metabolism. You've made it through the hardest part, the transition period. You've gotten familiar with new foods and recipes, and are well on the way to finding your groove. Over the next three to four weeks, if you stay on track, this metabolic state will become increasingly well established. Keep it up, and a lifetime of vital health and well-being, in body and mind, can be yours to claim.

Primal Fat Burning is a lifestyle, not a label. It doesn't matter if you see yourself as "paleo" or "primal" or having no label at all—adopting this way of eating is about returning to your fundamental human design. As such, it is universal, not niche. There isn't a different textbook of anatomy and physiology for each of us; there is but one design and basic set of foundational requirements. From there, we extrapolate from nuances and polymorphisms (individual genetic differences) . . . but those nuances do not necessarily change the solidly established foundations we all share in common.

This book has endeavored to identify and to strengthen those foundations, first and foremost.

You are now part of a unique tribe, standing side by side with all kinds of different people, many just like you—former vegetarians, animal lovers, ecologists, foodies, athletes, practitioners, and parents who want to give their kids a good start in life. What unites us all is a desire to throw off the shackles of bad dietary policy, substandard (and sickness-inducing) food systems, and corporate dictators pushing us (way) down the wrong paths. To forge better health, a better planet, you can now support the cycle of life the way nature intended, by sourcing foods from humane, healthy, and sustainable sources.

There are a host of resources to support you on your journey—I encourage you to explore some of the resources listed in this book, and follow me on my website www.primalfatburner.com.

As you may remember, my quest to discover the truth about the fat-burning metabolism was launched by my deep desire to know if there was indeed a single, universal, foundational way of eating that gave the human body everything it needed. I set out by following the footsteps of the Inuit people—those whose diet was the simplest and most basic (while still providing them with everything they needed to be superbly healthy), according to Dr. Weston A. Price. The diet of the Inuit essentially had the fewest "moving parts" of any other people group Price studied. Their menu was based almost solely on fats and meats (and salty broths made from these), with few add-ins—no grains, dairy, or starch of any kind. They were also among the healthiest of all peoples he had encountered, and they had the strongest character and most cheerful dispositions, while living and thriving ingeniously in one of the harshest climates on earth. They were a culture that had never known war or child abuse. Their physical prowess was unmatched. They were and still are my heroes—a people I deeply admire.

Today we are in the middle of a huge "real food" moment, returning to discovering a plethora of seemingly nutrient-rich foods, from more traditional schools of cooking and preparing. Much of this movement is inspired by the research of Dr. Price, who showcased a myriad of traditional and primitive diets. His amazing work inspires many people to broaden their diets to include all kinds of things from sourdough bread and soaked grains to raw cheese and milk. The *relative* balance was always seemingly toward health in these other cultures, but that was also a very different time. I suggest applying these ideas with considerable caution, if not hesitation. It is my hypothesis that Dr. Price's varied research subjects were better able to tolerate those foods back then (rather than benefit from them, particularly when it came to eating grains) precisely *because* their robust health was built on grass-fed animal foods and fat. I've seen way too many people compromised by gluten, dairy, or other inflammatory foods to trust that many of us can tolerate them in the same way. And although I have certainly seen persons who benefitted from the inclusion of pastured raw milk in their diets, I also increasingly see those whose immune systems absolutely cannot tolerate dairy proteins (not just the lactose) and who suffer from gluten-like effects with dairy in *any* form (the one immunologic exception for most, interestingly, being camel's milk). And most people having this health-compromising issue simply do not know it (until they get Cyrex Labs testing). I know I didn't! The inflammatory consequences can be devastating to those with these sensitivities, if not debilitating and lethal over time. We are simply not living in Weston Price's time anymore. Instead, I remind you to keep the humble Eskimo in mind, the man or woman whose primary caloric intake was at one time solely fat-rich meat and fat on its own, all from pure, uncontaminated sources. I believe that when it comes to the optimal human diet, this is our *universal* and most basic starting place. Now, by no means do I conclude from this that these are the only foods that any of us should be eating. Far from it. But based on this deduction, it *is* reasonable to conclude that their diet supplied the most foundational essentials. There is a key hidden foundational principle we simply cannot ignore. Their robust health, sound constitution, peaceful nature and communities, and attune-ment to nature is something we would do well to aspire to today. And I believe that this truly starts with food. Let *Primal Fat Burner* be your foundation, and keep it simple! In other words, we all share the same essential underlying necessary nutritional foundation. The rest is mere nuance. It's important that whatever dietary nuance you add to this basic underlying universal formula for health support your basic foundation and not compromise it in some way.

It is reasonable here and not too far out on a limb to say that *fat*—animal fat—is fundamentally meant to be the primary source of energy and nourishment for each and every one of us. It is what our body stores and burns the most efficiently. Fat in general supplies at least twice the calories per gram that carbohydrates or protein do, for that matter, but it is able to supply at least four times more even-burning, clean, and safe lasting energy! It's like a form of solar energy powering our cells, instead of the dirty petroleum and nuclear-type fuel sugar provides.

Becoming a primal fat burner is not a program for dietary dilettantes. It is really for the person seriously committed to restoring or maximizing his or her health for the long haul, and someone who isn't afraid of challenging the status quo. It is also for the person morally and ethically committed to seeking and demanding optimally healthy foods and sustainability. It is for the rabble-rouser and Robin Hood intent on shifting economic reward from corrupt, misanthropic multinational corporate interests into the pockets of hardworking, honest, and ethical farmers and smaller family companies working hard to do the right things. Nutritionally speaking (and borrowing from the movie *The Matrix*), primal fat burning is the proverbial "red pill" of health and diet pursuits. Once you take this step, you will never be the same again—you will never be able to walk into a conventional grocery store or convenience market and see things in exactly the same way as before. This approach automatically triggers a fundamental shift in and evolution of consciousness and civil responsibility. Once your eyes are opened to the myriad of benefits this way of life offers on multiple levels, together with the skewed politics that have clouded these truths and consistently compromised your health, there is no going back. Far beyond being some "fad diet" designed to merely change your dress size, this is a dietary health approach that is hell-bent on changing the world and the health of everyone in it who is willing to listen and has the courage to take that luscious, juicy red pill.

But also know that you are anything but alone. This process of awakening is already well under way and inspiring positive changes and activism everywhere as you read this. There are many hands to hold yours. There is a form of "tribal" consciousness emerging that inspires a greater sense of community and purpose and that recognizes the central importance of food and the manner in which it is produced. Welcome to the tribe!

The ultimate rewards of this highly conscious dietary lifestyle approach go well beyond energy, clarity, and relief from a myriad of pains and other symptoms. Once you get this ball rolling, the results you will experience will speak for themselves and will naturally and automatically inspire the determination and passion to stick with it. Note that this is absolutely doable; not only that, but with the right approach it is even more affordable than the standard American diet so many (erroneously) feel their economic restrictions doom them to. Another myth bites the dust! Health is not only for the wealthy. It is accessible now . . . and it is absolutely your primal birthright.

The Primal Fat Burner Plan is a win-win for you, your pocketbook, and the health and sustainable welfare of the entire planet!

This brings us to one final principle inherent in the "primal perspective": that of mutual cooperation and tribal community. Although those reading this may differ in their "tribal" ideological and political leanings, we are all as a human species more alike than unalike in our basic evolutionary history, anatomy, and physiology. The fact that you have been reading this book suggests to me that we also share some common passionate interests and goals. In fact, I think it's even safe to assume the same of most vegetarians and vegans. What we all share is far more, and far more important, than what we don't, and it is upon these things that we absolutely must unwaveringly focus:

- We all care passionately about our health and the health of those we love.
- We recognize the heavily compromised state of our food supply and the largely misanthropic nature of the political and economic forces controlling it.
- We all care deeply about the environment and the welfare of all living things.
- We all want a sustainably and humanely based food supply.
- We all want to empower and support farmers and companies working hard to do the right thing.
- We all want to see an end to the monopolies held by Big Agribusiness (and its unholy alliance with Big Oil), along with the monopolies and political control held by the biotech industry, chemical industries, industrial fertilizer

strip-mining operations, Big Pharma, and the medical industry behemoth, which remains blind to the concept of true health care while profiting from disease management.

- We all believe in our right to self-determination when it comes to our own health care and transparency when it comes to food labeling. I also think we all agree that labeling simply isn't enough and that *GMOs have got to go!*
- Most of us understand that the kind of changes we envision will never be handed to us from the top down. It is up to us to make this happen in a very grassroots-oriented way. It's time to take our health and our future as a species into our own hands for the benefit of all future generations.

This is why we all need to be working together. The world is polarized enough. *Enough already!* And that polarization serves only the interests of those who stand to benefit from seeing us divided and conquered. In the end, it is the things we have in common that are foundational to the solution of both our planetary and health woes. Nothing meaningful, optimal, or lasting will ever be accomplished without this recognition and its application.

And with that in mind, together we have the collective potential to move mountains.

The Sacred Cows of Yesteryear (and How Eating This Way Can Literally Save the World!)

I know you're all asking this question silently in your own heads right now . . .

Is this way of eating even sustainable?

How can we *possibly* feed the planet this way?

The current conventions of feedlot meat and GMO- and chemically driven agricultural production are simply not healthy, natural, or sustainable. These methods have never once proven capable of meeting the challenge of feeding the world (much less keeping anyone healthy). Our domesticated ruminants were never designed to eat grains, corn, or soybeans (much less many of the other shocking things they are often fed), either. They are designed to eat but one thing: natural grasses and forage. The health of the meat on our plates directly correlates to the health of the animal that meat came from. For tens of millions of years—long before humans ever came along—vast herds of wild ruminants (many utterly massive in size) filled the landscapes across the globe. It turns out that all grasslands and wild ruminants coevolved . . . and if you remove the ruminants from the grasslands, the grasslands die.

We are seeing unprecedented evidence of this today through the spread of desertification over two-thirds of Earth's land mass. Prior to the arrival of Europeans, North America once had sixty million bison thundering across the Great Plains; they are all but gone now. Prior to the last Ice Age, there were an additional forty species of large herbivores that coexisted with those massive bison numbers on the same continent. While they trod upon the land en masse, the land and the health of the soils thrived, as did natural ecological diversity. Today, though, 70 percent of the world's grasslands have been degraded. Today we are losing healthy topsoil and its minerals—so vital to our health—at an unprecedented rate. Soil is actually depleting 13 percent faster than it can be replaced, and we've lost 75 percent of the world's crop varieties in just the last one hundred years. More than a billion people in the world have no access to safe drinking water, while 80 percent of the world's precious freshwater supply (far more valuable than oil) is used for industrial agriculture.

Nothing about this is remotely sustainable (even as it is highly profitable for a select few). And our tax dollars literally subsidize this.

Feedlots *do* pose a grave environmental threat, as does industrial monoculture agriculture worldwide. A change in the way we do things is imminently needed, and the answer from a human health or environmental standpoint is clearly not veganism. The good news is that we have everything we need to turn things around today, in a completely affordable manner. The know-how and technology exist right now. The Savory Institute (www.savory.global) has trained thousands of livestock operations the world over in Holistic Management, a process that seeks to restore natural systems, healthy soils, healthy watersheds, and environmental diversity (plus a certain measure of global climate stability) through the healthy systematic restoration of ruminants to the land, where they belong. We should all be supporting this organization and its efforts. The exclusive grass feeding of animals (currently representing little more than 3 to 4 percent of all meat production worldwide) literally has the potential to turn *virtually every one of our health and environmental issues around*, while also feeding vast human populations across the world, particularly in the most impoverished places where agriculture simply isn't possible. Two-thirds of Earth's landmass (consisting of tundra, steppes, deserts, noncultivatable grasslands, mountainous regions, and other ecosystems) cannot be utilized for agriculture at all, yet there are sedges, forage, and grasses in all of these places capable of feeding large populations of ruminants and other herbivores (while simultaneously accommodating the natural diversity already existing there), all while improving the soils and even allowing for the development of symbiotic crop planting in many places. The appropriate management of these animals using the model of *natural systems* has the potential to solve many, many problems, including social and political instability and warfare in places throughout the world currently relegated to battling for dwindling resources, food, and water. Holistic Management has the potential to change all that. We need to change our thinking and our actions—and we need to change them now.

Our reward—apart from radically improved health—will be a world we are not ashamed to leave to future generations.

ACKNOWLEDGMENTS

I want to thank the following individuals for their dedication, loyalty, contributions, and support of my work, without whom this book would simply not be possible. Lisa Collins and Susie Arnett, I will never forget what you have done to help make this happen. A shout-out to Tracy Bosnian and Rosalyn Newhouse for all your help. Thanks, too, to Celeste Fine and Sarah Passick for all your help and for believing in this project! Amely Greeven—in the end, I couldn't have done it without you.

I also want to thank the following brilliant and wonderful researchers for their pioneering work, tireless passion, and inspiration: Ron Rosedale, David Perlmutter, Datis Kharrazian, Jay Wortman, Aristo Vojdani, the late George Cahill, Richard Veech, the late Mary Enig, the late Roger Mann, Gary Taubes, William R. Leonard, Josh Snodgrass and Marcia Robertson, Michael Eades, Peter Attia, Stephen Phinney, Richard Feinman, Alex Vasquez, John Briffa, Miki Ben-Dor, the late Weston A. Price, the late Francis Pottenger, the late Robert Ardrey, and the late Barry Groves.

Finally, I want to thank L. David Mech, Vilhjálmur Stefánsson, Farley Mowat, Will Steger, and Barry Lopez for helping to give me an appreciation (wittingly or unwittingly) of fat's importance and the profoundly inspiring lessons of Arctic peoples.

NOTES

DISCLAIMER

Poplawski MM, Mastitis JW, Isoda F, Grosjean F, Zheng F, Mobbs CV. "Reversal of Diabetic Nephropathy by a Ketogenic Diet." *PLoS ONE* (20 April 2011). http://dx.doi.org /10.1371/journal.pone.0018604.

INTRODUCTION

1 Pérez-Guisado J. [Ketogenic diets: additional benefits to the weight loss and unfounded secondary effects]. *Arch Latinoam Nutr* (2008); 58(4): 323–9.
2 Westman EC, Yancy WS, Mavropoulos JC, et al. "The effect of a low-carbohydrate, ketogenic diet versus a low-glycemic index diet on glycemic control in type 2 diabetes mellitus." *Nutr Metab* (London 2008); 5:36. doi: 10.1186/1743-7075-5-36.
3 Volek JS, Sharman MJ, Gomez AL, et al. "Comparison of energy-restricted, very low-carbohydrate and low-fat diets on weight loss and body composition in overweight men and women." *Nutrition & Metabolism* (2004); 1:13. doi:10.1186/1743-7075-1-13.
4 Bough KJ, Wetherington J, Hassel B, et al. "Mitochondrial biogenesis in the anticonvulsant mechanism of the ketogenic diet." *Ann Neurology* (2006); 60(2): 223–35.
5 Rosedale R, Westman EC, and Konhilas JP. "Clinical experience of a diet designed to reduce aging." *J Appl Res* (2009 Jan 1); 9(4): 159–65.

CHAPTER 1: From Lucy to Tribal Hunter

1 McPherron SP, Alemseged Z, Marean CW, et al. "Evidence for stone tool-assisted consumption of animal tissue before 3.39 million years ago at Dikika, Ethiopia" (2010 12 Aug); 466. doi: 10.1038/nature09248.
2 Schaller GB, Lowther G. "The relevance of carnivore behavior to the study of early hominids." *Southwest J Anthropology* (1969): 307–34.
3 Ferraro JV, Plummer TW, Pobiner BL, Oliver JS, Bishop LC, et al. "Earliest archaeological evidence of persistent hominin carnivory." *PLoS ONE* (2013); 8(4): e62174. doi:10.1371/journal.pone.
4 Milton K. "A hypothesis to explain the role of meat-eating in human evolution." *Evol Anthropol* (1999); 8: 11–21. doi:10.1002/(SICI)1520-6505(1999).
5 DeAnna EB, Koltz AM, Lambert JE, Fierer N, Dunn RR. "The evolution of stomach acidity and its relevance to the human microbiome." *PLoS ONE* (2015); 10(7): e0134116. doi: 10.1371/journal.pone.0134116.
6 Bothwell TH, Charlton RW. "A general approach to the problems of iron deficiency and iron overload in the population at large." *Semin Haematol* (1982); 19: 54–67.
7 Speth J. "Early hominid hunting and scavenging: the role of meat as an energy source." *J Hum Evol* (1989); 18: 329–43. Mann NJ. "Meat in the human diet: An anthropological perspective." *Nutrition & Dietetics* (2007); 64 (Suppl. 4): S102–S107. doi: 10.1111/j.1747-0080.2007.00194.x.
8 Richards MP, Hedges REM, Jacobi R, Current A, Stringer C. "Focus: Gough's Cave and Sun Hole Cave human stable isotope values indicate a high animal protein diet in the British Upper Palaeolithic." *J Archeolog Sci* (2000); 27(1): 1–3.
9 Foley R. "The evolutionary consequences of increased carnivory in hominids." In: Stanford CB, Bunn HT, eds. *Meat-Eating and Human Evolution* (Oxford: Oxford

University Press, 2001); 305–31. Anton SC, Leonard WR, Robertson ML. "An ecomorphological model of the initial hominid dispersal from Africa." *J Hum Evol* (2002); 43: 773–85. doi:10.1006/jhev.2002.0602.

10 Bonsall C, Lennon R, McSweeney K, Stewart C, Harkness D, Boroneant V, Barto-siewicz V, Payton R, Chapman J. "Mesolithic and early Neolithic in the Iron Gates: A palaeodietary perspective." *J Eur. Archaeol* (1997); 51: 50–92.

11 Stanford DJ, Day JS. *Ice Age Hunters of the Rockies.* (Niwot: University Press of Colorado, 1992).

12 Enig M, Fallon S. "Cave man diet." *Price-Pottenger Nutrition Foundation Health Journal* (1999); 21(2).

13 Speth JD. *The Paleoanthropology and Archaeology of Big-Game Hunting: Protein, Fat, or Politics?* (New York: Springer, 2010).

14 Mann NJ. "Human evolution and diet: A modern conundrum of health versus meat consumption, or is it?" *Animal Production Science* (2013 Jan); 53(11): 1135.

15 Kinzie C, Que Hee SS, Stich A, et al. "Nanodiamond-rich layer across three continents consistent with major cosmic impact at 12,800 Cal BP." *J Geology* (2014); 122: 475–506.

16 Brink J. *Imagining Head Smashed In: Aboriginal Buffalo Hunting on the Northern Plains.* (Edmonton: Athabasca University Press, 2008).

17 Ben-Dor M, Gopher A, Hershkovitz I, Barkai R. "Man the fat hunter: The demise of *Homo erectus* and the emergence of a new hominin lineage in the Middle Pleistocene (ca. 400 kyr) Levant." *PLoS ONE* (2011 Dec); 6(12): e28689. Speth JD. "Early hominid hunting and scavenging: the role of meat as an energy source." *J Hum Evolution* (1989); 18(4): 329–43.

CHAPTER 2: Think Fat

1 George F. Cahill Jr. "Fuel Metabolism in Starvation." *Ann Rev Nutr* (2006) 26: 1–22. doi:10.1146/annurev.nutr.26.061505.111258.

2 Leonard WR, Robertson ML. "Evolutionary perspectives on human nutrition: the influence of brain and body size on diet and metabolism." *Am J Human Biol* (1994); 6: 77–88.

3 Aiello LC. "Brains and guts in human evolution: the expensive tissue hypothesis." *Brazilian J Genetics* (1997); 20: 141–8.

4 Cahill GF Jr, Veech RL. "Ketoacids? Good medicine?" *Trans Am Clin Climatol Assoc* (2003); 114: 149–61; discussion 162–3.

5 Boyd R, Silk JB. *How Humans Evolved.* 7th ed. (New York: W. W. Norton, 2014).

6 Henneberg M. "Decrease of human skull size in the Holocene." *Human Biology* (1988); 395–405.

7 Ben-Dor M, Gopher A, Hershkovitz I, Barkai R. "Man the fat hunter: The demise of *Homo erectus* and the emergence of a new hominin lineage in the Middle Pleistocene (ca. 400 kyr) Levant." *PLoS ONE* (2011 Dec); 6(12): e28689.

8 Cahill GF. "Survival in starvation." *Am J Clin Nutr* (1998); 68: 1–2.

9 Crawford M. "The role of dietary fatty acids in biology: their place in the evolution of the human brain." *Nutr Rev* (1992); 50: 3–11. Chamberlain JG. "The possible role of long-chain omega-3 fatty acids in human brain phylogeny." *Perspect Biol Med* (1996); 39: 436–45.

10 Emken RA, Adlof RO, Rohwedder WK, et al. "Comparison of linolenic and linoleic acid metabolism in man: influence of dietary linoleic acid." In: Sinclair A, Gibson R, eds. *Essential Fatty Acids and Eicosanoids, Invited Papers from the Third International Congress* (Champaign, IL: AOCS Press, 1992), 23–5.

11 Chamberlain JG. "The possible role of long-chain omega-3 fatty acids in human brain phylogeny." *Perspect Biol Med* (1996); 39: 436–45.

12 Girao H, Mota C, Pereira P. "Cholesterol may act as an antioxidant in lens membranes." *Curr Eye Res* (1999 Jun); 18(6): 448–54.

13 Smith LL. "Another cholesterol hypothesis: cholesterol as antioxidant." *Free Radic Biol Med* (1991); 11(1): 47–61.

14 Hardy K, Brand-Miller J, Brown KD, Thomas NG, Copeland L. "The importance of dietary carbohydrate in human evolution." *Quarterly Rev Biology* (2015); 90(3): 251. doi: 10.1086/682587.

15 Sorensen A, Roebroeks W, van Gijn A. "Fire production in the deep past? The expedient strike-a-light model." *J Archaeol Sci* (2014); 42: 476–86.

16 Cordain L. "Ancestral fire production: Implications for contemporary 'paleo' diets." *The Paleo Diet* (2014 Apr 20). http://thepaleodiet.com/ancestral-fire-production -implications-contemporary-paleo-diets.

17 Richards MP. "Stable isotope evidence for European Upper Paleolithic human diets." In: Hublin JJ, Richards MP, eds. *The Evolution of Hominin Diets Integrating Approaches to the Study of Palaeolithic Subsistence.* 251–57 (Netherlands: Springer 2009). Richards MP, Trinkaus E. "Isotopic evidence for the diets of European Neanderthals and early modern humans." *Proc Natl Acad Sci* USA (2009); 106(38):16034–9. Lee-Thorp JA, Sponheimer MB. "Contributions of biogeochemistry to understanding hominin dietary ecology." *Yearbook of Physical Anthropology* (2006): 49: 131–48.

18 Perry GH, Dominy NJ, Claw KG, Lee AS, Fiegler H, et al. "Diet and the evolution of human amylase gene copy number variation." *Nature Genetics* (2007): 39(10): 1256–60.

19 Leonard WR, Robertson ML, Snodgrass JJ, Kuzawa CW. "Metabolic correlates of hominid brain evolution." *Comp Biochem Physiol A Mol Integr Physiol* (2003): 136: 5–15.

20 Maalof MA, Rho JM, Matteson MP. "The neuroprotective properties of calorie restriction, the ketogenic diet, and ketone bodies." *Brain Res Rev* (2009 Mar): 59(2): 293–315. doi: 10.1016/j.brainresrev.2008.09.002.

21 Siegell GJ, Agranoff BW, Albers RW, et al. *Basic Neurochemistry: Molecular, Cellular and Medical Aspects,* 6th ed. (Windermere, FL: American Society for Neurochemistry).

22 Cahill GF Jr. "Fuel Metabolism in Starvation." *Ann Rev Nutr* (2006); 26: 1–22. doi: 10.1146/annurev.nutr.26.061505.111258

23 Cunnane SC, Crawford MA. "Survival of the fattest: fat babies were the key to evolution of the large human brain." *Comp Biochem Physiol A Mol Integr Physiol* (2003 Sep); 136(1): 17–26.

24 Henneberg M. "Decrease of human skull size in the Holocene." *Hum Biol* (1988); 60: 395–405.

25 Childers M, Herzog H. "Motivations for meat consumption among ex-vegetarians." Annual Meeting of the International Society for Anthrozoology (2009).

CHAPTER 3: A is for Agriculture and Adapting to Glucose

1 Diamond J. "The worst mistake in the history of the human race." *Discover* (May 1987).

2 Seiler R, Spielman AI, Zink A, Rühli, F. "Oral pathologies of the Neolithic Iceman, c. 3300 BC." *European J Oral Sci* (2013); 1–5.

3 Acsádi GY, Nemeskeri J. "History of human life span and mortality (Akademiai Kiado, Budapest)." *Current Anthropology* (1974 Dec); 15(4): 495–507. Cohen MN. *Health and the Rise of Civilization.* (New Haven: Yale University Press, 1989). Diamond J. *Guns, Germs, and Steel: The Fates of Human Societies.* (New York: Norton, 1997). Wesidorf JL. "From foraging to farming: Explaining the Neolithic revolution." *J Economic Surveys* (2006); 19: 561–86.

4 Pinhasi R, Eshed V, von Cramon-Taubadel N. "Incongruity between affinity patterns based on mandibular and lower dental dimensions following the transition to agriculture in the Near East, Anatolia and Europe." *PLoS ONE* (2015); 10(2):e0117301. doi: 10.1371/journal.pone.0117301.

5 "Malocclusion and dental crowding arose 12,000 years ago with earliest farmers." *Science Daily* (2015 Feb 4).

6 Cordain L. "Cereal grains: Humanity's double-edged sword." *World Rev Nutr Diet* (1999); 84: 19–73.

7   Hulsegge G, Susan H, Picavet J, et al. "Today's adult generations are less healthy than their predecessors: generation shifts in metabolic risk factors: the Doetinchem Cohort Study." *Eur J Preventive Cardiology* (2014 Sep); 21(9): 1134–44.

8   Murray CJL, Lopez AD. *The Global Burden of Disease: A Comprehensive Assessment of Mortality and Disability from Diseases, Injuries and Risk Factors in 1990 and Projected to 2020.* Geneva: World Health Organization (1996).

9   Dantzer R, O'Connor JC, Freund GG, Johnson RW, Kelley KW. "From inflammation to sickness and depression: When the immune system subjugates the brain." *Nature Rev Neurosci* (2008 Jan); 9(1): 46–56.

10 Hallert C, et al. "Evidence of poor vitamin status in coeliac patients on a gluten-free diet for ten years." *Alimentary Pharmacol Therapeutics* (2002 Jul); 16(7): 1333–9.

11 Addolorato G, et al. "Regional cerebral hypoperfusion in patients with celiac disease." *Am J Medicine* (2004); 116(5): 312–7.

12 Taubes G. "What if it's all been a big fat lie?" *New York Times Magazine* (2002 Jul 7).

13 ———. "What if it's all been a big fat lie?" *New York Times Magazine* (2002 Jul 7).

14 Margutti P, Delunardo F, Ortona E. "Autoantibodies associated with psychiatric disorders." *Curr Neurovasc Res* (2006 May); 3(2): 149–57. Matsunagab H, Kimuraa M, Tatsumia K, et al. "Autoantibodies against four kinds of neurotransmitter receptors in psychiatric disorders." *J Neuroimmunology* (2003 Aug); 141(1–2): 155–64. Benros ME, Waltoft BL, Noprdentoft M, et al. "Autoimmune diseases and severe infections as risk factors for mood disorders: A nationwide study." *JAMA Psychiatry* (2013); 70(8): 812–820. doi:10.1001/jamapsychiatry.2013.1111.

15 Benros ME, Waltoft BL, Noprdentoft M, et al. "Autoimmune diseases and severe infections as risk factors for mood disorders: A nationwide study." *JAMA Psychiatry* (2013); 70(8): 812–20. doi:10.1001/jamapsychiatry.2013.1111. Eaton WW, Pedersen MG, Nielsen PR, Mortensen PB. "Autoimmune diseases, bipolar disorder, and non-affective psychosis." *Bipolar Disord* (2010 Sep); 12(6): 638–46. doi: 10.1111/j.1399-5618.2010.00853.x.

16 King S, Chambers CT, Huguet RC, et al. "The epidemiology of chronic pain in children and adolescents revisited: A systematic review." *PAIN* 152, issue 12 (Dec 2011) pub by Elsevier. doi:10.1016/j.pain.2011.07.016.

17 "Vegetables without vitamins." *Life Extension Magazine* (2001 Mar). *Composition of Foods (Raw, Processed, Prepared): Agriculture Handbook No. 8.* USDA Agricultural Research Service (1963).

18 Senate Document #264; Presented by Rex Beach, June 1936. (United States GPO, Washington, D.C., 1936).

19 Heinrich E. "The root of all disease." *TRC* 4th ed. (Tulsa: The Rockland Corporation, 2000).

20 "Vegetables without vitamins." *Life Extension Magazine* (2001 Mar).

21 Diez-Gonzalez F, et al. "Grain-feeding and the dissemination of acid-resistant *Escherichia coli* from cattle." *Science* (1998); 281: 1666–8.

22. International Food Policy Research Institute, 2016. Global Nutrition Report 2016: From Promise to Impact; Ending Malnutrition by 2030. Washington DC.

23 Health at a Glance, 2013: OECD Indicators. OECD Publishing. http://dx.doi.org/10.1787/health_glance-201.

24 Hammond RA, Levine R. "The economic impact of obesity in the United States." *DovePress Journal: Diabetes, Metabolic Syndrome and Obesity: Targets and Therapy.* 2010; 3: 285–95. doi: 10.2147/DMSOTT.S7384.

25 Robert Preidt (Healthday). "Cost of obesity approaching $300 billion a year." *USA Today*, Your Life (2011).

26 Ryan Maslow. "Obesity to affect 42% of Americans by 2030 with $550 billion in costs, say researchers." CBS News (May 8, 2012).

27 Tumulty K. "The health care crisis hits home." *Time* (2009 Mar 5).

CHAPTER 4: You Can Choose Your Fuel (Just Please Don't Choose Glucose)

1   Wortman J. "The story so far." Dr. Jay's Blog. www.drjaywortman.com/blog/word press/about.

2   http://www.dummies.com/how-to/content/how-your-body-turns-carbohydrates-in to-energy.html.

3   Alberts B. *Molecular Biology of the Cell.* 4th ed. (New York: Garland Science, 2002); 93.

4   Welsh JA, Sharma A, Abramson JL, Vaccarino V, Gillespie C, Vos MB. "Caloric sweetener consumption and dyslipidemia among US adults." *JAMA* (2010 Apr 21); 303(15): 1490–7.

5   Johnson RK et al. "Dietary sugars intake and cardiovascular health: A scientific statement from the American Heart Association." *Circulation* (2009); 120: 1011–20.

6   Voss MB, et al. "Dietary fructose consumption among US children and adults: The Third National Health and Nutrition Examination Survey." *Medscape J Med* 208; 10: 160.

7   Wallace DC. "Mitochondrial DNA mutations in disease and aging." *Environ Mol Mutagen* (2010 Jun); 51(5): 440–50.

8   Mecocci P, MacGarvey U, Kaufman AE, et al. "Oxidative damage to mitochondrial DNA shows marked age-dependent increases in human brain." *Ann Neurol* (1993 Oct); 34(4): 609–16.

9   Shimazu T, et al., "Suppression of Oxidative Stress by β-Hydroxybutyrate, an Endogenous Histone Deacetylase Inhibitor." *Science* (2012) doi:10.1126/science.1227166

10 Shimazu T, et al. "Suppression of oxidative stress by B-hydroxybutyrate, an endogenous histone deacetylase inhibitor." *Science* (2013 Jan 11); 339(6116): 211–4. doi: 10.1126/science.1227166.

11 Cohen E, Cragg M, deFonseka J, et al. "Statistical review of US macronutrient consumption data, 1965–2011: Americans have been following dietary guidelines, coincident with the rise in obesity." *Nutrition* (2015 May); 31(5):727–32. doi: http:// dx.doi.org/10.1016/j.nut.2015.02.007.

12 Ogden CL, Carroll, MD; Lawman, HG, Fryar, CD, Kruszon-Moran, D, Kit, BK, and Flegal KM. (2016). "Trends in obesity prevalence among children and adolescents in the United States, 1988–1994 through 2013–2014." *JAMA*, 315(21), 2292–99.

13 Hite AH, Feinman RD, Guzman GE, Satin M, Schoenfeld PA, Wood RJ. "In the face of contradictory evidence: report of the Dietary Guidelines for Americans Committee." *Nutr Burbank Los Angel City Calif* (2010); 26: 915–24.

14 Zinn AR. "Unconventional wisdom about the obesity epidemic." *Am J Med Sci* (2010); 340: 481–91.

15 US Department of Agriculture, US Department of Health and Human Services. Report of the Dietary Guidelines Advisory Committee on the Dietary Guidelines for Americans, 2010. US Department of Agriculture, Washington DC (2010).

16 Pontzer H, et al. "Hunter-gatherer energetics and human obesity." *PLoS ONE* (2012); 7(7): e40503. doi:10.1371/journal.pone.0040503.

17 Manninen AH. "Low-carbohydrate diets: Misunderstood 'villains' of human metabolism." *Int Soc Sports Nutr.* 2004; 1(2): 7–11. doi:10.1186/1550-2783-1-2-7 http://www .ncbi.nlm.nih.gov/pmc/articles/PMC2129159.

18 Dietary Guidelines for Americans—2010. Food and Nutrition Information Center, Center for Nutrition Policy and Promotion. United States Department of Agriculture. http://fnic.nal.usda.gov/dietary-guidance/dietary-guidelines.

CHAPTER 5: Harnessing Your Superfuel

1   Cahill GF Jr. "Starvation in man." *N Engl J Med* (1970); 19: 668–75.

2   Landau BR, Brunengraber H. "The role of acetone in the conversion of fat to carbohydrate." *Trends in Biochemical Sciences* (1987); 12: 113–4.

3   Argiles JM. "Has acetone a role in the conversion of fat to carbohydrate in mammals?" *Trends in Biochemical Sciences* (1986); 11(2): 61–3.

4 Cahill GF Jr, Veech RL. "Ketoacids? Good medicine?" *Trans Am Clin Climatol Assoc* (2003); 114: 149–61; discussion 162–3.

5 Cahill GF Jr. "Fuel metabolism in starvation." *Annu Rev Nutr* (2006); 26: 1–22.

6 Klein S, Wolfe RR. "Carbohydrate restriction regulates the adaptive response to fasting. *Am J Physiol* (1992); 262: E631?E636.

7 Gibson AA, Seimon RV, Lee CM, et al. "Do ketogenic diets really suppress appetite? A systematic review and meta-analysis." *Ones Rev* (2015 Jan); 16(1): 64–76. doi: 10.1111 /obr.12230. Epub 2014 Nov 17.

8 Sumithran P, Prendergast, L A, Delbridge E, et al. "Ketosis and appetite-mediating nutrients and hormones after weight loss." *Eur J Clin Nutr* (2013 Jul); 67: 759–64. doi:10.1038/ejcn.2013.90.

9 Dashti HM, Mathew TC, Hussein T, et al. "Long-term effects of a ketogenic diet in obese patients." *Exp Clin Cardiol* (2004 Fall); 9(3): 200–5.

10 Hussain TA, Mathew TC, Dashti AA, Asfar S, Al-Zaid N, Dashti HM. "Effect of low-calorie versus low-carbohydrate ketogenic diet in type 2 diabetes." *Nutrition* (2012 Oct); 28(10): 1016–21. doi:10.1016/j.nut.2012.01.016.

11 Kraschnewski JL, Boan J, Esposito J, et al. "Long-term weight loss maintenance in the United States." *Int J Obes (Lond)* (2010); 34(11): 1644–54.

12 Douketis JD, Macie C, Thabane L, Williamson DF. "Systematic review of long-term weight loss studies in obese adults: clinical significance and applicability to clinical practice." *Int J Obes (Lond)* (2005); 29(10): 1153–67.

13 Cappello G, Franschelli A, Capello A, DeLuca P. "Ketogenic enteral nutrition as a treatment for obesity: short term and long term results from 19,000 patients." *Nutrition and Metabolism* (2012): 9: 96 doi:10.1186/1743-7075-9-96.

14 Cahill GF Jr. "Fuel Metabolism in Starvation." *Ann Rev Nutr* (2006): 26: 1–22. doi: 10.1146/annurev.nutr.26.061505.111258.

15 Bernstein, RK. "Dr. Bernstein's Diabetes Solution," 4th ed. (New York: Little Brown, 2011), 130

16 Noli D, Avery G. "Protein poisoning and coastal subsistence." *J Archaeol Sci* (1988); 15(4): 395–401.

17 Stefansson V. *Arctic Manual* (New York: Macmillan, 1944), 232–33.

18 Isner JM, Sours HE, Paris AL. "Unexpected death in avid dieters using the liquid protein-modified-fast diet." *Circulation* (1979 Dec); 60(6).

19 Witte AV, Fobker M, Gellner R, Knecht S, Flöel A. "Caloric restriction improves memory in elderly humans." *PNAS* (2009); 106(4): 1255–60.

20 Klein S, Wolfe RR. "Carbohydrate restriction regulates the adaptive response to fasting." *Am J Physiol.* 1992; 262: E631–E636. Cahill GF Jr. "Fuel metabolism in starvation." *Ann Rev Nutr* (2006); 26:S.1–22. doi:10.1146/annurev.nutr.26.061505.111258.

CHAPTER 6: Becoming a Lifelong Fat Burner

1 Haenisch B, von Holt K, Wiese B, et al. "Risk of dementia in elderly patients with the use of proton pump inhibitors." *Eur Arch Psychiatry Clin Neurosci* (2015 Aug); 265(5): 419–28. doi:10.1007/s00406-014-0554-0.

2 Festi D, Colecchia A, Orsini M, et al. "Gallbladder motility and gallstone formation in obese patients following very low calorie diets. Use it (fat) to lose it (well)." *Int J Obes Relat Metab Disord* (1998 Jun); 22(6): 592–600.

3 Tsai C-J, Leitzmann MF, Willett WC, Giovannucci EL. "Dietary carbohydrates and glycaemic load and the incidence of symptomatic gall stone disease in men." *Gut* (2005); 54: 823–28 doi:10.1136/gut.2003.031435.

4 Festi D, Colecchia A, Orsini M, et al. "Gallbladder motility and gallstone formation in obese patients following very low calorie diets. (Use it) fat or lose it (well)." *Int J Obes Relat Metab Disord* (1998 Jun); 22(6): 592–600.

5 Bloomfield PH, Chopra R, Sheinbaum RC, et al. "Effects of Ursodeoxycholic Acid and Aspirin on the Formation of Lithogenic Bile and Gallstones during Loss of Weight." *N Engl J Med* (1988); 319: 1567–72. doi:10.1056/NEJM198812153192403.

6 Kerl ME. "Diabetic ketoacidosis: Treatment recommendations." *Compend Contin Educ Pract Vet* (2001); 23: 330–40.

CHAPTER 7: A Field Guide to Fat-Soluble Nutrients
1 Fletcher R, Fairfield KM. "Vitamins for chronic disease prevention in adults." *JAMA* (2002); 287(23): 3127–9.
2 Borrowed and modified from: Gedgaudas N. "Why Paleo?" The Paleo Way. www .thepaleoway.com.
3 Sullivan K. *Naked at Noon: Understanding Sunlight and Vitamin D* (Laguna Beach, CA: Basic Health Publications, 2003).
4 Sanchez-Martinez R, Castillo A, Steinmeyer A, Aranda A. "The retinoid X receptor ligand restores defective signaling by the vitamin D receptor." *EMBO Rep* (2006 Oct); 7(10): 1030–4. Epub 2006 Aug 25.
5 Berkner KL, Runge W. "The physiology of vitamin K nutriture and vitamin K-dependent protein function in atherosclerosis." *J Thromb Haemost* (2004); 2(12): 2118–32.
6 Masterjohn C. "Vitamin D toxicity redefined: Vitamin K and the molecular mechanism." *Med Hypotheses* (2006) [Epub ahead of print].
7 Russell RM. "The vitamin A spectrum: from deficiency to toxicity." *Am J Clin Nutr* (2000); 71: 878–84.
8 Institute of Medicine. Food and Nutrition Board. *Dietary Reference Intakes for Vitamin A, Vitamin K, Arsenic, Boron, Chromium, Copper, Iodine, Iron, Manganese, Molybdenum, Nickel, Silicon, Vanadium, and Zinc* (Washington, DC: National Academy Press; 2001).
9 Fallon S, Enig MG. "Vitamin A saga." Weston A. Price Foundation (2002 Mar 30). www.westonaprice.org/health-topics/abcs-of-nutrition/vitamin-a-saga.
10 Fletcher RH. "Review: vitamin D3 supplementation may reduce mortality in adults; vitamin D2 does not." *Ann Intern Med* (2014 Jul 15); 161(2): JC5. doi:10.7326 /0003-4819-161-2-201407150-02005. Logan VF, Gray AR, Peddie MC, Harper MJ, Houghton LA. "Long-term vitamin D3 supplementation is more effective than vitamin D2 in maintaining serum 25-hydroxyvitamin D status over the winter months." *Br J Nutr* (2013 Mar 28); 109(6): 1082–8. doi: 10.1017/S0007114512002851. Mistretta VI, Delanaye P, Chapelle JP, Souberbielle JC, Cavalier E. "[Vitamin D2 or vitamin D3?]." *Rev Med Interne* (2008 Oct); 29(10): 815–20. doi: 10.1016 /j.revmed.2008.03.003.
11 Veugelers PJ, Ekwaru JP. "A statistical error in the estimation of the Recommended Dietary Allowance for vitamin D." *Nutrients* (2014); 6(10): 4472–5. doi:10.3390/ nu6104472.
12 Rolf I, Muris AII, Hupperts R, Damoiseaux J. "Vitamin D effects on B cell function in autoimmunity." *Ann NY Acad Sci* (2014 May); 1317: 84–91. doi:10.1111/nyas.12440. Bjelakovic G, Gluud LL, Nikolova D, et al. "Vitamin D supplementation for prevention of mortality in adults." *Cochrane Database Syst Rev* (2014 Jan 10); 1: CD007470. doi: 10.1002/14651858.CD007470.pub3. Ceria CD, Masaki KH, Rodriguez BL, et al. "Low dietary vitamin D in mid-life predicts total mortality in men with hypertension: the Honolulu heart program." *J Am Geriatr Soc* (2001 Jun); 49(6): 725–31.
13 Bischoff-Ferrari HA. "Optimal serum 25-hydroxyvitamin D levels for multiple health outcomes." *Adv Exp Med Biol* (2008); 624: 55–71. doi: 10.1007/978-0-387-77574-6_5. Masterjohn C. "Vitamin D toxicity redefined: Vitamin K and the molecular mechanism." *Med Hypotheses* (2006) [Epub ahead of print].
14 Schurgers LJ, Teunissen KJF, Hamulyak K, Knapen MHJ, Hogne V, Vermeer C. "Vitamin K-containing dietary supplements: comparison of synthetic vitamin K1 and natto-derived menaquinone-7." *Blood* (2006) [Epub ahead of print].
15 Plaza SM, Lamson DW. "Vitamin K2 in bone metabolism and osteoporosis." *Altern Med Rev* (2005); 10(1): 24–35.
16 DiNicolantonio JJ, Bhutan J, O'Keefe JH. "The health benefits of vitamin K." *Open Heart (BMJ)* (2015); 2(1): e000300. doi: 10.1136/openhrt-2015-000300.

17 Berkner KL, Runge W. "The physiology of vitamin K nutriture and vitamin K-dependent protein function in atherosclerosis." *J Thromb Haemost* (2004); 2(12): 2118–32.

18 Thaweboon S, Thaweboon B, Choonharuangdej S, Chunhabundit P, Suppakpatana P. "Induction of type I collagen and osteocalcin in human dental pulp cells by retinoic acid." *Southeast Asian J Trop Med Public Health* (2005); 36(4): 1066–9.

19 Nimptsch K, Rohrmann S, Kaaks R, Linseisen J. "Dietary vitamin K intake in relation to cancer incidence and mortality: Results from the Heidelberg cohort of the European Prospective Investigation into Cancer and Nutrition (EPIC—Heidelberg)." *Am J Clin Nutr* (2009), doi:10.3945/ajcn.2009.28691.

20 Schurgers LJ, Vermeer C. "Determination of phylloquinone and menaquinones in Food." *Haemostasis* (2000); 30: 298–307.

21 Whitehouse MW, Turner AG, Davis CK, Roberts MS. "Emu oil(s): A source of nontoxic transdermal anti-inflammatory agents in aboriginal medicine." *Inflammopharmacology* (1998); 6(1): 1–8. Howarth GS, Lindsay RJ, Butler RN, Geier MS. "Can emu oil ameliorate inflammatory disorders affecting the gastrointestinal system?" *Austr J Experimental Agriculture* (2008); 48(10): 1276–9. doi:10.1071/EA08139.

22 Moon EJ, Lee YM, Kim KW. "Anti-angiogenic activity of conjugated linoleic acid on basic fibroblast growth factor-induced angiogenesis." *Oncol Rep* (2003 May–June); 10(3): 617–21.

23 Spronk HMH, Soute BAM, Schurgers LJ, Thijssen HHW, De Mey JGR, Vermeer C. "Tissue-specific utilization of menaquinone-4 results in the prevention of arterial calcification in warfarin-treated rats." *J Vascular Res* (2003); 40(6): 531–7. doi:10.1159/000075344. Yoshida H, Shiratori Y, Kudo M, et al. "Effect of vitamin K_2 on the recurrence of hepatocellular carcinoma." *Hepatology* (2011); 54: 532–40. doi:10.1002/hep.24430.

24 Geleijnse JM, Vermeer C, Grobbee DE, et al. "Dietary intake of menaquinone is associated with a reduced risk of coronary heart disease: The Rotterdam Study." *J Nutr* (2004 Nov); 134(11): 3100–5.

25 Mizuta T, Ozaki I, Eguchi Y, et al. "The effect of menatetrenone, a vitamin K_2 analog, on disease recurrence and survival in patients with hepatocellular carcinoma after curative treatment: a pilot study." *Cancer* (2006); 106: 867–72. doi:10.1002/cncr.21667.

26 Mayo Clinic. "Vitamin K may protect against developing non-Hodgkin's lymphoma, say Mayo Clinic researchers." *ScienceDaily* (2010 Apr 21).

27 Habu D, Shiomi S, Tamori A, et al. "Role of vitamin K_2 in the development of hepatocellular carcinoma in women with viral cirrhosis of the liver." *JAMA* (2004); 292: 358–61, doi:10.1001/jama.292.3.358. Hotta N, Ayada M, Sato K, et al. "Effect of vitamin K_2 on the recurrence in patients with hepatocellular carcinoma." *Hepatogastroenterology* (2007); 54: 2073–7.

28 Liu M, Liu F. "Regulation of adiponectin multimerization, signaling and function." *Best Pract Res Clin Endocrinol Metab* (2014); 28: 25–31.

29 Knights AJ, Funnell AP, Pearson RC, Crossley M, Bell-Anderson KS. "Adipokines and insulin action: a sensitive issue." *Adipocyte* (2014); 3: 88–96.

30 Moreno-Aliaga MJ, Lorente-Cebrian S, Martinez JA. "Regulation of adipokine secretion by n-3 fatty acids." *Proc Nutr Soc* (2010); 69: 324–32.

31 Theuwissen E, Smit E, Vermeer C. "The role of vitamin K in soft-tissue calcification." *Adv Nutr* (2012 Mar 1); 3(2): 166–73. doi:10.3945/an.111.001628.

32 Ford ES, Sowell A. "Serum alpha-tocopherol status in the United States population: Findings from the Third National Health and Nutrition Examination Survey." *Am J Epidemiol* (1999 Aug 1); 150: 290–300.

33 Mahabir S, Schendel K, Dong YQ, et al. "Dietary alpha-, beta-, gamma- and delta-tocopherols in lung cancer risk." *Int J Cancer* (2008 Sep 1); 123(5): 1173–80. doi:10.1002/ijc.23649. Luk SU, Yap WN, Chiu Y-T, et al. "Gamma-tocotrienol as an effective agent in targeting prostate cancer stem cell-like population." *Int J Cancer* (2011 May); 128(9): 2182–91.

34 Jiang Q, Elson-Schwab I, Courtemanche C, Ames BN. "Gamma-tocopherol and its

major metabolite, in contrast to alpha-tocopherol, inhibit cyclooxygenase activity in macrophages and epithelial cells." *Proc Natl Acad Sci USA* (2000 Oct); 10; 97(21): 11494–9.

35 Chiu CJ, Milton RC, Klein R, et al. "Dietary compound score and risk of age-related macular degeneration in the age-related disease study." *Ophthalmology* (2009 May); 116(5): 939–46. doi: 10.1016/j.ophtha.2008.12.025.

36 Yachi R, Muto C, Ohtaka N, et al. "Effects of tocotrienols on tumor necrosis factor -α/d-galactosamine-induced steatohepatitis in rats." *J Clin Biochem Nutr* (2013 Mar); 52(2): 146–53. doi:10.3164/jcbn.12–101.

37 Dysken MW, Sano M, Asthana S, et al. "Effect of vitamin E and Mementine on functional cognitive decline in Alzheimer's disease." *JAMA* (2014); 311(1).

38 "The effect of vitamin E and beta carotene on the incidence of lung cancer and other cancers in male smokers. The Alpha-Tocopherol, Beta Carotene Cancer Prevention Study Group." *N Engl J Med* (1994 Apr 14); 330(15): 1029–35.

39 Kappus H, Diplock AT. "Tolerance and safety of vitamin E: A toxicological position report." *Free Radic Biol Med* (1992); 13(1): 55–74.

40 "Epigenetics." Icahn School of Medicine at Mount Sinai. The Friedman Brain Institute. http://icahn.mssm.edu/research/friedman/research/epigenetics.

41 "Influence of pasture or grain-based diets . . . on antioxidant/oxidative balance of Argentine beef." *Meat Science* (2005); 70: 35–44.

42 Mercier, Y., P. Gatellier, M. Renerre. "Lipid and protein oxidation in vitro, and antioxidant potential in meat from Charolais cows finished on pasture or mixed diet." *Meat Science* (2004); 6: 467–3.

43 Daley CA, Abbott A, Doyle PS, et al. "A review of fatty acid profiles and antioxidant content in grass-fed and grain-fed beef." *Nutr J* (2010); 9:10. doi:10.1186/1475-2891-9-10.

44 Levine I. "Cancer among the American Indians and its bearing upon the ethnological distribution of the disease." *J Cancer Res Clin Oncol* (1910); 9: 422–35.

45 Brown GM, Cronk LB, Boag TJ. "The occurrence of cancer in an Eskimo." *Cancer* (1952); 5: 142–43.

CHAPTER 8: Primal Fat Burning May Help Prevent and Alleviate Disease

1 Dedkova EN, Blatter LA. "Role of B-hydroxybutyrate, its polymer poly-B-hydroxybutyrate and inorganic polyphosphate in mammalian health and disease." *Frontiers I Physiology* (2014); 5: 260. doi:10.3389/fphys.2014.00260.

2 Kashiwaya Y, Sato K, Tsuchiya S, Thomas S, Fell DA, et al. "Control of glucose utilization in the perfused rat heart." *J. Biol. Chem* (1994); 269: 25502–14.

3 Foster GD, et al. "A randomized trial of a low carbohydrate diet for obesity." *N Eng J Med* (2003 May 22); 348: 2082–90. Hays JH. "Effect of a high saturated fat and no-starch diet on serum lipid subfractions in patients with documented atherosclerotic cardiovascular disease." *Mayo Clinic Proceedings* (2003); 78: 1331–6. Aude YW, Agatston AS, Lopez-Jimenez F, et al. "The National Cholesterol Program Diet vs a diet lower in carbohydrates and higher in protein and saturated fat: a randomized trial." *Arch Intern Med* (2004); 164(19): 2141–6. doi:10.1001/archinte.164.19.2141.

4 McBride PE. "Triglycerides and risk for coronary heart disease." *JAMA* (2007); 298(3): 336–8. doi:10.1001/jama.298.3.336.

5 Noakes M, et al. "Comparison of isocaloric very low carbohydrate/high saturated fat and high carbohydrate/low saturated fat diets on body composition and cardiovascular risk." *Nutrition & Metabolism* (2006); 3:7.

6 DiNicolantonio JD, Lucan SC. "The wrong white crystals: not salt but sugar as aetiological in hypertension and cardiometabolic disease." *Open Heart* (2014); 1. doi:10.1136/openhrt-2014-000167. Bjerregaard P, Dewailly E, Young TK, et al. Blood pressure among the Inuit (Eskimo) populations in the Arctic. *Scand J Public Health* (2003); 31(2): 92–9.

7 Mann GV. "Coronary Heart Disease: Dietary Sense and Nonsense" (Janus Publishing, 1993).

8   Siri-Tarino PW, Sun Q, Hu FB, Krauss RM. "Meta-analysis of prospective cohort studies evaluating the association of saturated fat with cardiovascular disease." *Am J Clin Nutr* (2010 Mar); 91(3):535–46. doi: 10.3945/ajcn.2009.27725. Epub 2010 Jan 13. Krumholz HM, Seeman TE, Merrill SS, et al. "Lack of association between cholesterol and coronary heart disease mortality and morbidity and all-cause mortality in persons older than 70 years." *JAMA* (1994); 272: 1335–40.

9   Ramadan CE, Zamora D, Majchrzak-Hong S, et al. "Re-evaluation of the traditional diet-heart hypothesis: Analysis of recovered data from Minnesota Coronary Experiment (1968–73)." *BMJ* (2016); 353: i1246.

10 Malhotra A. "Saturated fat is not the major issue." *BMJ* (2013); 347: f6340. doi: http://dx.doi.org/10.1136/bmj.f6340.

11 Rose GA, et al. "Corn oil in treatment of ischaemic heart disease." *BMJ* (1965); 1: 1531–3. DiNicolantonio JJ. "The cardiometabolic consequences of replacing saturated fats with carbohydrates or Ω-6 polyunsaturated fats: Do the dietary guidelines have it wrong?" *Open Heart* (2014); 1. doi:10.1136/openhrt-2013-000032. Howard BV, Van Horn L, Hsia J, et al. "Low-fat dietary pattern and risk of cardiovascular disease: The Women's Health Initiative randomized controlled dietary modification trial." *JAMA* (2006); 295: 655–66. Chowdhury R, Warnakula S, Kunutsor S, et al. "Association of dietary, circulating, and supplement fatty acids with coronary risk: A systematic review and meta-analysis." *Ann Intern Med* (2014); 160(6): 398–406. doi:10.7326/M13-1788. Siri-Tarino PW, Sun Q, Hu FB, Krauss RM. "Meta-analysis of prospective cohort studies evaluating the association of saturated fat with cardiovascular disease." *Am J Clin Nutr* (2010); 91: 535–46.

12 Girao H, Mota C, Pereira P. "Cholesterol may act as an antioxidant in lens membranes." *Curr Eye Res* (1999 Jun); 18(6): 448–54. Smith LL. "Another cholesterol hypothesis: Cholesterol as antioxidant." *Free Radic Biol Med* (1991); 11(1): 47–61.

13 Champeau, R. "Most heart attack patients' cholesterol levels did not indicate cardiac risk." *UCLA Newsroom* (2009). http://newsroom.ucla.edu/portal/ucla/majority-of -hospitalized-heart-75668.aspx.

14 Okuyama H, Hamazaki T, Ogushi Y; Committee on Cholesterol Guidelines for Longevity, Japan Society for Lipid Nutrition. "New cholesterol guidelines for longevity." *World Rev Nutr Diet* (2011); 102: 124–36. Epub 2011 Aug 5. Petursson H, Sigurdsson JA, [. . .], Getz L. "Is the use of cholesterol in mortality risk algorithms in clinical guidelines valid? Ten years prospective data from the Norwegian HUNT 2 study." *J Eval Clin Practice* (2012 Feb); 18(1): 159–68.

15 Ravnskov U. "High cholesterol may protect against infections and atherosclerosis." *Quart J Med* (2003); 96: 927–34.

16 Anderson KM, Castelli WP, Levy D. "Cholesterol and mortality: 30 years of follow-up from the Framingham Study." *JAMA* (1987); 257(16): 2176–80. doi:10.1001/jama.1987.03390160062027.

17 Ravnskov U, Diamond DM, Hama R, et al. "Lack of an association or an inverse association between low-density-lipoprotein cholesterol and mortality in the elderly: A systematic review." *BMJ Open* (2016); 6:e010401. doi:10.1136/bmjopen-2015-010401.

18 Mazza A, Casiglia E, Scarpa R, et al. "Predictors of cancer mortality in elderly subjects." *Eur J Epidemiol* (1999); 15: 421–7.

19 Wannamethee G, Shaper AG, Whincup PH, Walker M. "Low serum total cholesterol concentrations and mortality in middle-aged British men." *BMJ* (1995); 311: 409–13.

20 Felton CV, Crook D, Davies MJ, Oliver MF. "Dietary polyunsaturated fatty acids and composition of human aortic plaques." *Lancet* (1994 Oct 29); 344 (8931): 1195–6.

21 Santos FL, et al. "Systematic review and meta-analysis of clinical trials of the effects of low carbohydrate diets on cardiovascular risk factors." *Obesity Rev.* Epub 21 Aug 2012. Bjornholt JV, Erikssen G, Aaser E, et al. "Fasting blood glucose: an underestimated risk factor for cardiovascular death. Results from a 22-year follow-up of healthy nondiabetic men." *Diabetes Care* (1999 Jan); 22(1): 45–9. Batty GD, Kivimäki M, Smith GD, Marmot MG, Shipley MJ. "Post-challenge blood glucose concentration and stroke mortality rates in non-diabetic men in London: 38-year follow-up

of the original Whitehall prospective cohort study." *Diabetologia* (2008 Jul); 51: 1123–6. Wilson PWF, Cupples LA, Kannel WB. "Is hyperglycaemia associated with cardiovascular disease? The Framingham Study." *Am Heart J* (1991 Feb); 121 (2 Pt 1): 586–90.

22 McMaster University. "Trans fats, but not saturated fats like butter, linked to greater risk of early death and heart disease." *ScienceDaily* (2015 Aug 11). De Souza RJ, Mente A, Maroleanu A, et al. "Intake of saturated and trans unsaturated fatty acids and risk of all cause mortality, cardiovascular disease, and type 2 diabetes: Systematic review and meta-analysis of observational studies." *BMJ* (2015); 351:h3978. doi: http://dx .doi.org/10.1136/bmj.h3978.

23 Sundram K, Karupaiah T, Hayes KC. "Stearic acid-rich interesterified fat and trans-rich fat raise the LDL/HDL ratio and plasma glucose relative to palm olein in humans." *Nutr Metab* (2007); 4:3. doi:10.1186/1743-7075-4-3.

24 DiNicolantonio JJ. "The cardiometabolic consequences of replacing saturated fats with carbohydrates or Ω-6 polyunsaturated fats: Do the dietary guidelines have it wrong?" *Open Heart* (2014); 1. doi:10.1136/openhrt-2013-000032.

25 Donsky A. "Worst ingredients in food." *Naturally Savvy.* 2013 Jun 1. Kobylewski S, Jacobson MF. "Food dyes: A rainbow of risks." *CSPI* (2010 Jun).

26 Samsel A, Seneff S. "Glyphosate suppression of cytochrome P450 enzymes and amino acid biosynthesis by the gut microbiome: Pathways to modern diseases." *Entropy* (2013); 15(4): 1416–63. doi:10.3390/c15041416.

27 Vojdani A, Tarash I. "Cross-reaction between gliadin and different food and tissue antigens." *Food Nutri Sci* (2013); 4: 20–32.

28 Mayr M, Yusuf S, Weir G., Chung YL, Mayr U, Yin X, et al. "Combined metabolomic and proteomic analysis of human atrial fibrillation." *J. Am. Coll. Cardiol* (2008); 51: 585–94.

29 Malhotra A. "Saturated Fat Is Not the Major Issue." *BMJ* (2013); 347:f6340, doi:10.1136/bmj.f6340.

30 Yang X, Cheng B. "Neuroprotective and anti-inflammatory activities of ketogenic diet on MPTP-induced neurotoxicity." *J Molec Neurosci* (2010 Oct); 42(2): 145–53. Dressler A, Reithofer E, Trimmel-Schwahofer P, Klebermasz K, Prayer D, Kasprian G, Rami B, Schober E, Feucht M. "Type 1 diabetes and epilepsy: Efficacy and safety of the ketogenic diet." *Epilepsia* (2010 Jun); 51(6): 1086–9.

31 Evangeliou A, Viachonikolis I, Mihailidou H, et al. "Application of a ketogenic diet in children with autistic behavior: Pilot study." *J Child Neurol* (2003 Feb); 18(2): 113–18. doi:10.1177/08830738030180020501.

32 Millichap JG, Yee MM. "The diet factor in attention-deficit/hyperactivity disorder." *Pediatrics* (2013 Feb); 129(2): 330–7. doi: 10.1542/peds.2011-2199.

33 Prins ML, Fujima LS, Hovda DA. "Age-dependent reduction of cortical contusion volume by ketones after traumatic brain injury." *J Neurosci Res* (2005); 82: 413–20.

34 Kashiwaya Y, Takeshima T, Mori N, Nakashima K, Clarke K, Veech RL. "D-beta-hydroxybutyrate protects neurons in models of Alzheimer's and Parkinson's disease." *Proc Natl Acad Sci USA* (2000); 97: 5440–4.

35 Siva N. "Can ketogenic diet slow progression of ALS?" *Lancet Neurol.* 2006; 5: 476. Zhao Z, Lange DJ, Voustianiouk A, MacGrogan D, Ho L, Suh J, et al. "A ketogenic diet as a potential novel therapeutic intervention in amyotrophic lateral sclerosis." *BMC Neurosci* (2006); 7:29.

36 Zhou W, Mukherjee P, Kiebish MA, et al. "The calorically restricted ketogenic diet, an effective alternative therapy for malignant brain cancer." *Nutr Metab* (2007); 4: 5. doi:10.1186/1743-7075-4. Seyfried TN, Shelton LM. "Cancer as a metabolic disease." *Nutr Metab.* 2010; 7: 7. Seyfried TN, Marsh J, Mukherjee P, et al. "Could metabolic therapy become a viable alternative to the standard of care for managing glioblastoma?" *Oncol Hematol Rev* (2014); 10(1): 13–20.

37 Newport M. "Ketones as an alternative fuel for Alzheimer's disease and other disorders." Hippocrates Institute presentation, May 2014. www.charliefoundation.org /images/open-access/Mary_Newport_MD_Presentation_May_2014.pdf. Henderson

ST. "Ketone bodies as a therapeutic for Alzheimer's disease." *J Am Soc Experimental NeuroTherapeutics* (2008 Jul); 5: 470–80.

38 Elias PK et al. "Serum cholesterol and cognitive performance in the Framingham Heart Study." *Psychosomatic Medicine.* (2005); 67(1): 24–30.

39 Burns CM, Chen K, Kaszniak AW, et al. "Higher serum glucose levels are associated with cerebral hypometabolism in Alzheimer regions." *Neurology* (2013 Apr 23); 80(17): 1557–64.

40 Krikorian R, Shidler MD, Dangelo K, Couch SC, Benoit SC, Clegg DJ (2010). Dietary ketosis enhances memory in mild cognitive impairment. *Neurobiology of aging* PMID: 21130529.

41 Reger MA, Henderson ST, Hale C, et al. "Effects of beta-hydroxybutyrate on cognition in memory-impaired adults." *Neurobiol Aging* (2004 Mar); 25(3): 311–4. PMID: 15123336.

42 Laugerette F, Furet JP, Debard C, et al. "Oil composition of high-fat diet affects metabolic inflammation differently in connection with endotoxin receptors in mice." *Am J Physiol Endocrinol Metab* (2012 Feb 1); 302(3): E374–86. doi: 10.1152/ajpendo.00314.2011.

43 Read TE, Harris HW, Grunfeld C, et al. "The protective effect of serum lipoproteins against bacterial lipopolysaccharide." *Eur Heart J* (1993); 14 (suppl K): 125–9.

44 Youm YH, Nguyen KY, Grant RW, et al. "The ketone metabolite B-hydroxybutyrate blocks NLRP3 inflammasome-mediated inflammatory disease." *Nat Med* (2015).

45 Yang X, Cheng B. "Neuroprotective and anti-inflammatory activities of ketogenic diet on MPTP-induced neurotoxicity." *J Mol Neurosci* (2010); 42(2): 145–53.

46 Ahmad AS, Ormiston-Smith N and Sasieni PS. "Trends in the lifetime risk of developing cancer in Great Britain: Comparison of risk for those born in 1930 to 1960." *British Journal of Cancer* (2015). doi:10.1038/bjc.2014.606 and Greg Jones. "Why Are Cancer Rates Increasing?" Cancer Research UK. (2015 Feb 4).

47 World Health Organizantion, "Cancer, Fact sheet N° 297. Updated Feb 2015.

48 Vazquez A, Liu J, Zhou Y, Oltvai Z. "Catabolic efficiency of aerobic glycolysis: The Warburg effect revisited." *BMC Systems Biol* (2010); 4:58. doi:10.1186/1752-0509-4-58.

49 Digirolamo M. *Diet and Cancer: Markers, Prevention and Treatment.* (New York: Plenum Press, 1994), 203.

50 Volk T, et al. "pH in human tumor xenografts: Effect of intravenous administration of glucose. "*Br J Cancer* (1993 Sep); 68(3): 492–500.

51 Boyle P, Koechlin A, Pizot C, et al. "Blood glucose concentrations and breast cancer risk in women without diabetes: A meta-analysis." *Eur J Nutr* (2013 Aug); 52(5): 1533–40. Osaki Y, Taniguchi S, Tahara A, et al. "Metabolic syndrome and incidence of liver and breast cancers in Japan." *Cancer Epidemiol* (2012); 36(2): 141–7.

52 Vander Heiden MG, Cantley LC, Thompson CB. "Understanding the Warburg effect: The metabolic requirements of cell proliferation." *Science* (2009 May 22); 324(5930): 1029–33. doi:10.1126/science.1160809. Vazquez A, Liu J, Zhou Y, Oltvai ZN. "Catabolic efficiency of aerobic glycolysis: The Warburg effect revisited." *BMC Systems Biol* (2010); 4: 58. Seyfried TN, Shelton LM. "Cancer as a metabolic disease." *Nutrition and Metabolism* (2010); 7: 7.

53 Onodera Y, Nam JM, Bissell MJ. "Increased sugar uptake promotes oncogenesis via EPAC/RAP1 and O-GlcNAc pathways." *J Clin Invest* (2014 Jan 2); 124(1): 367–384. doi: 10.1172/JCI63146.

54 King MC, Marks JH, Mandell JB; New York Breast Cancer Study Group. "Breast and ovarian cancer risks due to inherited mutations in BRCA1 and BRCA2." *Science* (2003 Oct 24); 302(5645): 643–6.

55 Klement RJ, Kämmerer U. "Is there a role for carbohydrate restriction in the treatment and prevention of cancer?" *Nutr Metab (Lond)* (2011); 8: 75. doi:10.1186/1743-7075-8-75.

56 "Simple sugar, lactate, is like 'candy for cancer cells': Cancer cells accelerate aging and inflammation in the body to drive tumor growth." *Science News* (2011 May 28).

57 Daye D, Wellen KE. "Metabolic reprogramming in cancer: Unraveling the role of glu-

tamine in tumorigenesis." *Semin Cell Dev Biol* (2012 Jun); 23(4): 362–9. doi: 10.1016 /j.semcdb.2012.02.002. Epub 2012 Feb 11.

58 Pollak M, Russell-Jones D. "Insulin analogues and cancer risk: Cause for concern or cause célèbre?" *Int J Clin Pract* (2010 Apr); 64(5): 628–36. doi:10.1111/j.1742-1241.2010.02354.x.

59 Seccareccia E, Brodt P. "The role of the insulin-like growth factor-I receptor in malignancy: An update." *Growth Horm IGF Res* (2012 Dec); 22(6): 193–9. doi:10.1016 /j.ghir.2012.09.003.

60 Levine ME, Suarez JA, Brandhorst S, Balasubramanian P, Cheng CW, Madia F, Fontana L, Mirisola MG, Guevara-Aguirre J, Wan J, Passarino G, Kennedy BK, Wei M, Cohen P, Crimmins EM, Longo VD. "Low protein intake is associated with a major reduction in IGF-1, cancer, and overall mortality in the 65 and younger but not older population." *Cell Metabol* (2002); 19(3): 407–7. doi:10.1016/j.cmet.2014.02.006.

61 http://www.health.harvard.edu/diseases-and-conditions/glycemic_index_and _glycemic_load_for_100_foods

62 Seyfried TN, Sanderson TM, El-Abbadi MM, McGowan R, Mukherjee P. "Glucose and ketone bodies in the metabolic control of experimental brain cancer." *Br J Cancer* (2003 Oct 6); 89(7): 1375–82.

63 Ip, C., JA Scimeca, et al. (1994). "Conjugated linoleic acid. A powerful anticarcinogen from animal fat sources." *Cancer* 74(3 Suppl): 1050–4.

64 Wang M. "The role of glucocorticoid action in the pathophysiology of the metabolic syndrome." *Nutr Metabol* (2005); 2:3. doi: 10.1186/1743-7075-2-3.

65 Jabekk P. "High fat diets and endurance exercise performance." *Ramblings of a Carnivore* (2010 Sep 5); http://ramblingsofacarnivore.blogspot.com/2010/09/high-fat -diets-and-endurance-exercise.html.

66 Cameron-Smith D, Burke LM, Angus DJ, et al. "A short-term, high-fat diet up-regulates lipid metabolism and gene expression in human skeletal muscle." *Am J Clin Nutr* (2003 Feb); 77(2): 313–8.

67 Rosedale R. "Diabetes is not a disease of blood sugar." Ron Rosedale MD. http:// drrosedale.com/Diabetes_is_NOT_a_disease_of_blood_sugar#axzz3q69J9aU3.

68 Qu J, Wang Y, Wu X, et al. "Insulin resistance directly contributes to androgenic potential within ovarian theca cells." *Fertil Steril* (2009 May); 91(5 Suppl): 1990–7. doi: 10.1016/j.fertnstert.2008.02. Wu S, Divall S, Nwaopara A, et al. "Obesity-induced infertility and hyperandrogenism are corrected by deletion of the insulin receptor in the ovarian theca cell." *Diabetes* (2014 Apr); 63(4): 1270–82. doi:10.2337/db13-1514.

69 Mavropoulos JC, Yancy WS, Hepburn J, Westman EC. "The effects of a low-carbohydrate, ketogenic diet on the polycystic ovary syndrome: A pilot study." *Nutr Metabol* (2005); 2:35. doi:10.1186/1743-7075-2-35.

70 Perel E, Killinger DW. "The interconversion and aromatization of androgens by human adipose tissue." *J Steroid Biochem* (1979 Jun); 10(6): 623–7.

71 Accurso A, Bernstein RK, Dahlqvist A, Draznin B, et al. "Dietary carbohydrate restriction in type 2 diabetes mellitus and metabolic syndrome: Time for a critical appraisal." *Nutr Metabol* (2008); 5: 9. doi:10.1186/1743-7075-5-9.

CHAPTER 9: Carbovore No More

1 "Type 2 diabetes—Steve's story." *NHS Choices* (UK). http://www.nhs.uk/Conditions /Diabetes-type2/Pages/SteveRedgrave.aspx.

2 Manninen AH. "Very-low carbohydrate diets and preservation of muscle mass." *Nutr Metabol* (2006); 3:9. doi:10.1186/1743-7075-3-9.

3 Neely JR, Morgan HE. Relationship between carbohydrate and lipid metabolism and the energy balance of heart muscle. *Ann Rev Physiol* (1974); 36: 413–59.

4 Bastone K. "The paleo proposal." *Runner's World* (2014 Jul 18).

5 "Strongwoman Maureen Quinn!" *The Wellness Blog*, US Wellness Meats. June 19, 2015. http://blog.grasslandbeef.com/bid/92930/Strongwoman-Maureen-Quinn.

6 Sherwin RS, Hendler RG, Felig P. "Effect of ketone infusions on amino acid and nitrogen metabolism in man." *J Clin Invest* (1975); 55(6): 1382–90.

7   Brederode J, Rho JM. "Ketone bodies are protective against oxidative stress in neo-cortical neurons." *J Neurochem* (2007); 101(5): 1316–26.
8   Jarrett SG, Milder JB, Liang LP, Patel M. "The ketogenic diet increases mitochondrial glutathione levels." *J Neurochem* (2008); 106(3): 1044–51.
9   Manninen AH. "Very-low carbohydrate diets and preservation of muscle mass." *Nutr Metabol* (2006); 3:9. doi:10.1186/1743-7075-3-9.
10 Sherwin RS, Hendler RG, Felig P. 1975. "Effect of ketone infusions on amino acid and nitrogen metabolism in man." *J Clin Invest* (1975); 55(6): 1382–90.
11 Phinney SD, Bistrian BR, Wolfe RR, Blackburn GL. "The human metabolic response to chronic ketosis without caloric restriction: physical and biochemical adaptation." *Metabolism* (1983 Aug); 32(8): 757–68.
12 Fernandez ML, Feinman RD, Volek JS, et al. "Comparison of low fat and low carbohydrate diets on circulating fatty acid composition and markers of inflammation." *Lipids* (2008); 43(1): 65–67.
13 Long W, Wells K, Englert V, et al. "Does prior acute exercise affect postexercise substrate oxidation in response to a high carbohydrate meal?" *Nutr Metab (Lond)* (2008); 5: 2.
14 Stephens BR, Braun B. "Impact of nutrient intake timing on the metabolic response to exercise." *Nutr Rev.* 2008; 66(8): 473–6. Holtz KA, Stephens BR, Sharoff CG, et al. "The effect of carbohydrate availability following exercise on whole-body insulin action." *Appl Physiol Nutr Metab* (2008); 33(5): 946–56.
15 Koopman R, Wagenmakers AJ, Manders RJ, et al. "Combined ingestion of protein and free leucine with carbohydrate increases post exercise muscle protein synthesis in vivo in male subjects." *Am J Physiol Endocrinol Metab* (2005); 288(4): D645–53.
16 Smith TJ, Schwarz JM, Montain SJ, et al. "High protein diet maintains glucose production during exercise-induced energy deficit: a controlled trial." *Nutr Metabol* (2011); 8:26. doi: 10.1186/1743-7075-8-26.

CHAPTER 10: Setting Up for Success
1   Carolyn Rush: "Primal Tightwad" at www.primaltightwad.com.

CHAPTER 11: The Primal Fat Burning Food Guide
1   Vojdani A, Tarash I. "Cross-reaction between gliadin and different food and tissue antigens." *Food Nutri Sci* (2013); 4: 20–32. Karjalainen J, et al. "A bovine albumin peptide as a possible trigger of insulin-dependent diabetes mellitus." *N Engl J Med* (1992); 327: 302–7. Riemekasten G, et al. "Casein is an essential cofactor in autoantibody reactivity directed against the C-terminal SmD1 peptide AA83–119 in systemic lupus erythematosus." *Immunobiology* (2002); 206: 537–45. Kristjánsson G, et al. "Mucosal reactivity to cow's milk protein in celiac disease." *Clin Exp Immunol* (2007); 147: 449–55. Vojdani A, et al. "Immune response to dietary proteins, gliadin and cerebellar peptides in children with autism." *Nutr Neurosci* (2004); 7(3): 151–61.
2   Guggenmos J, et al. "Antibody cross-reactivity between MOG and the milk protein butyrophilin in multiple sclerosis." *J Immunol.* 2004; 172: 661–8. Lauer K. "Diet and multiple sclerosis." *Neurology* (1997); 49(Suppl 2): S55–S61.
3   www.cyrexlabs.com.
4   De Matos Feijo F, Ballard CR, Foletto KC, et al. "Saccharin and aspartame, compared with sucrose, induce greater weight gain in adult Wistar rats, at similar total caloric intake levels." *Appetite.* 60: 203–7. Stellman SD, Garfinkel L. "Artificial sweetener use and one-year weight change among women." *Prev Med* (1986 Mar); 15(2): 195–202.
5   Anton SD, Martin CK, Han H, et al. "Effects of stevia, aspartame, and sucrose on food intake, satiety, and postprandial glucose and insulin levels." *Appetite* (2010 Aug); 55(1): 37–43.
6   Laugerette F, Furet JP, Debard C, et al. "Oil composition of high-fat diet affects metabolic inflammation differently in connection with endotoxin receptors in mice." *Am J Physiol Endocrinol Metab* (2012 Feb 1); 302(3): E374–86. doi:10.1152/ajpendo.00314.2011.

INDEX

ABOUT THE AUTHOR

Nora Gedgaudas, a widely recognized expert on what is popularly referred to as the paleo diet, is a highly successful, experienced nutritional consultant, speaker, and educator. Her popular podcasts are widely listened to on iTunes, and her website provides numerous free articles and helpful resources. She maintains a private practice in Portland, Oregon, as both a board-certified nutritional consultant and a board-certified clinical neurofeedback specialist. She is the author of *Primal Body, Primal Mind* and *Rethinking Fatigue: What Your Adrenals Are Really Telling You and What You Can Do About It.*

H. pylori
Helicobacter
manuka Honey
Maca powder.